THE LEARNING
ROUNDTABLE ON VALUE

DIGITAL INFRASTRUCTURE FOR THE LEARNING HEALTH SYSTEM

The Foundation for Continuous Improvement in Health and Health Care

Workshop Series Summary

Claudia Grossmann, Brian Powers, and J. Michael McGinnis,
Rapporteurs and Editors

INSTITUTE OF MEDICINE
OF THE NATIONAL ACADEMIES

THE NATIONAL ACADEMIES PRESS
Washington, D.C.
www.nap.edu

THE NATIONAL ACADEMIES PRESS   500 Fifth Street, N.W.   Washington, DC 20001

NOTICE: The project that is the subject of this report was approved by the Governing Board of the National Research Council, whose members are drawn from the councils of the National Academy of Sciences, the National Academy of Engineering, and the Institute of Medicine.

This project was supported by the Office of the National Coordinator for Health Information Technology. Any opinions, findings, conclusions, or recommendations expressed in this publication are those of the author(s) and do not necessarily reflect the view of the organizations or agencies that provided support for this project.

International Standard Book Number-13: 978-0-309-15416-1
International Standard Book Number-10: 0-309-15416-2

Additional copies of this report are available from the National Academies Press, 500 Fifth Street, N.W., Lockbox 285, Washington, DC 20055; (800) 624-6242 or (202) 334-3313 (in the Washington metropolitan area); Internet, http://www.nap.edu.

For more information about the Institute of Medicine, visit the IOM home page at: www.iom.edu.

Copyright 2011 by the National Academy of Sciences. All rights reserved.

Printed in the United States of America

The serpent has been a symbol of long life, healing, and knowledge among almost all cultures and religions since the beginning of recorded history. The serpent adopted as a logotype by the Institute of Medicine is a relief carving from ancient Greece, now held by the Staatliche Museen in Berlin.

Suggested citation: IOM (Institute of Medicine). 2011. *Digital Infrastructure for the Learning Health System: The Foundation for Continuous Improvement in Health and Health Care: Workshop Series Summary.* Washington, DC: The National Academies Press.

*"Knowing is not enough; we must apply.
Willing is not enough; we must do."*
—Goethe

INSTITUTE OF MEDICINE
OF THE NATIONAL ACADEMIES

Advising the Nation. Improving Health.

THE NATIONAL ACADEMIES
Advisers to the Nation on Science, Engineering, and Medicine

The **National Academy of Sciences** is a private, nonprofit, self-perpetuating society of distinguished scholars engaged in scientific and engineering research, dedicated to the furtherance of science and technology and to their use for the general welfare. Upon the authority of the charter granted to it by the Congress in 1863, the Academy has a mandate that requires it to advise the federal government on scientific and technical matters. Dr. Ralph J. Cicerone is president of the National Academy of Sciences.

The **National Academy of Engineering** was established in 1964, under the charter of the National Academy of Sciences, as a parallel organization of outstanding engineers. It is autonomous in its administration and in the selection of its members, sharing with the National Academy of Sciences the responsibility for advising the federal government. The National Academy of Engineering also sponsors engineering programs aimed at meeting national needs, encourages education and research, and recognizes the superior achievements of engineers. Dr. Charles M. Vest is president of the National Academy of Engineering.

The **Institute of Medicine** was established in 1970 by the National Academy of Sciences to secure the services of eminent members of appropriate professions in the examination of policy matters pertaining to the health of the public. The Institute acts under the responsibility given to the National Academy of Sciences by its congressional charter to be an adviser to the federal government and, upon its own initiative, to identify issues of medical care, research, and education. Dr. Harvey V. Fineberg is president of the Institute of Medicine.

The **National Research Council** was organized by the National Academy of Sciences in 1916 to associate the broad community of science and technology with the Academy's purposes of furthering knowledge and advising the federal government. Functioning in accordance with general policies determined by the Academy, the Council has become the principal operating agency of both the National Academy of Sciences and the National Academy of Engineering in providing services to the government, the public, and the scientific and engineering communities. The Council is administered jointly by both Academies and the Institute of Medicine. Dr. Ralph J. Cicerone and Dr. Charles M. Vest are chair and vice chair, respectively, of the National Research Council.

www.national-academies.org

ROUNDTABLE ON VALUE & SCIENCE-DRIVEN HEALTH CARE[1]

Mark B. McClellan (*Chair, 2011-Present*), Director, Engelberg Center for Healthcare Reform, The Brookings Institution
Denis A. Cortese (*Chair, 2006-2011*), Emeritus President and Chief Executive Officer, Mayo Clinic; Foundation Professor, ASU
Donald Berwick, Administrator, Centers for Medicare & Medicaid Services (*ex officio*)
Bruce G. Bodaken, Chairman, President, and Chief Executive Officer, Blue Shield of California
David R. Brennan, Chief Executive Officer, AstraZeneca PLC
Paul Chew, Chief Science Officer and CMO, sanofi-aventis U.S., Inc.
Carolyn M. Clancy, Director, Agency for Healthcare Research and Quality (*ex officio*)
Michael J. Critelli, Chief Executive Officer, Dossia
Helen Darling, President, National Business Group on Health
Thomas R. Frieden, Director, Centers for Disease Control and Prevention (*designee*: **Chesley Richards**) (*ex officio*)
Patricia A. Gabow, Chief Executive Officer, Denver Health & Hospital Authority
Atul Gawande, General and Endocrine Surgeon, Brigham and Women's Hospital
Gary L. Gottlieb, President and CEO, Partners HealthCare System
James A. Guest, President, Consumers Union
George C. Halvorson, Chairman and Chief Executive Officer, Kaiser Permanente
Margaret A. Hamburg, Commissioner, Food and Drug Administration (*ex officio*)
James Heywood, Chairman, PatientsLikeMe
Carmen Hooker Odom, President, Milbank Memorial Fund
Ardis Hoven, Immediate Past Board Chair, American Medical Association
Brent James, Chief Quality Officer and Executive Director, Institute for Health Care Delivery Research, Intermountain Healthcare
Michael M. E. Johns, Chancellor, Emory University
Craig Jones, Director, Vermont Blueprint for Health
Cato T. Laurencin, Director, Regenerative Engineering, University of Connecticut
Stephen P. MacMillan, President and Chief Executive Officer, Stryker

---

[1] Formerly the Roundtable on Evidence-Based Medicine. Institute of Medicine forums and roundtables do not issue, review, or approve individual documents. The responsibility for the published workshop summary rests with the workshop rapporteur and the institution.

Sheri S. McCoy, Vice Chair, Executive Committee, Johnson & Johnson
Farzad Mostashari, National Coordinator, Office of the National Coordinator for Health IT (*ex officio*)
Elizabeth G. Nabel, President, Brigham and Women's Hospital
Mary D. Naylor, Professor and Director, NewCourtland Center, University of Pennsylvania
Peter Neupert, Corporate Vice President, Health Solutions Group, Microsoft Corporation
William D. Novelli, Former CEO, AARP; Professor, Georgetown University
Jonathan B. Perlin, President, Clinical and Physician Services (Health), HCA, Inc.
Robert A. Petzel, Under Secretary (Health), Department of Veterans Affairs (*ex officio*)
Richard Platt, Professor and Chair, Population Medicine, Harvard Medical School
John C. Rother, Group Executive Officer, AARP
John W. Rowe, Professor, Mailman School of Public Health, Columbia University
Susan Shurin, Acting Director, National Heart, Lung, and Blood Institute (*ex officio*)
Mark D. Smith, President and CEO, California HealthCare Foundation
Glenn D. Steele, President and Chief Executive Officer, Geisinger Health System
Reed D. Tuckson, Executive VP and Chief of Medical Affairs, UnitedHealth Group
Frances M. Visco, President, National Breast Cancer Coalition
Jonathan Woodson, Assistant Secretary for Health Affairs (Acting), Department of Defense (*designee*: **Michael Dinneen**) (*ex officio*)

Workshop Planning Committee[2]

Laura L. Adams (*Chair*), Rhode Island Quality Institute
Kenneth Buetow, National Institutes of Health
Janet Corrigan, National Quality Forum
Gregory Downing, Health and Human Services
Christopher Greer, Office of Science and Technology Policy
John Halamka, Beth Israel Deaconess Medical Center
Rebecca Kush, Clinical Data Interchange Standards Consortium
Martin LaVenture, Minnesota Department of Health

---

[2] Institute of Medicine planning committees are solely responsible for organizing the workshop, identifying topics, and choosing speakers. The responsibility for the published workshop summary rests with the workshop rapporteurs and the institution.

Kenneth Mandl, Children's Hospital Boston
Daniel Masys, Vanderbilt University
David McCallie, Cerner Corporation
Anthony Rodgers, Centers for Medicare & Medicaid Services
David Ross, Public Health Informatics Institute
Edward Shortliffe, American Medical Informatics Association
Jonathan Silverstein, University of Chicago (former, now NorthShore University Health System)
James Walker, Geisinger Health System
Jon White, Agency for Healthcare Research and Quality

Roundtable Staff

Neha Agarwal, Intern (through August 2010)
Christie Bell, Financial Associate
Malcolm Biles, Program Assistant (through October 2010)
Greta Gorman, Editorial Projects Manager
Claudia Grossmann, Program Officer
J. Michael McGinnis, Senior Scholar and Executive Director
Brian Powers, Senior Program Assistant
Elizabeth Rach, Research Assistant (through November 2010)
Valerie Rohrbach, Program Assistant
Julia Sanders, Program Assistant
Robert Saunders, Program Officer
Leigh Stuckhardt, Program Associate
Kate Vasconi, Senior Program Assistant (through January 2011)
Isabelle Von Kohorn, Program Officer

Reviewers

This report has been reviewed in draft form by individuals chosen for their diverse perspectives and technical expertise, in accordance with procedures approved by the National Research Council's Report Review Committee. The purpose of this independent review is to provide candid and critical comments that will assist the institution in making its published report as sound as possible and to ensure that the report meets institutional standards for objectivity, evidence, and responsiveness to the study charge. The review comments and draft manuscript remain confidential to protect the integrity of the deliberative process. We wish to thank the following individuals for their review of this report:

Robert Califf, Duke University
Art Davidson, Denver Public Health
Shelley A. Hearne, The Pew Charitable Trusts
Carl Kesselman, University of Southern California
Kristen Rosati, Coppersmith Schermer & Brockelman PLC

Although the reviewers listed above have provided many constructive comments and suggestions, they were not asked to endorse the final draft of the report before its release. The review of this report was overseen by **Christopher Forrest,** Children's Hospital of Philadelphia. Appointed by the National Research Council and the Institute of Medicine, he was responsible for making certain that an independent examination of this report was carried out in accordance with institutional procedures and that all review comments were carefully considered. Responsibility for the final content of this report rests entirely with the editors and the institution.

Institute of Medicine
Roundtable on Value & Science-Driven Health Care
Charter and Vision Statement

The Institute of Medicine's Roundtable on Value & Science-Driven Health Care has been convened to help transform the way evidence on clinical effectiveness is generated and used to improve health and health care. Participants have set a goal that, by the year 2020, 90 percent of clinical decisions will be supported by accurate, timely, and up-to-date clinical information, and will reflect the best available evidence. Roundtable members will work with their colleagues to identify the issues not being adequately addressed, the nature of the barriers and possible solutions, and the priorities for action, and will marshal the resources of the sectors represented on the Roundtable to work for sustained public–private cooperation for change.

* *

The Institute of Medicine's Roundtable on Value & Science-Driven Health Care has been convened to help transform the way evidence on clinical effectiveness is generated and used to improve health and health care. We seek the development of a *learning health system* that is designed to generate and apply the best evidence for the collaborative healthcare choices of each patient and provider; to drive the process of discovery as a natural outgrowth of patient care; and to ensure innovation, quality, safety, and value in health care.

Vision: Our vision is for a healthcare system that draws on the best evidence to provide the care most appropriate to each patient, emphasizes prevention and health promotion, delivers the most value, adds to learning throughout the delivery of care, and leads to improvements in the nation's health.

Goal: By the year 2020, 90 percent of clinical decisions will be supported by accurate, timely, and up-to-date clinical information, and will reflect the best available evidence. We feel that this presents a tangible focus for progress toward our vision, that Americans ought to expect at least this level of performance, that it should be feasible with existing resources and emerging tools, and that measures can be developed to track and stimulate progress.

Context: As unprecedented developments in the diagnosis, treatment, and long-term management of disease bring Americans closer than ever to the promise of personalized health care, we are faced with similarly unprecedented challenges to identify and deliver the care most appropriate for individual needs and conditions. Care that is important is often not delivered. Care that is delivered is often not important. In part, this is due to our failure to apply the evidence we have about the medical care that is most effective—a failure related to shortfalls in provider knowledge and accountability, inadequate care coordination and support, lack of insurance, poorly aligned payment incentives, and misplaced patient expectations. Increasingly, it is also a result of our limited capacity for timely generation of evidence on the relative effectiveness, efficiency, and safety of available and emerging interventions. Improving the value of the return on our healthcare investment is a vital imperative that will require much greater capacity to evaluate high-priority clinical interventions, stronger links between clinical research and practice, and reorientation of the incentives to apply new insights. We must quicken our efforts to position evidence development and application as natural outgrowths of clinical care—to foster health care that learns.

Approach: The IOM Roundtable on Value & Science-Driven Health Care serves as a forum to facilitate the collaborative assessment and action around issues central to achieving the vision and goal stated. The challenges are myriad and include issues that must be addressed to improve evidence development, evidence application, and the capacity to advance progress on both dimensions. To address these challenges, as leaders in their fields, Roundtable members will work with their colleagues to identify the issues not being adequately addressed, the nature of the barriers and possible solutions, and the priorities for action, and will marshal the resources of the sectors represented on the Roundtable to work for sustained public–private cooperation for change.

Activities include collaborative exploration of new and expedited approaches to assessing the effectiveness of diagnostic and treatment interventions, better use of the patient care experience to generate evidence on effectiveness, identification of assessment priorities, and communication strategies to enhance provider and patient understanding and support for interventions proven to work best and deliver value in health care.

Core concepts and principles: For the purpose of the Roundtable activities, we define evidence-based medicine broadly to mean that, *to the greatest extent possible, the decisions that shape the health and health care of Americans—by patients, providers, payers, and policy makers alike—will be grounded on a reliable evidence base, will account appropriately for individual variation in patient needs, and will support the generation of new insights on clinical effectiveness.* Evidence is generally considered to be information from clinical experience that has met some established test of validity, and the appropriate standard is determined according to the requirements of the intervention and clinical circumstance. Processes that involve the development and use of evidence should be accessible and transparent to all stakeholders.

A common commitment to certain principles and priorities guides the activities of the Roundtable and its members, including the commitment to the right health care for each person; putting the best evidence into practice; establishing the effectiveness, efficiency, and safety of medical care delivered; building constant measurement into our healthcare investments; the establishment of healthcare data as a public good; shared responsibility distributed equitably across stakeholders, both public and private; collaborative stakeholder involvement in priority setting; transparency in the execution of activities and reporting of results; and subjugation of individual political or stakeholder perspectives in favor of the common good.

Foreword

Marshaling the best information has always been fundamental to the success of all aspects of health and health care—medical diagnosis and treatment, quality improvement, public health and health research. What is different today—and what makes this field so exciting—is the possibility, through digital data systems, to have information that is not only relevant to actions and decisions for the delivery of care, but is available, accessible, transferable, usable, and manipulatable in a way that integrates information from a number of sources and provides unprecedented opportunity for learning and improvement.

Improvement is clearly vital. In 2001, the Institute of Medicine issued its landmark report, *Crossing the Quality Chasm*, which drew the nation's attention sharply to the fact that health care in the United States was falling far short of its potential. The central lesson in that report was, in effect, that the nation needed a continuously improving learning health system that reliably delivered the best outcome. In 2006, the Institute of Medicine chartered the Roundtable on Evidence-Based Medicine, now the Roundtable on Value & Science-Driven Health Care, to engage key stakeholders in a discussion of ways to ensure that better information is available and used to transform healthcare delivery in this country. The Roundtable brings together patients, consumers, providers, researchers, health product manufacturers, payers, employees, and policy makers to discuss health reform priorities in a neutral venue and identify key impediments to progress toward a patient-centered learning health system. The Roundtable's vision of a learning health system describes a health infrastructure characterized by evidence-based care that ensures proper decision making for each patient and provider, and generates scientific evidence as a natural by-product of the care process.

Building on previous efforts to characterize, develop, and implement the infrastructure for a learning health system, and with generous support from the Office of the National Coordinator for Health Information Technology, the Roundtable convened stakeholders from across the healthcare and information technology fields in a series of workshops whose discussions are summarized in this volume, *Digital Infrastructure for the Learning Health System: The Foundation for Continuous Improvement in Health and Health Care.*

This compilation summarizes the presentations and discussions from the series, which look at the role of the digital health data systems and how they can be used to provide the information backbone for a learning health system. Participants worked to identify the opportunities, challenges, and priorities represented by the application of new information systems to health care and to consider strategy options that could further the development of a learning health system.

I would like to extend my personal thanks especially to David Blumenthal and his Office of the National Coordinator for Health Information Technology, its Chief Scientist, Charles Friedman, to the Planning Committee assembled for the series, to the Roundtable membership for their continued leadership and commitment to advancing health care in this nation, and to the Roundtable staff for their contributions in coordinating and supporting the meeting series and ongoing Roundtable activities.

Harvey V. Fineberg, M.D., Ph.D.
President, Institute of Medicine

Preface

Spurred by the growing potential of the availability of large amounts of digital health information to improve the quality of health care in this country, the Roundtable on Value & Science-Driven Health Care, with the support of the Office of the National Coordinator for Health Information Technology, convened the three-part workshop series summarized in this volume, *Digital Infrastructure for the Learning Health System: The Foundation for Continuous Improvement in Health and Health Care*. Stakeholders from across the health system—including patient advocates, providers, researchers, privacy experts, computer scientists, and policy makers—met to discuss the opportunities and challenges presented by the application of advanced information technology systems to health and health care. This summary of the workshop presentations and discussions conveys the thoughts of field leaders, and the views they shared on important strategy elements and next steps to transform the information infrastructure of the American health system into one characterized by patient engagement and continuous improvement.

The vision of the Institute of Medicine (IOM) Roundtable on Value & Science-Driven Health Care is to help advance the development of a learning health system in which evidence is generated in a timely manner by capturing results of the care process, and applied effectively and efficiently to ensure best care practices. Since its inception in 2006, the Roundtable has set out to advance this vision through collaborative initiatives, public workshops, and published proceedings that involve senior leadership from key healthcare stakeholders. Building on previous work of the Roundtable to identify the structural components of a learning health system, this workshop considered the transformational power of digital technology in health and health care.

Workshop participants focused their discussion on four important cross-cutting dimensions of the opportunities and challenges: promoting technical advances and innovation, knowledge generation and use, engaging patients and the public, and fostering stewardship and governance. Initial discussions focused on mapping the current state of play with respect to these areas and on the ways in which a developed digital infrastructure presents challenges and opportunities within each realm. Next, participants worked together to envision innovative approaches to the way in which a learning health system would be supported by a powerful, nimble, and secure digital infrastructure. The final stages of the series were centered on developing concrete strategy options whereby specific actors could work to accelerate the effective implementation of advances in building this learning health system.

Numerous organizations and individuals devoted their time and efforts in developing this workshop summary. We, of course, also wish to acknowledge and offer strong appreciation for the contributors to this volume for their insightful perspectives and observations. In this respect, we should emphasize that this workshop summary is intended to convey only the views and opinions of individuals participating in this workshop. As such, it is not intended to express or reflect the opinions of the Roundtable on Value & Science-Driven Health Care, its sponsors, or IOM.

In particular, we are indebted to the members of the expert IOM Planning Committee, who worked to guide and shape a series of productive and insightful workshop discussions. We were privileged to have the following individuals represented on the committee: Laura Adams (*Chair*) (Rhode Island Quality Institute), Ken Buetow (National Institutes of Health), Janet Corrigan (National Quality Forum), Greg Downing (U.S. Department of Health and Human Services), Chris Greer (Office of Science and Technology Policy), John Halamka (Beth Israel Deaconness Medical Center), Rebecca Kush (Clinical Data Interchange Standards Consortium), Martin LaVenture (Minnesota Department of Health), Ken Mandl (Children's Hospital Boston), Dan Masys (Vanderbilt University), David McCallie (Cerner Corporation), Anthony Rodgers (Centers for Medicare & Medicaid Services), David Ross (Public Health Informatics Institute), Edward Shortliffe (American Medical Informatics Association), Jonathan Silverstein (University of Chicago), James Walker (Geisinger Health System), and Jon White (Agency for Healthcare Research and Quality).

Under the leadership of IOM Program Officer Claudia Grossmann, a number of Roundtable staff played instrumental roles in coordinating the workshops and translating the workshop proceedings into this summary, including Neha Agarwal, Christie Bell, Malcolm Biles, Brian Powers,

Elizabeth Rach, Robert Saunders, and Kate Vasconi. We would also like to acknowledge National Academy of Sciences colleagues Jon Eisenberg and Herb Lin who participated in the meetings and provided valuable counsel on the technical components of these issues. Finally, we would also like to thank Greta Gorman, Christine Stencel, Vilija Teel, and Jordan Wyndelts for helping to coordinate the various aspects of review, production, and publication.

Successfully developing and implementing the next generation of the digital infrastructure for the learning health system will require considerable additional effort and collaboration. We believe the perspectives summarized in *Digital Infrastructure for the Learning Health System: The Foundation for Continuous Improvement in Health and Health Care* will be a very important resource not only with respect to the vision of the possible, but to the practical near-term decisions and actions of leaders and stakeholders in many quarters.

Laura L. Adams
Planning Committee Chair

Denis A. Cortese
Chair, Roundtable on Value & Science-Driven Health Care
(2006-2011)

Mark B. McClellan
Chair, Roundtable on Value & Science-Driven Health Care
(2011-Present)

J. Michael McGinnis
Executive Director,
Roundtable on Value & Science-Driven Health Care

Contents

Abbreviations and Acronyms	xxiii
Synopsis and Highlights	1
1 Introduction	53

The Learning Health System, 54
The Digital Health Infrastructure, 55
About the Digital Infrastructure Meetings, 67

2 Visioning Perspectives on the Digital Health Utility	71

Introduction, 71
Informed and Empowered Patients: Moving Beyond a
   Bystander in Care, 73
   Adam M. Clark
Building a Learning Health System Clinicians Will Use, 78
   James Walker
Improving Quality and Safety, 81
   Janet M. Corrigan
Clinical Research in the Information Age, 85
   Christopher G. Chute
Integrating the Public Health Perspective, 90
   Martin LaVenture, Sripriya Rajamani, and Jennifer Fritz

3 Technical Issues for the Digital Health Infrastructure — 99
Introduction, 99
Building a Standards and Interoperability Framework, 101
  Douglas Fridsma
Interoperability for the Learning Health System, 108
  Rebecca D. Kush
Promoting Secure Data Liquidity, 114
  Jonathan C. Silverstein
Innovative Approaches to Information Diversity, 119
  Shaun Grannis

4 Engaging Patient and Population Needs — 125
Introduction, 125
Electronic Health Data for High-Value Health Care, 127
  Mark McClellan
Engaging Individuals in Population Health Monitoring, 134
  Kenneth D. Mandl
Optimizing Chronic Disease Care and Control, 138
  Sophia W. Chang
Targeting Population Health Disparities, 141
  M. Christopher Gibbons

5 Weaving a Strong Trust Fabric — 149
Introduction, 149
Demonstrating Value to Secure Trust, 151
  Edward H. Shortliffe
Policies and Practices to Build Public Trust, 155
  Deven McGraw
HIPAA and a Learning Healthcare System, 157
  Bradley Malin
Building a Secure Learning Health System, 161
  Ian Foster

6 Stewardship and Governance in the Learning Health System — 167
Introduction, 167
Governance Coordination, Needs, and Options, 169
  Laura Adams
Consistency and Reliability in Reporting for Regulators, 172
  Theresa Mullin
Complying with Patient Expectations for Data De-Identification, 176
  Shawn N. Murphy
Information Governance in the National Health Service (UK), 180
  Harry Cayton

7 Perspectives on Innovation — 185
Introduction, 185
Conceptualizing a U.S. Population Health Record, 186
  Daniel J. Friedman
Accelerating Innovation Outside the Private Sector, 190
  Molly J. Coye
Combinatorial Innovation in Health Information Technology, 193
  Michael Liebhold

8 Fostering the Global Dimension of the Health Data Trust — 197
Introduction, 197
TRANSFoRm: Translational Medicine and Patient Safety in Europe, 198
  Brendan Delaney
Healthgrids, the SHARE Project, and Beyond, 202
  Tony Solomonides
A Global Perspective on the Importance of Systematic Data to Drive Improvements in Care, 211
  Ashish K. Jha
Informatics and the Future of Infectious Disease Surveillance, 216
  David L. Buckeridge and John S. Brownstein

9 Growing the Digital Health Infrastructure — 223
Introduction, 223
Technical Progress, 225
Knowledge Generation and Use, 227
Patient and Population Engagement, 230
Governance, 231
Common Themes and Principles, 233

10 Accelerating Progress — 239
Introduction, 239
Stakeholder Engagement, 241
Technical Progress, 241
Infrastructure Use, 243
Governance, 244
Opportunities in the Next Stages of Meaningful Use, 245
Stakeholder Responsibilities and Opportunities, 247

Appendixes

A	The Learning Health System and the Digital Health Utility	251
B	Case Studies for the Digital Health Infrastructure	255
C	Example Stakeholder Responsibilities and Opportunities	277
D	Summary Overview of Meaningful Use Objectives	279
E	PCAST Report Recommendations	281
F	Workshop Agendas	285
G	Workshop Participants	297

Abbreviations and Acronyms

ADE	adverse drug event
AHRQ	Agency for Healthcare Research and Quality
AMI	acute myocardial infarction
API	Application Programming Interface
ARB	antinogensin receptor blocker
ARRA	American Reinvestment and Recovery Act (2009)
ASTER	Adverse Drug Event Spontaneous Triggered Events Recording
ATM	automated teller machine
BIRN	Biomedical Informatics Research Network
BRIDG	Biomedical Research Integrated Domain Group
caBIG	cancer Biomedical Informatics Grid
CAMD	Coalition Against Major Diseases
CC	Coordinating Committee
CCD	Continuity of Care Document
CDASH	Clinical Data Acquisition Standards Harmonization
CDC	Centers for Disease Control and Prevention
CDISC	Clinical Data Standards Interchange Consortium
CER	comparative effectiveness research
CHCF	California HealthCare Foundation
CMMI	Center for Medicare & Medicaid Innovation
CMS	Centers for Medicare & Medicaid Services
CTSA	Clinical and Translational Science Award

CVRG	CardioVascular Research Grid
DALY	disability-adjusted life year
DOD	Department of Defense
ED	emergency department
EHR	electronic health record
EISA	Energy Independence and Security Act
ELSE	ethical, legal, social, and economic issues
EMA	European Medicines Agency
EU	European Union
EVS	Enterprise Vocabulary Services
FCC	Federal Communications Commission
FDA	Food and Drug Administration
FDAAA	Food and Drug Administration Amendments Act
FERC	Federal Energy Regulatory Commission
FHA	Federal Health Architecture
FPC	Federal Partners' Collaboration
GE	General Electric
GWAS	genome-wide association study
HHS	U.S. Department of Health and Human Services
HIE	health information exchange
HISB	American National Standards Institute's Healthcare Informatics Standards Board
HISPP	Health Information Standards Planning Panel
HITECH	Health Information Technology for Economic and Clinical Health Act
HITSC	Healthcare Information Technology Standards Committee
HITSP	Healthcare Information Technology Standards Panel
HMO	health maintenance organization
HMORN	HMO Research Network
HRSA	Health Resources and Services Administration
ICD	International Classification of Diseases
ICT	information and communications technology
IEEE	Institute of Electrical and Electronics Engineers
IEPD	Information Exchange Package Documentation
IETF	Internet Engineering Task Force

ABBREVIATIONS AND ACRONYMS

IHE	Integrating the Healthcare Enterprise
INPC	Indiana Network for Patient Care
IOM	Institute of Medicine
IRB	institutional review board
ISO	independent system operator
IT	information technology
KP	Kaiser Permanente
LOINC	Logical Observation Identifiers Names and Codes
MSCC	Mini-Sentinel Coordinating Center
NCI	National Cancer Institute
NCVHS	National Committee on Vital and Health Statistics
NDA	new drug application
NHS	National Health Service (UK)
NIEM	National Information Exchange Model
NIGB	National Information Governance Board for Health and Social Care (UK)
NIH	National Institutes of Health
NIST	National Institute of Standards and Technology
NLM	National Library of Medicine
NQF	National Quality Forum
NWHIN	Nationwide Health Information Network
OMB	Office of Management and Budget
ONC	Office of the National Coordinator for Health Information Technology
PCAST	President's Council on Science and Technology
PCHR	personally controlled health record
PCORI	Patient-Centered Outcomes Research Institute
PHI	protected health information
PHIN-NCMT	Public Health Information Network Notifiable Condition Mapping Table
PHR	personal health record
PopHR	Population Health Record
RDF	Resource Description Framework
RFD	Retrieve Form for Data Capture
RTO	regional transmission organization
RWJF	Robert Wood Johnson Foundation

SDK	Software Development Kit
SDTM	Study Data Tab Model
SHARP	Strategic Health Information Technology Advanced Research Projects
SNOMED	Systematized Nomenclature of Medicine
SWRL	Semantic Web Rule Language
TATRC	Telemedicine and Advanced Technology Research Center
TC	Technical Committee
UK	United Kingdom
ULS	ultra-large-scale
VA	Department of Veterans' Affairs
VHA	Veterans Health Administration
VistA	Veterans Health Information Systems and Technology Architecture
VLER	Virtual Lifetime Electronic Record
VPN	virtual private network
WHO	World Health Organization
XACML	eXtensible Access Control Markup Language

Synopsis and Highlights

INTRODUCTION AND OVERVIEW

Health and health care are going digital. As multiple intersecting platforms evolve to form a novel operational foundation for health and health care—the nation's digital health utility—the stage is set for fundamental and unprecedented transformation. Most changes will occur virtually out of sight, and the pace and profile of the transformation will be determined by stewardship that fosters alignment of technology, science, and culture in support of a continuously learning health system. In the context of growing concerns about the quality and costs of care, the nation's health and economic security are interdependently linked to the success of that stewardship.

Progress in computational science, information technology (IT), and biomedical and health research methods have made it possible to foresee the emergence of a learning health system that enables both the seamless and efficient delivery of best care practices and the real-time generation and application of new knowledge. Increases in the complexity and costs of care compel such a system. With rapid advances in approaches to diagnosis (such as molecular diagnostics), therapeutics, genetic insights into individual variation, and emerging measurement modalities (such as within proteomics and imaging), clinicians and patients must sort through exponentially increasing numbers of factors with each clinical decision. At the same time, healthcare costs are draining the purchasing power of consumers and handicapping the competitiveness of U.S. businesses, yet health outcomes are falling far short of the possible.

Against this backdrop of opportunity and urgency, the Institute of Medicine (IOM) of the National Academies, sponsored by the Office of the National Coordinator for Health Information Technology (ONC), convened a series of expert meetings to explore strategies for accelerating the development of the digital infrastructure for the learning health system. Presentations and major elements of those discussions are summarized in this publication, *Digital Infrastructure for the Learning Health System: The Foundation for Continuous Improvement in Health and Health Care.*

The Learning Health System

In 2001, the IOM report *Crossing the Quality Chasm* called national attention to untenable deficiencies in health care, noting that every patient should expect care that is *safe, effective, patient-centered, timely, efficient, and equitable* (IOM, 2001). Based on the determination that health care is a complex adaptive system—one in which progress on its central purpose is shaped by tenets that are few, simple, and basic—the report identified several rules to guide health care. In particular, these rules underscore the importance of issues related to the locus of decisions, patient perspectives, evidence, transparency, and waste reduction. The report envisioned, in effect, engaging patients, providers, and policy makers alike to ensure that every healthcare decision is guided by timely, accurate, and comprehensive health information provided in real time to ensure constantly improving delivery of the right care to the right person for the right price.

The release of the IOM *Chasm* report stimulated broad activities related to clinical quality improvement and the effectiveness of health care, including the eventual creation by the IOM of the Roundtable on Value & Science-Driven Health Care. Begun in 2006 as the IOM Roundtable on Evidence-Based Medicine, it has explored ways to improve the evidence base for medical decisions and sought the development of a learning health system "designed to generate and apply the best evidence for collaborative health choices of each patient and provider; to drive the process of discovery as a natural outgrowth of patient care; and to ensure innovation, quality, safety, and value in health care." From its inception, the Roundtable has conducted *The Learning Health System Series* of public meetings to consider the capture of emerging innovations—such as those occurring in IT, research methods, and care delivery—as building blocks in the foundation of a learning health system. Characteristics of such a system are noted in Box S-1 and in matrix form in Appendix A. In broad terms, they represent delivery of best practice guidance at the point of choice, continuous learning and feedback in both health and health care, and seamless, ongoing communication among participants, all facilitated through the application of IT.

> **BOX S-1**
> **Learning Health System Characteristics**
>
> *Culture*: participatory, team-based, transparent, improving
>
> *Design and processes*: patient-anchored and tested
>
> *Patients and public*: fully and actively engaged
>
> *Decisions*: informed, facilitated, shared, and coordinated
>
> *Care*: starting with the best practice, every time
>
> *Outcomes and costs*: transparent and constantly assessed
>
> *Knowledge*: ongoing, seamless product of services and research
>
> *Digital technology*: the engine for continuous improvement
>
> *Health information*: a reliable, secure, and reusable resource
>
> *The Data utility*: data stewarded and used for the common good
>
> *Trust fabric*: strong, protected, and actively nurtured
>
> *Leadership*: multi-focal, networked, and dynamic
>
> SOURCE: Adapted from *The Learning Healthcare System* (IOM, 2007).

Because IT serves as the functional engine for the continuous learning system, this ONC-commissioned exploration was broadly conceived to consider the issues and strategies required for the emergence of a digital infrastructure that allows data collected during activities in various settings—clinical, research, and public health—to be integrated, analyzed, and broadly applied ("collect once, use for multiple purposes") to inform and improve clinical care decisions, promote patient education and self-management, design public health strategies, and support research and knowledge development efforts in a timely manner.

The Digital Health Infrastructure

The digital infrastructure for the learning health system will not solely be the result of features designed and built *de novo*. Existing initiatives and resources are actively in play at multiple levels—including electronic health records (EHRs); personal health records (PHRs); telehealth; health information portals; electronic monitoring devices; biobanks; health information databases maintained by large health systems, private insurers, and regulatory agencies; and advances in molecular diagnostics. Each adds important capacity for clinical care, clinical and health services research, public health surveillance and intervention, patient education and self-management, and safety and cost monitoring.

Still, these capacities are relatively early in their development, and progress depends on improvements on several dimensions. As of 2009, only about 12% of hospitals and 6% of clinician offices had an EHR in place (DesRoches et al., 2008; Jha et al., 2010) and only about 1 in 14 Americans had electronic access to any patient-oriented version of their health record (CHCF, 2010). On the other hand, since 2000, the number of Americans who have access to the internet has jumped from 46% to 74%, and the number of American adults who have looked online for health information has jumped from 25% to 61% (Fox, 2010). Wireless technology is quickening the pace of change. With 6 in 10 American adults using wireless capability with a laptop or mobile device (Smith, 2010), mobile applications are rapidly developing the potential for remote site access to health information, as well as diagnostic and even treatment services.

This developing potential presents opportunities and challenges for stewardship. Issues related to interoperability, governance, patient and public engagement, and privacy and security concerns, among others, will need to be better addressed for successful progress toward a learning health system. Approaches and lessons from sectors outside health include those from energy and the financial sector, two examples discussed in the meetings and summarized in this publication (see Appendix B). VISA used a minimalist approach, crafted on the combination of mutual self-interest and basic rules-of-play, to build its platform for a global credit card network. Consumer Energy's work in the Smart Grid Initiative applied an analytically driven approach to accommodate and network a wide variety of legacy nodes in growing the electronic platform operating the nation's energy system. Background on the Smart Grid Initiative is presented in Box S-2.

Regardless of the model, a key rationale for the workshop discussions was the reality that effective and efficient progress in the growth and development of our national and global digital health infrastructure requires active cooperation, collaboration, and role delineation among many organizations, companies, and agencies—private and public—at the cutting edge of using health IT to improve health and health care.

The striking, and accelerating, progress in the capacity and transformative influences of IT on society over the past three decades is a blended product of interrelated initiatives arising from within the commercial, in-

> **BOX S-2**
> **Case: The Smart Grid**
>
> The Smart Grid is a long-term, complex systems development project to grow the electronic platform operating the nation's energy system using an engineering approach to accommodate a wide variety of legacy nodes that are organic—constantly growing and evolving, much like a biological system. This continuous evolution allows the Smart Grid's architecture to preserve and encourage the capacity of each node to innovate locally and deal with complexity in a way that suits local and grid needs. As conceived, the Smart Grid will
>
> - Enable active participation by consumers
> - Accommodate all generation and storage options
> - Enable new products, services, and markets
> - Provide power equality for the digital economy
> - Optimize asset utilization and operate efficiently
> - Anticipate and respond to system disturbances (self-heal)
> - Operate resiliently against attack and natural disaster
>
> Because there is no need for consensus among the nodes on how they should operate within local boundaries, the Smart Grid development methodology is not based on comprehensive internal design and operating standards for each node on the Grid to follow. Instead, the approach accommodates highly diverse nodes connecting to the Smart Grid using open data translation protocols that standardize information management, rather than using the internal workings of each node. The Grid becomes a communications bus to which each node must be able to write, and from which each node must be able to read. This architecture preserves capacities for local operating autonomy and innovation throughout the Smart Grid. It also manages a standardized communications capacity among complex, and otherwise noninteroperable, legacy nodes on the Grid. These features are all characteristics of ultra-large-scale (ULS) software-intensive systems.

dependent, and public sectors. Leaps in the speed, power, and efficiency of information processing, the development of the Internet and World Wide Web, and its use to facilitate near-universally available real-time access to information, have spawned a new economy and new vehicles for progress.

Health information vendors, large and small, have emerged to meet the growing demand for capacity to manage the retrieval, storage, and delivery of information for agencies, institutions, professionals, and individuals in virtually every aspect of health and health care. The range of newly digitalized services—and the growth of vendors to provide them—is startling. Through technologies developed by companies such as Google, Microsoft, and Yahoo, the amount of web-based health information accessed daily by individuals and clinicians is already transforming the care process. Beyond the publicly available digital resources, a vast array of specialized care management products have emerged for activities such as scheduling and billing; claims processing and payment; supply and equipment inventory maintenance; individual patient charting; medication prescribing and tracking; family and personal health records; clinician-patient communication; clinician and patient decision support; robotics-assisted procedures; telehealth for remote site diagnosis and treatment; disease surveillance; vital statistics reporting; postmarket product monitoring; safety and hazard exposure monitoring; clinical research protocols; disease and intervention registries; and data aggregation, analysis, and modeling.

Various large academic health centers and healthcare delivery organizations—Veterans Health Administration (VHA), Kaiser Permanente (see Box S-3), Geisinger Health System, Vanderbilt, MD Anderson, Palo Alto Medical Foundation, Group Health Cooperative, several Harvard facilities, Children's Hospital of Philadelphia, Virginia Mason, and the Mayo Clinic, to name a few—have invested substantially in the creation of advanced digital resources for administrative, patient care, and research functions. Additionally, some related collaborative research networks have begun to develop. Nonetheless, the diversity and limited compatibility of the products, and the lack of economic incentives for their use have, to date, restrained the broader uptake, application, and functional utility of digital capacity across the system.

A number of public, private, and independent sector initiatives have emerged to accelerate stakeholder action on various dimensions important to progress. To supplement the relatively limited pre-2009 public investments, independent sector leadership has come from foundations such as the Markle Foundation, the Robert Wood Johnson Foundation, and the California HealthCare Foundation. Furthermore, in addition to the formation of capacity-building resources such as the Health Information Exchanges, a number of facilitative stakeholder groups have emerged—for example, the eHealth Initiative, the Clinical Data Interchange Standards Consortium (CDISC), and the National eHealth Collaborative. On the professional advancement dimension, the American Medical Informatics Association has developed as a growing resource for the contributions of biomedical and health informaticians working in activities to organize, manage, analyze, and use information in health care. An example of the coordinative potential of these groups is found in the development of integration profiles by Integrating the Healthcare Enterprise and CDISC to support the use of EHRs for clinical research, quality, and public health, and the testing and demonstration of these profiles by several vendors including Cerner, Allscripts, Greenway Medical, and General Electric Healthcare.

At the federal level, ONC was created in 2004 in the U.S. Department

> **BOX S-3**
> **Case: Kaiser Permanente**
>
> In 2003, Kaiser Permanente (KP) launched a $4 billion health information system called KP HealthConnect that links its facilities and clinicians throughout their delivery system and represents the largest civilian installation of electronic health records in the United States. The EHR at the heart of KP HealthConnect provides a reliably accessible longitudinal record of member encounters across clinical settings including laboratory, medication, and imaging data; as well as supporting:
>
> - Electronic prescribing and test ordering (computerized physician-order entry) with standard order sets to promote evidence-based care
> - Population and patient-panel management tools such as disease registries to track patients with chronic conditions
> - Decision support tools such as medication-safety alerts, preventive-care reminders, and online clinical guidelines
> - Electronic referrals that directly schedule patient appointments with specialty care physicians
> - Personal health records providing patients with the ability to view their personal clinical information including lab results, plus linkage with pharmacy, physician scheduling, and secure and confidential e-mail messaging with clinicians.
> - Performance monitoring and reporting capabilities
> - Patient registration and billing functions
>
> Physician leaders report that access to the EHR in the exam room is helping to promote compliance with evidence-based guidelines and treatment protocols, eliminate duplicate tests, and enable physicians to handle multiple complaints more efficiently within one visit. Ongoing evaluation by Kaiser indicates that patient satisfaction with outpatient physician encounters has increased and that the combination of computerized physician-order entry, medication bar coding, and electronic documentation tools is helping to reduce medication administration errors in hospital care.
> Overall, Kaiser's experience suggests that use of the EHR and online portal to support care management and new modes of patient encounters is having positive effects on utilization of services and patient engagement. For example, three-quarters or more of online users surveyed agreed that the portal enables them to manage their health care effectively and that it makes interacting with the healthcare team more convenient.

of Health and Human Services (HHS) to stimulate progress in the field. Since 2009, with the enactment of the Health Information Technology for Economic and Clinical Health Act (HITECH) as part of the American Recovery and Reinvestment Act, the federal government leadership profile has become especially prominent. This has included the commitment of unprecedented resources for health information technology (HIT), administered through the leadership of ONC. Under HITECH, ONC was granted $2 billion to facilitate the adoption and meaningful use of HIT. In addition, an estimated $27 billion was designated for the Centers for Medicare & Medicaid Services (CMS) to distribute as incentive payments for physicians and hospitals to become meaningful users of HIT.

Designed as a set of staged requirements to qualify for CMS incentive payments, the first-stage elements of "meaningful use" were released by CMS on July 13, 2010. These established a core set of requirements for eligible professionals and hospitals, as well as a menu of additional choices, from which five are to be chosen. The stage 1 meaningful use target elements are listed in summary fashion in Box S-4, and details are contained in Appendix D. The subsequent stages of meaningful use are currently under development and are presented later in this summary, along with an indication of related issues flagged in workshop discussions.

In addition to the meaningful use requirements, ONC has funded a series of grant programs through HITECH, including the Beacon Community grants, aimed at demonstrating community-wide digital infrastructure capacity and use for health improvement, and the Strategic Health Information Technology Advanced Research Projects Program, to foster the capture of technological advances to improve system performance. At the broader level, ONC is pursuing a series of initiatives to foster health information exchange among stakeholders, including the regional health information exchanges and under the Nationwide Health Information Network (NWHIN).

Several additional HHS agencies have activities important to the development of the digital learning health system. CMS, in addition to establishing rules for meaningful use and requirements for uniform condition identifiers central to healthcare payment and research, recently created the Center for Medicare and Medicaid Innovation to test innovative payment and program service delivery methods. Within the National Institutes of Health (NIH), the National Library of Medicine serves as the central coordinating body for clinical terminology standards, and other NIH programs, such as the Clinical and Translational Science Awards Program, and the National Cancer Institute's Enterprise Vocabulary Series and cancer Biomedical Informatics Grid (caBIG®, see Box S-5 and Appendix B for additional information) serve as key contributors to building the capacity to derive scientific discovery from patient care. Through its National Resource Center for Health IT and capacity initiatives on patient registries, the Agency for Healthcare Research and Quality (AHRQ) supports a number of programs to advance the digital utility for healthcare quality and safety.

At the Food and Drug Administration (FDA), the Sentinel Initiative (see Box S-6 and Appendix B) has been designed to build and implement a national electronic system for postmarket surveillance of approved drugs

> **BOX S-4**
> **Meaningful Use Requirement Categories**
>
> Core structured personal data (age, sex, ethnicity, smoking status)
>
> Core list of active problems and diagnoses
>
> Core structured clinical data (vital signs, meds, [labs])
>
> Outpatient medications electronically prescribed
>
> Automated medication safeguard/reconciliation
>
> Clinical decision support
>
> Care coordination support/interoperability
>
> Visit-specific information to patients
>
> Automated patient reminders
>
> e-Record patient access (copy or patient portal)
>
> Embedded measures for clinical quality reporting
>
> Security safeguards
>
> Examples of optional elements:
>   Advance directives for ages >65
>   Condition-specific data retrieval capacity
>   Public health reporting (reportable conditions)
>
> SOURCE: Adapted from Blumenthal and Tavenner (2010). See Appendix D for details.

and other medical products. The Centers for Disease Control and Prevention (CDC) supports several IT-based public health data collection and surveillance programs and serves as the primary agency responsible for these tracking efforts, response and public health links to domestic and international public health data systems, and the Health Resources and Services Administration (HRSA) has developed initiatives introducing HIT to improve care access and coordination in rural areas and for underserved populations.

Efforts to promote the development, implementation, and widespread adoption of HIT also build on a wide array of digital learning leadership efforts by other federal agencies. In particular, important contributions stem

> **BOX S-5**
> **Case: The National Cancer Institute's caBIG® Initiative**
>
> The National Cancer Institute of the National Institutes of Health has developed an informatics program designed to improve patient care and accelerate scientific discoveries by enabling the collection and analysis of large amounts of biological and clinical information and facilitating connectivity and collaboration among biomedical researchers and organizations. More than 700 different organizations are actively engaged in caBIG®, including basic and clinical researchers, consumers, physicians, advocates, software architects and developers, bioinformatics specialists and executives from academe, medical centers, government, and commercial software, pharmaceutical, and biotechnology companies from the United States and in 15+ countries around the globe.
>
> At the heart of the caBIG® program is caGrid, a model-driven, service-oriented architecture that provides standards-based core "services," tools, and interfaces so the community can connect to share data and analyses efficiently and securely. More than 120 organizations are connected to caGrid. In partnership with the American Society of Clinical Oncology, caBIG® is developing specifications and services to support oncology-extended EHRs that are being deployed in community practice and hospital settings. caBIG® tools and technology are also being used by researchers working on cardiovascular health, arthritis, and AIDS. In addition, pilot projects have successfully connected caGrid to other networks, including the Nationwide Health Information Network, the CardioVascular Research Grid, and the computational network TeraGrid.

from responsibilities and activities of the VHA—for example, the highly regarded Veterans Health Information Systems and Technology Architecture system of IT supporting better care, as well as personal tools such as "My HealtheVet" and the Virtual Lifetime Electronic Record programs—the Department of Defense (DOD), the Federal Communications Commission (FCC), and the National Science Foundation (NSF). The VHA and the DOD have formed the Telemedicine and Advanced Technology Research Center as a joint program to advance research and applications in health informatics, telemedicine, and mobile health monitoring systems. Because of the deep and broad set of capabilities and initiatives collectively sponsored by federal agencies, their coordination and interface with private sector activities offers a vital strategic opportunity to accelerate the development of a learning health system.

Testament to the compelling priority of the prospects, in December 2010, the President's Council of Advisors on Science and Technology (PCAST) issued its report, *Realizing the Full Potential of Health Information Technology to Improve Healthcare for Americans: The Path Forward* (PCAST, 2010). The PCAST report examines the opportunities and needs

> **BOX S-6**
> **Case: The FDA's Sentinel Initiative**
>
> In 2008, the Department of Health and Human Services and the Food and Drug Administration (FDA) announced the launch of FDA's Sentinel Initiative, a long-term program designed to build and implement a national electronic system—the Sentinel System—for monitoring the safety of FDA-approved drugs and other medical products. Data partners in the Sentinel System will include organizations such as academic medical centers, healthcare systems, and health insurance companies. As currently envisioned, participating data partners will access, maintain, and protect their respective data, functioning as part of a "distributed system."
>
> In a related pilot activity, FDA is working with Harvard Pilgrim Health Care, Inc. to develop a smaller working version of the future Sentinel System, dubbed "Mini-Sentinel." Through this pilot, FDA will learn more about some of the barriers and challenges, both internal and external, to establishing a Sentinel System for medical product safety monitoring. The Mini-Sentinel Coordinating Center (MSCC) represents a consortium of more than 20 collaborating institutions, working with participating data partners to use a common data model as the basis for their approach. Data partners transform their data into a standardized format, based upon which the MSCC will write a single analytical software program for a given safety question and provide it to each of the data partners. Each partner will conduct analyses behind its existing, secure firewall and send only summary results to the MSCC for aggregation and further evaluation.
>
> As this pilot is being implemented, a governance structure is being developed to ensure the activity encourages broad collaboration within appropriate guidelines for the conduct of public health surveillance activities. In order to accomplish that, the MSCC is developing a Statement of Principles and Policies that will include descriptions of the organizational structure and policies related to communication, privacy, confidentiality, data usage, conflicts of interest, and intellectual property.

for the use of HIT to improve healthcare quality and reduce cost, as well as the activities and aligment of current federal programs with relevant responsibilities. It sets out a series of recommendations intended to facilitate private, entrepreneurial initiatives through governmental action to speed development of a "universal exchange language" for health information, the application of which would maximize the ability to use existing and developing electronic record systems. Specifically, it recommends action by the federal government, especially ONC and CMS, in accelerating the identification of standards required for health information exchange using metadata-tagged data elements; mapping various existing semantic taxonomies onto the tagged elements; developing incentives for product use of tagged elements; fostering use of metadata for security and safety protocols;

bringing federal program capacity and policy leverage to bear in implementing and guiding the efforts; and developing metrics to assess progress. The PCAST recommendations are included as Appendix E.

About the Digital Infrastructure Meetings

It was in this general context of opportunity and challenge that the IOM workshops on the digital health infrastructure were organized. Since the inaugural workshop in 2006, the IOM has conducted 15 workshops in the *Learning Health System Series*, with 10 reports published and in production:

- *The Learning Healthcare System*
- *Leadership Commitments to Improve Value in Health Care: Finding Common Ground*
- *Evidence-Based Medicine and the Changing Nature of Health Care*
- *Redesigning the Clinical Effectiveness Research Paradigm: Innovation and Practice-Based Approaches*
- *Clinical Data as the Basic Staple of Healthcare Learning: Creating and Protecting a Public Good*
- *Engineering a Learning Healthcare System: A Look at the Future*
- *Learning What Works: Infrastructure Required for Comparative Effectiveness Research*
- *Value in Health Care: Accounting for Cost, Quality, Safety, Outcomes, and Innovation*
- *The Healthcare Imperative: Lowering Costs and Improving Outcomes*
- *Patients Charting the Course: Citizen Engagement and the Learning Health System*

This publication considers what has been variously described as the system's nerve center, its circulation system, and the engine to drive the progress envisioned in the *Learning Health System Series*: the digital infrastructure. To explore the range of issues necessary to engage if that infrastructure is to develop as effectively and efficiently as possible, ONC requested that the IOM, through the Roundtable on Value & Science-Driven Health Care, organize the series of expert meetings summarized in this publication, *Digital Infrastructure for the Learning Health System: The Foundation for Continuous Improvement in Health and Health Care*.

As the title indicates, the primary intent of the meetings was to identify and explore strategic opportunities for accelerating the evolution of a digital infrastructure that will support and drive continuous improvement in health and health care. Three meetings were held in the summer and fall of 2010, bringing together researchers, computer scientists, privacy experts, clinicians, health care administrators, HIT professionals, representatives of

SYNOPSIS AND HIGHLIGHTS 13

patient advocacy groups, healthcare policy makers, and other stakeholders. Building on the existing foundations of HIT, the main objectives were to foster a shared understanding of the vision for the digital infrastructure, explore the current state of the system, identify key priorities for future work, and consider strategy elements and priorities for accelerating progress on improving the infrastructure to build a more seamless learning enterprise that will improve health and health care in America.

Aims and Planning

A planning committee,[1] composed of leading authorities on various aspects of the digital health learning process, shaped the workshop series around the following aims:

- Foster a shared understanding of the vision for the digital infrastructure for continuous learning and quality-driven health and healthcare programs.
- Explore current capacity, approaches, incentives, and policies; and identify key technological, organizational, policy, and implementation priorities for the development of the digital infrastructure.
- Discuss the characteristics of potentially disruptive breakthrough developments.
- Consider strategy elements and priorities for accelerating progress on the approach to the infrastructure and for moving to a more seamless learning enterprise.

Contextual considerations informing the Committee's development of the agenda included

- Rapid developments in IT exponentially facilitating the potential of health data for knowledge generation and care improvement.
- Policy initiatives leading eventually to the digital capture and storage of virtually all clinical and related health data for use in performance improvement.
- Promising potential in federated and distributed research approaches allows data to remain local while enabling querying and virtual pooling across systems.

---

[1] Institute of Medicine planning committees are solely responsible for organizing the workshop, identifying topics, and choosing speakers. The responsibility for the published workshop summary rests with the workshop rapporteurs and the institution.

- Ongoing innovation in search technologies with the potential to accelerate use of available data from multiple sources for new insights.
- Meaningful use criteria and health reform provisions that provide starting points, incentives, and guidance, while retaining the flexibility necessary to accommodate breakthrough capacities.
- Appreciation of the need to limit the burden for health data collection to the issues most important to patient care and knowledge generation.
- Requirement for governance policies that foster strengthening the data utility as a core resource to advance the common good; in particular by cultivating the trust fabric among stakeholders and accelerating collaborative progress.
- Developing standards that will facilitate distributed access to large datasets for comparative effectiveness research, biomarker validation, disease modeling, and research process improvement.

Structure and Thematic Arc

The three workshops in the series progressed from a broad exploration of the state of play and various stakeholder perspectives on a learning health system, to a more specific identification of strategic approaches to the challenges, and concluded with detailed discussions of strategic elements, stakeholder responsibilities, and key cross-cutting challenges. To maximize identification and sharing of perspectives, expert presentations were followed by open discussion among participants and separate small group discussion sessions were built into each of the meetings.

The first workshop, "Opportunities, Challenges, Priorities," considered the overall vision of the digital infrastructure for the learning health system as well as some of the prominent issues and opportunities related to technical progress, ensuring commitment to population and patient needs, development of the necessary trust fabric, stewardship and governance, and the implications of the global character of the health data trust. The second meeting, "The System After Next," went deeper into three cross-cutting areas identified during the first workshop: engaging the patient and population, promoting technical advances, and fostering stewardship and governance structures. The third and final meeting of the series, "Strategy Scenarios," reviewed the common themes and information from the previous workshops and extended into deeper consideration of strategy elements, opportunities, responsibilities, and next steps for progress on four key focus areas: technical progress, knowledge generation and use, patient and population engagement, and governance.

COMMON THEMES AND PRINCIPLES

Several common themes recurred throughout the rich and varied discussions. These themes, included in Box S-7 and summarized below, were reflected in discussions of each of the four focus areas (technical progress, knowledge generation and use, patient and population engagement, and governance), as well as the discussions around various strategic elements. They ranged from issues related to the culture and environment for learning, to the centrality of the patient and the importance of flexibility and trust.

- *Build a shared learning environment.* HIT provides an opportunity to change the current environment in which health decisions are made to one of shared input and active participation from patients, caregivers, and the population at large. Discussed approaches to developing this shared learning environment include the direct involvement and support of patient and population roles in the generation of knowledge through the incorporation of user-generated data; understanding the benefits of information use in patient care and population health improvement; and improving patient access to health information to allow for a more active role in care decisions.
- *Engage health and health care, population and patient.* Many participants reiterated that in order to improve health outcomes for the nation, thinking must extend beyond clinical encounters, and even beyond the individual patient, to the population as a whole. This shift of scope brought into clearer focus several issues discussed, including the opportunity to use HIT and its associated informa-

---

BOX S-7
Common Themes and Principles

- Build a shared learning environment
- Engage health and health care, population and patient
- Leverage existing programs and policies
- Embed services and research in a continuous learning loop
- Anchor in an ultra-large-scale systems approach
- Emphasize decentralization and specifications parsimony
- Keep use barriers low and complexity incremental
- Foster a sociotechnical perspective, focused on the population
- Weave a strong and secure trust fabric among stakeholders
- Provide continuous evaluation and improvement

tion to build a concept of health that is about more than medical care and draws on seamless interface with information from non-medical health-related sources to generate knowledge that allows for a more inclusive view of population health improvement.

- *Leverage existing programs and policies.* A foundational assumption during the discussions was the advantage provided by building on and accelerating the substantial recent progress, both nationally and internationally, with an emphasis on the importance of fostering coordination among these efforts to capture efficiencies and prevent unnecessary duplication and waste going forward. Participants often noted that recent policies and legislation have laid a foundation for this work, and that the resulting investments and progress can be leveraged to move toward long-term system goals.

- *Embed services and research in a continuous learning loop.* Meeting participants often underscored that a digital infrastructure that supports both the generation and use of knowledge cannot be effective unless it is integrated seamlessly within the processes from which it draws and is meant to support care delivery, research, quality improvement, and population health monitoring. Ease of use for health system stakeholders, attention to the effects on workflow, and the delivery of useful decision support at point of care were often mentioned in discussions.

- *Anchor in an ultra-large-scale systems approach.* One of the most prominent features of the discussions was the notion that the health system is a complex, sociotechnical ecosystem, needing a unique conceptual approach. Grounding this approach to coordination and integration of the digital infrastructure for the learning health system in the principles of an ultra-large-scale (ULS) systems approach was suggested by several workshop participants from the computer science community (see Box S-8). The term "ultra-large-scale system" refers to the existence of a virtual system that has bearing on a social purpose—for example, improving health and health care—and in which a few key elements, such as interchange representation, may be standardized, but whose many participants have diverse and even conflicting goals, so adaptability is key. Institutions retain flexibility for innovation in their choices, and evolutionary functional change can be shaped by architectural precepts, incentives, and compliance assessment, but not by centralized control. ULS functionality is therefore facilitated by protocols that allow maximum practical flexibility for participants. Incorporating decentralization of data, development, and operational authority and control, this approach fosters local innovation, personaliza-

> **BOX S-8**
> **Ultra-Large-Scale (ULS) System Characteristics**
>
> The ULS approach can be best described by a set of characteristics that tend to arise as a result of the scale of the system (in this case health and health care) rather than a prescriptive set of required components. Previous work on the ULS concept has identified the following key characteristics of ULS systems:
>
> *Decentralization:* The scale of ULS systems means that they will necessarily be decentralized in a variety of ways—decentralized data, development, evolution, and operational control.
>
> *Inherently conflicting, unknowable, and diverse requirements:* ULS systems will be developed and used by a wide variety of stakeholders with unavoidably different, conflicting, complex, and changing needs.
>
> *Continuous evolution and deployment:* There will be an increasing need to integrate new capabilities into a ULS system while it is operating. New and different capabilities will be deployed, and unused capabilities will be dropped; the system will be evolving not in phases, but continuously.
>
> *Heterogeneous, inconsistent, and changing elements:* A ULS system will not be constructed from uniform parts: there will be some misfits, especially as the system is extended and repaired.
>
> *Erosion of the people/system boundary:* People will not just be users of a ULS system; they will be elements of the system, affecting its overall emergent behavior.
>
> *Normal failures:* Software and hardware failures will be the norm rather than the exception.
>
> *New paradigms for acquisition and policy:* The acquisition of a ULS system will be simultaneous with the operation of the system and require new methods for control.
>
> SOURCE: Northrop et al. (2006).

tion, and emergent behaviors. Participants felt that this approach was well suited to the complex adaptive characteristics of the health system, and that it could serve as an anchoring framework for approaching both the social and technical components of the overall infrastructure.

- *Emphasize decentralization and specifications parsimony.* In line with the complex adaptive qualities of the health system outlined in the *Quality Chasm* (IOM, 2001) report and reiterated during the workshops, both the social and technical components of the digital health infrastructure require a framework that allows for tailoring to specific needs, local innovation, and evolvability. In this respect, the commonly repeated refrain was a call for the principle of parsimony and minimizing centralization that might constitute a barrier to entry: specify only the minimal set of standards or requirements necessary for key functional utility and push the maximum amount of control to the periphery. This approach is in line with strategies such as those suggested in the PCAST report for use of metadata for wrapping individual information packets to facilitate interoperability and health information exchange, in which a primary focus would be on development of the metadata standards.

- *Keep use barriers low and complexity incremental.* Similarly, incentives for broad participation in the digital infrastructure by all stakeholders was discussed as a crucial factor to its success. The proposal to keep the barriers for use of the infrastructure, such as deployment and operational complexity, low was articulated by workshop participants in order to allow for maximum participation at a baseline level, and allow for incremental complexity and sophistication where possible or necessary.
- *Foster a sociotechnical perspective, focused on the population.* From the outset of the discussions, participants pointed out that the major barriers to technical progress often lie in social and cultural domains. Acknowledging and engaging this fact were described as being crucial to success, with discussions centering on an approach that reorients future efforts to engage the patient more directly in the collection and use of information in a way that is most useful to them.
- *Weave a strong trust fabric among stakeholders.* Security and privacy concerns represent a strong threat to participation in, and therefore the success of, the sociotechnical ecosystem. Accordingly, they must be dealt with from both the social and technical perspectives. Participants emphasized the need for systems security to comply with all current requirements and regulations and retain an ability to evolve to meet future needs. In addition, continued honest communication to the public and other involved stakeholders about risks and benefits will be crucial to building a foundation of trust.
- *Provide continuous evaluation and improvement.* A learning system is one that assesses its own performance against a set of goals and uses the results of that evaluation to change future behaviors. Workshop participants articulated the importance that all compo-

nents of a digital infrastructure must themselves function as learning systems.

OPPORTUNITIES, CHALLENGES, AND PRIORITIES

During the first meeting, field authorities were invited to set the stage with overview perspectives summarized below on stakeholder views of the vision, data capture and use strategies, patient and population engagement, security and the trust fabric, stewardship and governance, and the global opportunities.

Visioning Perspectives on the Digital Health Utility

Building an effective learning health system requires arriving at a shared vision from sometimes highly varied perspectives. The initial discussion session brought out several of such perspectives, including those of the patient, clinician, quality and safety community, clinical research, and population health.

Informed and Empowered Patients: Moving Beyond a Bystander in Care

Adam Clark, formerly of the Lance Armstrong Foundation (now at FasterCures), shared his vision of a learning health system characterized by bidirectional exchange of health information (individuals as both donors and consumers). In order to support this vision, he described the need to develop appropriate interfaces to encourage and facilitate participation. This includes not only providing the most appropriate information to consumers in an accessible format, but accommodating the participation of family members and caregivers. Dr. Clark highlighted the value of including consumers as information donors in the learning health system, pointing to their ability to contribute types of information—such as accounts of fatigue or depression—and provide a level of context that would otherwise not be captured. He cited data from the Armstrong Foundation indicating that individuals want to share this information as long as their privacy concerns are addressed. Dr. Clark concluded by noting that the escalating complexity of medicine demands new kinds of relationships between patients, clinicians, and researchers, and that the digital infrastructure can serve as a platform for this going forward.

Building a Learning Health System Clinicians Will Use

The perspective of the healthcare team was explored by Jim Walker of Geisinger Health System. He defined a learning health system as one of goal-oriented feedforward and feedback loops that create actionable information with the potential to effect marked improvements in population health and decreases in the cost of evidence-based care if implemented correctly. Dr. Walker described the steps to building a learning health system, including defining system learning needs and associated questions, identifying the right information to answer those questions and the best methods to collect that information. He noted that an effective learning health system must be useful and useable to all healthcare team members. Dr. Walker described his experiences with health IT implementation at Geisinger and highlighted the complex, sociotechnical nature of the challenge—requiring that as much attention be given to the social aspects as is currently being given to technical capacity. Citing examples of healthcare system learning needs—such as the proper second-line therapy for diabetes—Walker laid out the potential for a learning system to address these questions and feed that information back to healthcare team members. However, he noted, this goal will require fundamental health IT systems redesign in order to support healthcare team decision making.

Improving Quality and Safety

Janet Corrigan from the National Quality Forum (NQF) noted that little progress had been made to improve quality and safety since the publication of the *Quality Chasm* report (IOM, 2001), and that value has concurrently decreased. She stated that increases in the safety, quality, and effectiveness of health care will require investments in a digital infrastructure capable of collecting information across the longitudinal "patient-focused episode," and feeding back performance results along with clinical decision support to patients and clinicians. Dr. Corrigan described the framework used by NQF to develop measures for reporting and value-based purchasing, and explored how a digital infrastructure could support capturing the relevant data. Finally, she stated that achieving better health outcomes will require collecting information from, and enabling communication with, individuals both within and outside of traditional healthcare settings.

Clinical Research in the Information Age

The growing information intensity of modern medicine and biomedical research, coupled with advances in computing capabilities, defined the clinical research perspective articulated by Christopher Chute from the Mayo Clinic. He observed that given these concurrent conditions, the technical requirements for information and knowledge management in health care should be high-priority issues. Drawing from examples of "big science" disciplines such as astronomy and physics, he suggested that the future of biology and medicine will be characterized by collaborative efforts and shared data and knowledge. As such, he pointed to the need for standardization in order to allow for comparability and consistency in health information. Reviewing the historical state of standards uptake and development efforts, he suggested that meaningful use may be a transformative effort that moves health care in this direction.

Integrating the Public Health Perspective

Martin LaVenture, Sripriya Rajamani, and Jennifer Fritz from the Minnesota State Department of Health shared his account of the opportunities and challenges surrounding a digital platform that supports population health activities. Acknowledging that the learning health system holds great promise for improving health at the population level, he described the need to bolster the capacity and capabilities of population health services in order to realize this potential. The principal challenge, he noted, is the lack of an integrated, modernized digital health infrastructure that is used by a trained workforce and stewarded by public health leaders who understand the potential benefits for population health. Accordingly, he articulated the need for a more unified vision of a digital infrastructure for population health, including the development of a population health approach to data standards; aggregation and infrastructure; and intelligent, bidirectional messaging for patients and consumers.

Technical Issues for the Digital Health Infrastructure

IT constitutes the core of the digital learning health system, and technological innovation in several key areas will be crucial in meeting future needs for security, healthcare quality, and clinical and public health applications. Many of the issues center on interoperability, a feature of IT systems that allows for efficient and useful exchange of a core set of data among an array of systems. Ensuring that data collected in one system can be utilized by other systems for a variety of different uses (e.g., quality, research, public health) is necessary if clinical data are to be collected and analyzed across the entire learning health system to improve health and health care.

Building on the Foundation of Meaningful Use

Douglas Fridsma from the Office of Standards and Interoperability at ONC provided an update on the current standards and interoperability framework being developed. He reviewed several lessons learned in past standards development efforts that are currently informing their approach. Dr. Fridsma described the priorities shaping the work of the Office of

Standards and Interoperability, highlighting the need to manage the lifecycle of standards and interoperability activities by providing mechanisms for continuous refinement. He detailed the model being used in the development of the standards and interoperability framework, which consists of interplay between community engagement, harmonization of core concepts with other exchange models, development of implementation specifications, reference implementation, and incorporation into certification and testing initiatives. Dr. Fridsma emphasized the need to leverage existing work, coordinate capacity, and integrate successful initiatives into the framework.

Interoperability for the Learning Health System

Rebecca Kush from the CDISC suggested that one approach to defining interoperability within the digital infrastructure of the learning health system might be the exchange and aggregation of information upon which trustworthy healthcare decisions can be made. Dr. Kush cited existing enablers that will contribute to this goal, including the Coalition Against Major Diseases's Alzheimer's initiative to share and pool clinical trial data across pharmaceutical companies. Furthermore, she noted that a standardized core dataset of EHR information that could be repurposed for research, safety monitoring, quality reporting, and population health would help facilitate an interoperable digital platform for health. Dr. Kush shared several examples of existing standards initiatives that could be leveraged as a foundation for the learning health system—for example, increasing adverse drug event (ADE) reporting through the implementation of the ADE Spontaneous Triggered Events Recording.

Promoting Secure Data Liquidity

Building from the notion of health care as a complex adaptive system, Jonathan Silverstein, formerly of the University of Chicago (now at NorthShore University Health System), asserted that current technological failures of the healthcare system are a result of incompatibility between the technology employed and the nature of the system. He suggested that what is needed is secure data liquidity, supported by a functional architecture that enables ever-expanding secure uses of health data. According to Dr. Silverstein, this can be achieved by employing provable electronic policy enforcement in regard to access, provenance, and logging, as well, through scalable data transport mechanisms and transformations that make data unambiguous and computable. He predicted that the increasing scale and complexity of medicine and biology will lead to more collaborative endeavors and sharing of resources—both data and technical. As a result, he noted, approaches to sharing technical resources through federated hosted services such as grids and clouds—which provide scalable ways to leverage existing distributed data, transport standards, and individual expertise—promise to be a crucial part of the digital infrastructure.

Innovative Approaches to Information Diversity

Drawing on his experiences with the Indiana Network for Patient Care, Shaun Grannis of the Regenstrief Institute shared his thoughts on what will be needed to mitigate data heterogeneity in a learning health system. Because information needed to support the functions of a learning health system must be compiled from a number of diverse data sources, integrating these data becomes a major barrier to learning. Dr. Grannis suggested that efforts to specify standards for vocabularies, messaging, and data transactions through interoperability specifications, standards, and use cases have not been sufficient to address this issue, and new approaches are needed. He noted that new strategies to deal with patient and provider identity management, vocabulary standardization, and value set maintenance by addressing elements, including patient- and provider-level aggregation, and health system metadata, should be prioritized.

Engaging Patient and Population Needs

The success of the digital infrastructure in improving health will require appreciation, support, enthusiasm, and active involvement from patients and the population. In this respect, measures were discussed on how the case can be best made on the value proposition for patients in terms that matter to them—for example, improved outcomes, enhanced efficiency, better satisfaction, more active participation, and greater equity.

Electronic Health Data for High-Value Health Care

Mark McClellan from the Brookings Institution detailed the essential components of a digital infrastructure that can more closely align quality measurement and improvement in order to achieve high-value health care. He stressed that patient-centered measures, repurposing data already being used to coordinate care for performance measurement, and alignment of these processes with other reform efforts—namely, value incentives—will be necessary to improve care and lower costs. Dr. McClellan used the example of diabetes care coordination to highlight ways in which information could be used to help providers improve care in a timely way, help patients obtain better care, and serve as the basis for driving value-based reforms. He noted that pilots such as accountable care organizations and ONC-funded Beacon

Communities will be instrumental in identifying best practices and aligning processes and incentives for systemwide improvement.

Engaging Individuals in Population Health Monitoring

Addressing the issue of engaging individuals in population health monitoring, Kenneth Mandl from Children's Hospital Boston observed that harnessing the knowledge possessed by populations through longitudinal studies of large, distributed, consented populations will become the focus of work in population health over the next decade. Based on his experience developing Indivo—a patient-centered health record that places patients in control of their own health information—and recent federal incentive initiatives, he predicted a shift in the health information economy from institutional to individual control. This shift will likely change population health research in a way already being seen through forums such as PatientsLikeMe. Finally, Dr. Mandl noted that a critical research question that needs to be addressed is how to achieve sustained engagement of patients in research.

Optimizing Chronic Disease Care and Control

Sophia Chang from the California HealthCare Foundation noted that a digital infrastructure provides important opportunities for informing and improving the care of patients with chronic disease. She discussed the potential to actively engage patients in the management of their conditions, but observed that, currently, this is not possible as the locus of control lies solely with healthcare providers and not patients. Additionally, Dr. Chang pointed to the lack of common nomenclature, data formats, and protocols for incorporating patient-generated information as barriers to aggregating and translating health data into useful decision support. Pointing to Kaiser Permanente and VHA as examples of institutions that have successfully used EHRs for population health management, she acknowledged that smaller institutions or individual physicians might have less opportunity for exposure, and therefore be less aware of the value. She noted that in order to maximize the value of EHRs, research paradigms should shift to real-time knowledge development and feedback. Finally, Dr. Chang highlighted several steps to move toward the goals of recentering the system around the patient, such as providing useful support for chronic disease management, aligning EHR data elements with patient priorities, and developing better paradigms for learning from patient data.

Targeting Population Health Disparities

M. Christopher Gibbons of the Johns Hopkins Urban Health Institute discussed opportunities for using a digitally supported learning health system to better comprehend and combat health disparities. Noting that understanding and treating health disparities requires integrating knowledge spanning many sources and disciplines, he pointed to several demographic trends that make this challenge ever more pressing—rising prevalence of chronic disease, an aging population, and the growing racial and ethnic diversity of the U.S. population. Dr. Gibbons introduced the terms "populomics" and "populovigilance" to describe the integrative, systems-oriented, and informatics-intensive approaches to understanding and monitoring the complex causes and manifestations of diseases and disparities. He suggested that as more and more data from diverse sources are collected and available for analysis, it will be important to adopt these new perspectives in order to enable advances in treatment, public health, and healthcare disparities.

Weaving a Strong Trust Fabric

Building trust among all the stakeholders—in particular, patients and the public—is vital to progress. The various dimensions of this issue include building confidence in the security safeguards for clinical data, deepening the appreciation for personal and population health, the fundamental value of sharing data for research purposes to support better care decisions, and economic advantages that result from a well-developed digital health infrastructure and clinical data utility.

Demonstrating Value to Secure Trust

Edward Shortliffe of the American Medical Informatics Association addressed the need to build a strong fabric of trust among stakeholders by communicating and demonstrating value. He stated that in order for health IT to meet its full potential, patient and provider participation must be secure. This sense of security depends on an appreciation of the value presented by HIT use as well as creating and maintaining proper security and safeguards. Sharing a personal anecdote about a provider who admitted that only patient demand would motivate him to adopt an EHR system, Dr. Shortliffe observed that sufficient patient demand may even obviate the need for federal incentives. Using electronic banking as an example, he suggested that educational programs are necessary to inform stakeholders about the risks and benefits of EHRs, and predicted that with the establishment of an environment of trust the increased convenience and quality offered by EHRs and data sharing would overcome concerns about privacy.

Currently, however, the risks of adopting an EHR system are both better understood and more effectively communicated. As a result, he suggested that the focus of stakeholder engagement activities going forward should be on communicating the benefits of EHR use—most importantly, better care and lower costs—to providers and the public.

Policies and Practices to Build Public Trust

The implementation of fair information practices to ensure privacy and security was the focus of the Center for Democracy and Technology's Deven McGraw's remarks. Citing surveys that show individuals desire electronic access to their health information even though they have significant privacy concerns, she suggested that providing individuals with meaningful choices around privacy is an important approach to addressing these concerns. Ms. McGraw pointed to a comprehensive approach to patient privacy and data security based on the Markle Common Framework for Secure and Private Health Information Exchange. Key elements of the framework include an open and transparent process, specification of purpose, individual participation and control, and accountability and oversight. Closing with a warning that overreliance on consent leads to weak protection—shifting the burden of privacy protection from the institution to the individual—and that existing regulations are insufficient to cover the privacy issues inherent in a learning health system, she underscored the need for a trust fabric based on fair information practices.

HIPAA and a Learning Health System

Since its passage in 1996 the Health Insurance Portability and Accountability Act (HIPAA), has served as the legal and policy framework for health information privacy. Bradley Malin of Vanderbilt University described the current state of play around health data de-identification and highlighted some of the relevant learning health system–related issues posed by HIPAA. Included among these were identity resolution (while maintaining privacy) and concerns that de-identification could cause modifications to patient information to the extent that they influence the meaning of clinical evidence. Dr. Malin noted, however, that these challenges are not insurmountable, and that efforts to quantify risk are an important first step to mitigation. He suggested that use cases to better define health information utility and improved capabilities for distributed query-based research will be important in moving to a privacy-assured learning health system.

Building a Secure Learning Health System

Ian Foster of Argonne National Laboratory addressed the technical components surrounding trust in the digital infrastructure for the learning health system. He laid out a number of challenges facing the establishment of a secure digital platform, for example, the fact that a learning health system requires data sharing on an unprecedented scale, and that the purpose of this sharing needs to be extended beyond individual patient care support to include research and population health. Highlighting the challenge of a highly complex system with an unclear definition of security, Dr. Foster suggested some basic principles and technology solutions that can form a basis for progress: auditabililty (information can be mapped to an individual and data can be mapped to its origin); scalability; and transparency in terms of data usage, policies, and enforcement. Methods to achieve these principles include attribute-based authorization, distributed attribute management, and end-to end (scalable) security.

Stewardship and Governance in the Learning Health System

The growth and development of the digital infrastructure for health will be determined in part by the effectiveness of the stewardship and governance instruments designed to facilitate its appropriate structure and function, as well as enlist and channel the engagement and balance of stakeholder interests.

Governance Coordination, Needs, and Options

Laura Adams of the Rhode Island Quality Institute identified and addressed fundamental questions posed in contemplating the governance of the digital health infrastructure. Focusing on the source and scope of authority; mission, purpose, and primary goals; and theoretical foundations for a governance structure, she laid out several governance options for consideration. Ms. Adams suggested that all of these potential models of governance structure and stakeholder participation should be considered, and that the scope of the governing body's authority should be succinctly communicated in a statement of purpose. This statement, she noted, should draw on guiding principles such as transparency and commitment to the common good, and that considering guiding theories—such as complexity theory—could aid in providing an ethical and legal framework. Pointing to some of the unique governance challenges posed by a learning health system, such as evolving privacy considerations and accommodating new sources of data, Ms. Adams suggested drawing on past successes and experiences while incorporating the widest array of viewpoints possible.

Consistency and Reliability in Reporting for Regulators

Theresa Mullin from FDA described ongoing efforts to implement a systematic strategy for data standards development and adoption. This process would address heterogeneity in new drug applications, improve regulatory efficiency, and contribute towards the agency's public health mandate by facilitating exploration of safety and efficacy issues. Dr. Mullin suggested that, through the standardization of clinical data in EHRs, this effort presents an opportunity to facilitate information exchange and analysis for learning, reduce costs, and reduce burdens on providers for adverse event reporting. Dr. Mullin also highlighted some of the overarching governance principles driving this effort: an open, transparent, and inclusive process, as well as the need for resulting requirements to be practical, user-oriented, sensitive to costs, and sustainable.

Complying with Patient Expectations for Data De-Identification

Shawn Murphy from Partners HealthCare explained that meeting patient expectations for privacy and security is central to developing a learning health system. He detailed how current limitations to privacy through de-identification could be overcome by a comprehensive security and privacy approach that does a better job of addressing patients' chief concerns around health information protection—avoiding embarrassment and economic risk. Citing an example of research program–based restrictions on physician access to data—whose risk to patient privacy is negligible given physicians' otherwise broad access to patient information—Dr. Murphy suggested that the certified trustworthiness of the recipient should be a component of access control. He went on to note that this, coupled with appropriate de-identification and secure data storage, provides a balanced approach to security that better matches the expectations of the patient while facilitating access for approved data users.

Information Governance in the National Health Service (UK)

Guidance for approaches to governing the digital health infrastructure can be gleaned by drawing from examples of similar efforts. Harry Cayton of the National Information Governance Board for Health & Social Care (NIGB) in the United Kingdom described the approach they have taken in dealing with information governance issues facing the National Health Service. Cayton detailed the role played by the NIGB as an independent statutory committee to advise the government on the use of patient-identifiable data for clinical audit and research. He described their philosophy that information governance (or stewardship) is the responsibility of every organization involved and provided a list of principles developed by the committee to guide their work. Stating that the purpose of the NIGB is to deal with the "wicked questions" that arise around use of health information, Cayton affirmed that there is no right or wrong answer, only the best answer at the time. In conclusion, he suggested that all governance systems need the same things: mechanisms for agreeing and applying consistent principles, checks for the practicality of guidance given, consistent procedures, and credibility with stakeholders.

Perspectives on Innovation

Especially in a field as rapidly evolving a HIT, innovation is the lifeblood of progress. Observations on innovative approaches to current obstacles and challenges were invited from several field innovators.

Conceptualizing a U.S. Population Health Record

Drawing from the assertion that population health is more than the aggregation of individual disease and that therefore, an understanding of population health cannot simply be gleaned by aggregating patient care data, Population and Public Health Information Services' Daniel Friedman advocated for the creation of a U.S. population health record. He emphasized that while the United States has large amounts of publicly accessible population-level disease-related data, challenges for population health include a lack of that same level of granularity for functional status and well-being as well as problems of data integration and integrity. In order to address these issues he proposed the establishment of a single source of population health data backed by an overarching data model and theoretical framework. In this model, data would be drawn from a number of different sources including those not typically integrated with clinical data such as environmental sampling and census data.

Accelerating Innovation Outside of the Private Sector

Molly Coye, formerly from the Public Health Institute (now with the University of California, Los Angeles), identified what she saw as three areas of opportunity for HIT innovation. Citing the need to improve the current state of clinical decision support, she suggested areas where innovation could help meet this goal: how to recognize and deal with incorrect or missing data, how to integrate a single patient's data from multiple sources, and how to turn data into clinical guidance. Dr. Coye cited the need for integrating research into care processes and for evidence generated to be fed back in a continuous, seamless process that supports informed, shared decision making. Additionally, she noted the movement of healthcare delivery to integrated models—such as accountable care organizations—which increase the need for remote data collection, diagnosis, consultation, and treatment. Dr. Coye concluded by stressing that many of these challenges are social rather than technical in nature, and successful approaches, therefore, will need to take into account the complex character of these systems.

Combinatorial Innovation in Health Information Technology

The growing prevalence of personal information ecologies provided the context for remarks made by the Institute for the Future's Michael Liebhold. He noted that these ecologies are composed of digital artifacts not only related to health and fitness, but also social activities, media use, and even civic life. Mr. Liebhold observed that citizens are ready and willing to collect and share their health information and, with the encouragement of industry and employers, to become more actively involved in their own health. However, he noted that effectively integrating information from all of these sources in a meaningful way presents a formidable challenge. Technologies such as those that underlie the semantic web hold much promise, but still face challenges, especially in the areas of privacy and security. Looking to the future, Mr. Leibhold stated the need for methods to curate web-based health information; interoperable health app stores; and the development of a web of linked, open healthcare information and knowledge interoperability.

Fostering the Global Dimension of the Health Data Trust

The ability to draw broadly from anywhere across the globe for lessons that can provide relevant insights for health and healthcare improvement is a long-term goal. Meanwhile, the ability to learn from the experiences of other countries, as well as to apply HIT for biosurveillance, can help facilitate progress. Several relevant activities were reviewed.

TRANSFoRm: Translational Medicine and Patient Safety in Europe

Brendan Delaney from Kings College London described the TRANSFoRm project, a European Union (EU) effort to develop a learning health system driven by HIT and aimed at improving patient safety as well as supporting and accelerating clinical research. Dr. Delaney outlined several of the challenges that have arisen, such as system interoperability, a need for advanced functionalities, and the support of knowledge translation. He also described several techniques being employed to address these challenges, including clinical research information models, service-based approaches to semantic interoperability and data standards, detailed clinical data element representations built on archetypes, and an effort to prioritize EHR workflow integration in the development of clinical decision support systems capable of capturing and presenting fine-grained clinical diagnostic cues.

Healthgrids, the SHARE Project, and Beyond

Drawing from his involvement with SHARE, an EU-funded project to define the path toward greater implementation of grid computing approaches to health, Tony Solomonides from the University of the West of England discussed his current work to automate policy and regulatory compliance to allow health information sharing. He described an approach to the implementation of attribute-based access controls to ensure enforcement of privacy obligations which, becuase of variations in their interpretation between EU countries, require a logic-based computed approach.

Systematic Data Collection for Global Improvements in Care

Health IT holds great promise to increase quality and improve patient safety in developing and transitional countries. Harvard University's Ashish Jha described how a dearth of reliable information has impeded efforts to both better understand and design solutions to higher rates of adverse event–associated morbidity in developing countries, as well as obtain an accurate calculation of global disease burden. Dr. Jha described an effort by the World Health Organization to maximize the impact of HIT in resource-poor settings through the development of a minimum dataset that would allow for systematic data collection of elements relating to safety issues.

Informatics and the Future of Infectious Disease Surveillance

David Buckeridge, from McGill University, described how HIT is enabling dramatic changes in domestic and international infectious disease surveillance. Detailing how the digital infrastructure can enhance existing systems through the use of automation and decision support, he explained novel approaches to surveillance enabled by recent informatics innovations. Using the DiSTRIBuTE project as an example of syndromic surveillance innovations that drastically improve coverage and speed, he called for a renewed science of disease surveillance that embraces IT—along with the potentially disruptive changes it brings—to improve disease control.

GROWING THE DIGITAL HEALTH INFRASTRUCTURE

Drawing on the collective expertise represented in the presentations and discussions of the first workshop, participants focused on four crosscutting priority domains in the two subsequent workshops: promoting technical advances and innovation, knowledge generation and use, engaging patients and the population, and fostering stewardship and governance. Encouraged to give due consideration to "out of the box" approaches and to use examples from health and nonhealth fields to illustrate and test key needs and opportunities through small group sessions, participants identified and presented for discussion a number of strategic elements important to progress in each domain. They are included in Box S-9 and described in more detail in the sections below.

Technical Progress

A *ULS system* is complex, constantly growing, and evolving, much like an organic, biological ecosystem. Introduced to the digital health information conversation by colleagues from the computer science field, hallmarks of a ULS system were described earlier under "Common Themes and Principles" (see Box S-8), and include its decentralization of data, development, and operational authority to foster local innovation, personalization, and emergent behaviors without requiring consensus from all nodes. The complexity, constant evolution, and enormous scale of the digital health infrastructure is consistent with the ULS system framework and terminology. During the discussions focused on developing a set of strategic scenarios for technical progress, the ULS system approach emerged as an appropriate framework.

In discussing the implications and issues surrounding this approach, participants identified the relevance and appeal of the engineering approach to health care—systems analyses, design, implementation, and evaluation plans—inherent to the ULS system perspective. Specifically, they noted the potential of a collaborative effort between the computer science and HIT communities to develop a deliberate and systematic engineering analysis—characterized by iterative testing and development of prototypes—to set technical and sociotechnical system goals, requirements, specifications, and architecture. This could be supported by a multidisciplinary research community, armed with clarified terminology for ease of collaboration, and with participation from a wide array of both private and public stakeholders (clinical, public health, computer science, health informatics, law, policy, ethics, etc). Similarly, workshop participants stressed the need for technical policies that support experimentation and innovation and allow for the

BOX S-9
Strategic Elements

TECHNICAL PROGRESS ... activities that advance:
- Ultra-large-scale system perspective
- Functionality focus
- System specifications/interoperability
- Workflow and usability
- Security and privacy safeguards
- System innovation

KNOWLEDGE GENERATION AND USE ... activities that advance:
- Shared learning environment
- Point of decision support and guidance
- Research-ready records for data reuse
- Patient-generated data
- Integration and use of data across sources
- Distributed data repositories
- Sentinel indicators
- Query capacity
- Analytic tools and methods innovation

PATIENT AND POPULATION ENGAGEMENT ... activities that advance:
- Value proposition and patient confidence
- Shared learning culture
- Patient–clinician outcomes partnerships
- Person-centric, lay-oriented health information access
- Closing the disparity gap
- Continuous evaluation

GOVERNANCE ... activities that advance:
- The vision
- Guiding principles
- Participant roles and responsibilities
- Process and protocol stewardship
- Implementation phasing
- Continuous evaluation

progressive adoption and evolution of system requirements, specifications, and architecture choices.

Participants pointed to a *focus on functionalities* consistent with ULS systems, and their application to the digital health system, as a potential starting point in advancing the ULS approach. Definition of the ULS principles and characteristics that support learning system functionalities, including the feedback and feedforward nature of the learning engine, such as identification strategies, privacy controls, the availability of a complete longitudinal record at the point of care, inferential capacity, and research readiness, were highlighted as critical foundational steps in the development of this technical enterprise. Noted as similarly important to system functionality was the mechanism for developing and maintaining an approach to information structure, classification, and storage.

Promoting these targeted functionalities requires advancing parsimonious *system specifications and interoperability*. Discussions centered on the need to specify the minimum set of standards to allow for partial interoperability. Semantic comparability, maintenance of context and provenance, architectural consistency, and transportability were discussed as potential starting points. In congruence with the priorities laid out subsequently in the PCAST report (see Appendix E), particular attention was paid to the use of metadata to facilitate interoperability and information exchange—including to maintain data context and provenance, authentication, and privacy. This, in concert with a fast-prototyping component, can allow for incremental specification and system growth with the opportunity for functional enhancement, such as refinement of semantic interoperability, to meet specific requirements depending on use.

Part and parcel with the need to address the technical specifications of the digital utility for the learning health system is consideration for how these interface with users. Considerations for *workflow integration* were discussed by workshop participants as important to ensure that the technology is not only innovative and useful but also usable. To date, this disjuncture between established workflow patterns and an unfamiliar, often awkward, overlay of HIT tools has proved a substantial barrier to adoption.

Security and privacy safeguards were an important consideration in all areas of discussion. Participants often pointed to a lack of trust as being one of the major impediments to health information exchange. Therefore, attendance to the technical aspects of these issues was emphasized as a crucial part of building trust among stakeholders. Discussions and presentations described technical approaches such as attribute-based authorization and distributed identity management, and provided examples of how they could be deployed to address these concerns and achieve a state of secure data liquidity. Additionally, innovations around data security and privacy in alternative environments such as hosted, web-based systems were suggested in order to build capacity.

Finally, the need for *continuous innovation* was a recurring theme in technical discussions. Participants suggested strategies such as creating a test-bed network for assessment of innovative system functionalities, the use of challenge problems to test ULS system issues and opportunities, and the cultivation of interdisciplinary research initiatives among academic, industry, and government stakeholders.

Knowledge Generation and Use

Discussions of the generation and use of knowledge fell into three areas: the availability and capture of reliable data, the tools to analyze the data, and seamless feedback of knowledge to the system. Research, quality improvement initiatives, and public health surveillance efforts are all examples of uses and drivers for these learning-associated processes.

A necessary precondition for successful progress on any of these dimensions is a *shared learning environment*. Technical advances and innovative research methods make it possible to bring clinical research and clinical practice much closer together. However, it was noted that the ability to take advantage of that opportunity depends on a healthcare culture in which both patients and clinicians are compelled by the prospects of clinical data to improve understanding, care delivery, and outcomes, as well as provide reliable, just-in-time information to assist decision making. For these reasons, participants highlighted the need for a learning environment that is supported, shared, and nurtured by both patients and clinicians.

Several tools and approaches currently exist to provide *point of decision support and guidance*. In the face of the number of interacting factors, competing priorities, and an ever-growing set of diagnostic and therapeutic options, "best practice" can only be a theoretical notion without the ability to bring the best available information to the decision process. On the other hand, it was noted that reminders and decision prompts not successfully engineered into natural workflow patterns will be little more than ignored distractions. Consequently, approaches are needed to better marshal reliable clinical information and guidelines in time, form, and content that is seamlessly accessed and used by clinicians and patients.

Participants identified a number of needs to be addressed in order for the digital health infrastructure to reach its full potential as a source of real-time clinical research insights. For example, clinical research activities require enlisting clinician support and involvement in *research-ready clinical records* on both quality and content dimensions for reuse in knowledge generation. The identification of a limited set of standardized core research-related components as basic elements across vendors and systems was one suggestion to facilitate individual and cooperative clinical research activities as well as sentinel event surveillance. Concerns over the reliability and heterogeneity of data in clinical records was underscored as an important rate-limiting factor for both quality of care and clinical research activities, again underscoring the importance of the mechanisms for information structure, classification, and storage. This is particularly important for repurposing data collected for other uses, such as FDA clinical trial–associated data, in order to maximally leverage efforts and investments already in place.

Discussions on the increased utility of clinical records for research went hand in hand with those on the need to take advantage of information from patients and other sources. *Patient-generated data* can provide a level of context that is impossible to capture through more traditional data collection methods. Initiatives to better develop, test, and improve the capture and use of these data so that they can be used to support research, quality improvement, public reporting, and patient care were suggested as priorities.

Similarly, efforts to promote the *integration and use of data across various sources*—clinical, public health, commercial—were emphasized as central to effectively leveraging the full range of information for progress in improving efforts aimed at populations as well as individuals. Included in this, and considered with a longer term vision, were growing information sources outside of "mainstream" health care, such as online forums and communities. In order for such proposals to be successful, it was noted that protocols must be developed to build interoperability as a natural and seamless element of data sources.

Storage and aggregation of data for the purpose of analysis and knowledge generation have been problematic given the security and privacy issues they entail. Discussions of current and ongoing efforts in the creation of *distributed data repositories*, such as those being used in FDA's Sentinel Initiative and the HMO Research Network, suggest a promising approach. Coordination between these ongoing efforts, additional support and incentives for their use for clinical research activities, and the support of coordinated intervention-specific patient registries were discussed as potential approaches moving forward. Prospects for the use of scalable, distributed, hosted, storage solutions—such as those used by Amazon—were also noted as promising future directions. These discussions, however, were often punctuated with caution around privacy and security, components that participants felt needed further exploration and development.

Finally, considerable attention was paid to the development of methods, tools, and *query capacity* for the generation of knowledge needed to sustain a digital learning health system. In line with the ULS system architecture approach, and the creation and support of distributed data repositories, the development of capacity for national, distributed query-based research— including the ability to identify and track *sentinel* events and indicators—was identified as a strategic priority. Challenges associated with the current state of public health IT infrastructure were cited as priorities for attention in order for these functionalities to be adequately sustained. To support this, and the continuing development and *innovation around other analytical approaches*, the importance of collaborative interdisciplinary networks of researchers was underscored. This was discussed not only for cooperative studies, but for cooperative engagement of issues such as strategies on consistent identifiers for patients, the use of modeling and simulation for knowledge generation, evaluation of approaches for the use of diverse data types and varying data quality, and development of methods for the use of information from mobile consumer devices and patient-generated data.

Patient and Population Engagement

Discussions on the roles of patients and the public in growing the digital infrastructure for the learning health system were anchored strongly in the concept of reengineering the care culture to ensure the centrality of the individual patient in the care process—a concept underscored in the *Quality Chasm* report (IOM, 2001) that remains elusive. Signs of change are only beginning to appear as appreciation increases for the use of web-based information and the clinical and outcome advantages of a patient who is better informed and more involved. Often referenced in the discussions was the need for the establishment of a "new norm" around engaging patients and the public in health—both theirs and that of the population—through the use of the digital infrastructure. Basic to this "renorming" is a deepened appreciation for the personal and public benefits that are likely to occur, as well as a strong measure of confidence in the security of the system.

The *value proposition* must be apparent to the stakeholders. Communication of the value of a digital health infrastructure in the improvement of care coordination, quality, and, ultimately, the health of the population at large, was identified in workshop discussions as a fundamental priority. Furthermore, participants pointed out that, in order to be successful, the value proposition should be approached in the context of transparent conversations about privacy, security, and other impeding concerns. The use of case studies and quantitative assessments of the contribution of HIT to improved patient experiences and outcomes was discussed as potential starting points.

A common theme across several workshop discussions was the value in fostering a *shared learning culture* among system stakeholders—in particular, a culture that recognizes the unique contributions that patients and the general population can make to the learning system as collaborators, not subjects. Activities that foster patient involvement in and support of knowledge generation, including illustrating the importance of patient preference information to improving care, were discussed as potential approaches to this issue.

Following the theme of "renorming" participation of patients and the population in health improvement, and building on the framework established by previous IOM work in this area, the opportunity for strengthening *patient–clinician outcome partnerships* through the digital infrastructure was discussed. The development of templates and protocols that support the use of HIT to engage patients in decision making as well as tools for more effective provider–patient communication were proposed. An important element in this respect is providing patients with secure access to and control of their health information. This includes further development of *patient portals*, building on technologies already widely accepted by consumers, and supporting efforts for increased information liquidity and control such as the VHA/CMS Blue Button initiative.

In concert with these efforts, participants discussed the need to increase the availability and access to *lay-oriented, user-friendly clinical and nonmedical health information*. Investing in templates for form and content of information for the lay consumer, as well as gathering patient-derived data for care and delivery improvement were suggested as areas of focus. Indeed, the "new norm" was discussed as involving a focus on improving patients' health, not just health care, by emphasizing health maintenance as a lifelong process that includes a patient's actions and decisions outside of the clinical care setting. To this end, many participants proposed providing individuals with useful information concerning their clinical encounters and the relevant state of evidence, as well as giving them more responsibility for utilizing this information in their own decision making.

HIT provides an opportunity for engaging populations not historically well served by the traditional healthcare community. For this reason, the potential of the digital health utility in the elimination of *health disparities* was discussed as a strategic priority for further attention and action. The impact of facilitating patient and population contribution to, and control of, their health information has the potential to address disparities in underserved populations.

The importance of a component of *continuous evaluation* and improvement in efforts for patient and population engagement in the digital health learning system was again emphasized. Areas of focus that were highlighted include ongoing assessment of patient preferences for use in tailoring of health plans, innovative approaches to confidentiality and privacy issues, and assessments of opportunities to use contemporary sociotechnological approaches (e.g., social networking and smart phones) for patient and population engagement.

Governance

Discussions of governance strategies for the digital infrastructure for the learning health system focused on facilitating activities to advance some very basic components and principles of the ULS digital health information system. Participants often struggled with the question "what are we proposing to govern?" and certainly the health information system as it exists now does not easily fit into most established governance models. On the other hand, upon applying the ULS lens to this issue, and considering innovative governance approaches in cases outside of health (such as VISA and the Smart GRID; see Appendix B for more information), certain governance-related strategic elements emerged. Several participants pointed to the example of the Internet Engineering Task Force as one example of a governance approach that, while created under different circumstances, reflects many of the same governing principles.

Of principal concern is the issue of the *vision*. As a means of establishing a reference point for progress, workshop participants articulated the need for work to establish a shared vision of the digital health utility for the learning health system. Prospective components noted for this vision include expectations, guiding principles, modus operandi, and an appreciation for the global perspective. Considerations of the differences between a structure that governs versus one that provides guidance were included in these discussions.

Participants noted that a governance model in line with the ULS approach would be one that identified and depended on a minimal set of *guiding principles* with which all stakeholders must comport, maximizing local autonomy over all other decisions. Tolerance of change and adaptability were additional characteristics that participants felt were important to incorporate. Exploring the most decentralized level at which these standards might be delegated and focusing standards on major functional requirements were proposed as starting points. Additionally, the importance of tailoring the governance approach to the local situation and needs was emphasized. A focus on the ability to use an inclusive (both/and) rather than a deterministic (either/or) approach was discussed as a foundational principle that encapsulated this thinking. A related issue discussed was the broader context of the governance enterprise. Participants discussed the need to include societal values such as trust, privacy, and fairness; fair information practices such as transparency and collection and data use limitation; goals of the health sector to improve quality of care and enhance clinical knowledge; technical concepts such as innovation; and economic aspects such as promoting efficiency and reducing costs.

Identification of possible *participant roles and responsibilities* in the governance structure were identified as an important early step, and different approaches were considered. These included broad participation by all stakeholders, which was pointed out to be logistically very difficult; very narrow participation, which participants felt was unlikely to be successful; or a hybrid model that incorporated both broad and narrow participation depending on the needs at that particular level. Some participants noted that multiple layers of governance were likely to be required to address concerns at the appropriate level, whether local, regional, national, or international.

Several approaches to the establishment of a governance model were considered and discussed by workshop participants. Leveraging lessons through collaborative discussions among ongoing efforts—at both the national and local levels—and establishing a working group to begin collecting initial input were suggested as starting points. To enhance the efficiency of deliberative efforts, participants suggested coordinating these activities, potentially through the ONC HIT Policy Committee's Governance Working Group; building upon and aligning existing policies, such as HIPAA, agency regulations, and informed consent processes to encourage learning health system activities; and nurturing the interfaces with the international community.

A potential responsibility discussed for the governance structure was the *stewardship of processes and protocols* associated with learning health system functionalities. Participants noted that developing processes for proposing, reviewing, and validating protocols on key elements including data gathering, security, and use is an integral part of this approach. Ongoing stewardship responsibilities for the governing entity will involve monitoring and maintaining protocols, managing variability across participants, and devising an approach to provide incentives to stakeholders to conform to stated goals and principles. A related element discussed as a governance challenge was that of *implementation phasing*, or sequencing protocol development activities so that barriers to progress in an entrepreneurial environment are not presented.

In the spirit of a continuously improving learning health system, a process for *continuous evaluation and improvement* of the governance entity and approach was emphasized as important. Areas highlighted included establishing an approach to ongoing assessment of progress and problems, systematic assessment of value realization for recognition and promotion of successful practices, and the support of research on governance and orchestration of the ULS digital health utility in the United States and globally.

ACCELERATING PROGRESS

Throughout the meetings—and especially at the third meeting—a number of specific cross-cutting action targets were identified as particularly pressing elements for attention. In several instances these involved seizing on the opportunities presented by ongoing efforts, and building upon them to include considerations or requirements specific to the learning capacity of the digital infrastructure. Those most frequently mentioned are presented in Box S-10 and described in more detail below.

> **BOX S-10**
> **Priority Action Targets Discussed**
>
> **Stakeholder Engagement**
>
> *The case:* Analyses to assess the potential returns on health and economic dimensions
>
> *Involvement:* Initiative on citizens, patients, and clinicians as active learning stakeholders
>
> **Technical Progress**
>
> *Functionality standards:* Consensus on standards for core functionalities—care, quality, public health, and research
>
> *Interoperability:* Stakeholder vehicle to accelerate exchange and interoperability specifications
>
> *ULS system test bed:* Identify opportunities, implications, and test beds for ULS system approach
>
> *Technical acceleration:* Collaborative vehicle for computational scientists and HIT community
>
> **Infrastructure Use**
>
> *Quality measures:* Consensus on embedded outcome-focused quality measures
>
> *Clinical research:* Cooperative network to advance distributed research capacity and core measures
>
> *Identity resolution:* Consortium to address patient identification across the system
>
> **Governance**
>
> *Governance and coordination:* Determination and implementation of governing principles, priorities, system specifications, and cooperative strategies

Priority Action Targets

The case: *Analyses to assess the potential returns on health and economic dimensions.* Because of the centrality of broad-based support to progress, and the "public good" nature of many of the activities, the need to demonstrate a value proposition or business case for participation by stakeholders in a digital learning health system was a topic of much discussion during the workshop series. This emphasis was reinforced by the approach taken by the PCAST report to encourage the development of a market around digital health information exchange. Support of methods that apply serious analytical rigor to these issues and generate both technical and policy suggestions were identified as being crucial to this effort. Researchers and organizations such as think tanks were discussed as likely being the best positioned to undertake the necessary analyses with support of a commissioning resource.

Involvement: *Initiative on citizens, patients, and clinicians as active learning stakeholders.* Many workshop discussions considered stakeholder investment to be a necessary component of any successful strategy. Participants identified the need to redefine the roles of citizens, patients, and clinicians in a way that activated their participation in their own health, and the health of the population at large, through the facilitative properties of the digital infrastructure. It was noted that patient and clinician groups can play a crucial role in this effort by helping to convey the value proposition and ensuring that the interests of their constituents are represented in the development and evolution of the system. Efforts that facilitate stakeholder participation—such as increased control of health information by patients and the use of patient-generated data in care plans and knowledge generating processes—were discussed as priority next steps in stakeholder engagement. Additionally, to attend to concerns around privacy, security, trust, and additional work burden, participants stressed the importance of honesty and transparency in facilitating support and understanding. Ultimately, discussions noted that demonstrating the value of a digital health infrastructure through the use of case studies that point to improved outcomes and efficiency was likely the most compelling strategy to appeal to stakeholders.

Functionality standards: *Consensus on standards for core functionalities— care, quality, public health, and research.* Progress on the technical standards necessary to support the core functionalities of the learning health system was continually referenced in workshop discussions. Participants focused on the standards necessary not only to improve, monitor, and guide care decisions but also to accelerate research, quality efforts, patient monitoring, and health surveillance. Related requirements include the ability to exchange information through the use of minimal standards (such as those to enable use of metadata-tagged information packets), query and analyze distributed repositories of data for research purposes, ensure care decision support, and enable quality improvement initiatives and public health surveillance and reporting. Discussions also touched on the need for the digital infrastructure to interface with next-generation systems including mobile health applications and the way in which these and other capacities could help engage patients and the public through improved information access. Participants also underscored the strategic importance of adhering to a minimal set of standards that support core functions but do not introduce unnecessary barriers to progress.

Interoperability: *Stakeholder vehicle to accelerate exchange and interoperability specifications.* System interoperability remains a major obstacle to realizing a digital learning health system. When applying the ULS system lens to this challenge, many participants stressed the need to develop a parsimonious set of standards—such as those for metadata—to allow for practical interoperability and information exchange across systems. Noting that this issue lies in the realm of both technical capacity and governance structure, several participants often compared this effort to the evolution and governance of the Internet. While the differences between the digital health infrastructure and the Internet were acknowledged, it was suggested that the establishment and work of the Internet Engineering Task Force might provide guidance for an industrial institution for the governance of interoperability-related standards. Additionally, leveraging and coordinating existing progress and ongoing efforts in the areas of standards development and facilitation were underscored as strategies to ensure that activities progress as efficiently as possible.

ULS system test bed: *Identify opportunities, implications, and test beds for ULS system approach.* As discussions focused on the characterization of the health system as a complex sociotechnical ecosystem, analysis was suggested on how the ULS approach might be applied to the health system in both the short and long term. Mapping of a key ULS system report (Northrop et al., 2006) to the learning health system through a collaborative effort between software engineers, computer scientists, medical informaticians, and clinicians was offered as a starting point for this effort. Furthermore, performing a rigorous engineering systems analysis leading to a concept paper was suggested to clarify further the opportunities and implications for the ULS system approach. Integral to the ULS approach is the need to support rapid prototyping for continuous innovation. It was suggested that test beds for the development, assessment, and dissemination of these prototypes would be central to continual innovation. In this vein, several participants pointed to the opportunity presented by the creation of the Center for Medicare & Medicaid Innovation (CMMI). Certain communities of excellence already provide some capacity in this area, and participants often referenced ongoing activities at these institutions (see Appendix B).

Technical acceleration: Collaborative vehicle for computational scientists and HIT community. Much of the work in the development of a digital learning health system will necessitate interdisciplinary collaboration between academic, public, and private partners across the computer science, HIT, science, and engineering communities. Participants suggested establishing a collaborative forum where these efforts can be initiated and developed. This forum could catalyze the interdisciplinary research program necessary to develop the digital health infrastructure, and some participants suggested that funding for such a forum and its associated activities might best be served by collaborative efforts across relevant federal agencies (such as NIH and NSF), relevant private sector partners, or both.

Quality measures: Consensus on embedded outcome-focused quality measures. Participants noted that the first step in determining the usefulness of data collected by the digital health infrastructure is to identify the necessary elements to collect. It was stated several times that in order to support the quality improvement and research activities required for a learning system, consensus around useful outcome-based measures is needed. Participants suggested that this would motivate vendors and users to incorporate these measures into their systems, driving seamless integration of quality measurement and reporting into the digital infrastructure. Work at the NQF, through the ONC HIT Policy Committee, and at CMS has already begun addressing these needs.

Clinical research: Cooperative network to advance distributed research capacity and core measures. Discussions often highlighted the centrality of ongoing and continuous generation of knowledge from clinical data as a central feature of the learning health system. Efforts to do research on data held in distributed repositories, such as the HMO Research Network and FDA's Mini-Sentinel program, were pointed to as important early-stage efforts in building systematic, larger scale capacity. Participants suggested that a multidisciplinary, cooperative network of the relevant stakeholders—principally computer scientists, clinical researchers, and data holders—could be a starting point in accelerating progress in this dimension. It was noted that this network would need to consider development of core datasets to facilitate research and quality efforts, fostering consensus on levels of consent and de-identification strategies necessary for effective reuse of data, development of methodologies for query-based and automated research and signal detection across distributed systems, development of standards for distributed queries across the system, implications for a ULS approach to existing and future distributed networks, and implications for distributed research from possible advances in data structure and packaging strategies for data interoperability and exchange across systems.

Identity resolution: Consortium to address patient identification across the system. One of the major barriers discussed for several key system functions—care appropriateness, continuity, quality assessment, and research—relates to the current inability to reliably track and link individual patients with their associated information across the health system. This poses a problem for issues around care coordination, including the goal of being able to make care decisions based on comprehensive health information, as well as the development of a useful knowledge generation engine that can incorporate all relevant information and deliver useful, accurate support. Privacy and system security are paramount, but participants noted that approaches are available to address these issues responsibly and the barrier appears to be one of cultural hesitancy rather than a lack of technical capability. Targeting this issue through a consortium approach was proposed as a way to provide the opportunity for stakeholder representation and engagement in an honest, transparent conversation about the component value issues involved.

Governance and coordination: Determination and implementation of governing principles, priorities, system specifications, and cooperative strategies. Workshop participants articulated the idea that governance principles and priorities for a learning health system will require breaking new ground both organizationally and functionally. Discussions identified the need to improve coordination among key stakeholders to accelerate progress in identifying and sharing lessons, examining commonalities, and exploiting opportunities for efficiencies. It was noted that broad agreement will need to be cooperatively marshaled to attend to principles and priorities that support learning system functionalities such as data integrity, policies for data use, human subjects research issues, and proprietary interests. In addition, discussions highlighted the role of governance in planning for and mitigating system failures, an inevitable occurrence in all systems, but one particularly well tolerated within the ULS system. Such failures would, of course, be opportunities for learning, but are potentially alarming in the context of health- and healthcare-associated information. An interdisciplinary consortium of computer scientists and health infomaticians, such as the one mentioned above, was suggested as a suitable place to engage this issue on a technical level. However, addressing system failures in the health system also has a deeply sociocultural component for which approaches that emphasize honesty and transparency with patients and the public were suggested. Education and outreach about this issue were identified as being crucial in preventing irreparable tears in the trust fabric necessary to support a digital learning health system. In this respect, participants noted the important contributions and potential of the Health IT Policy Committee's Governance Working Group. Discussions also underscored the potential advantages of establishing a novel nongovernmental or public–private venture to foster the necessary governance capacity in this country and to work with similar efforts internationally.

Opportunities in the Next Stages of Meaningful Use

In line with these priorities, discussions often focused on the ongoing meaningful use requirement development process. Workshop participants discussed the "beyond meaningful use" issue as key to increasing the utility of digitally embedded clinical records in a learning health system. Specifically, since meaningful use is now such a well-established benchmark process, elements of particular importance to the development of a learning health system might not otherwise be addressed in the meaningful use process if they are not called out for explicit attention in the upcoming stages. Depicted in Box S-11 is a brief description of the meaningful use stages, the current expected focus of the requirements for stages 2 and 3, and bullets highlighting some key possibilities proposed by workshop participants.

Stage 2. Items that workshop participants felt were of particular importance in enhancing the impact that stage 2 of meaningful use could have on the progress of the digital learning health system cut across several dimensions. Flagged as especially key were actions to accelerate standards for semantic interoperability and exchange, as well as approaches for consistent identification of patients. In order to further the utility of EHRs in clinical research and population health, participants suggested core data elements for EHRs, and seamless access to information from immunization registries. Reflecting the extensive discussion on the opportunity for using the digital infrastructure to better engage patients in their health care, participants suggested the addition of lay-interpretable language for patient-accessible information, and incorporation of patient-generated data. Finally, discussions emphasized the need for clinical decision support to be seamlessly integrated into HIT systems to speed adoption.

Stage 3. Looking ahead to stage 3 of meaningful use, workshop participants suggested deepening the focus on requirements related to demonstrating

BOX S-11
Meaningful Use and the Digital Learning Health System Infrastructure

STAGE 1: 2011–2012

Stage 1 of meaningful use established 14–15 (eligible hospitals or eligible professionals) required core functional components, focused on data capture and sharing, along with a menu set of 10 additional components, from which 5 are to be selected by the eligible hospitals or eligible professionals.

STAGE 2: 2013–2014

Stage 2 of meaningful use is under development by the HIT Policy Committee, including consideration of further focus on advanced clinical processes such as clinical decision support, disease management, patient access to health information, quality measurement, research, public health, and interoperability across IT systems. The following are items underscored in IOM discussions as being of particular and immediate importance to the impact of stage 2 enhancements on progress toward the Digital Infrastructure for the Learning Health System:

- Integration of semantic interoperability and exchange standards, including data provenance and context
- Elements fostering seamless integration of clinical decision support
- Use of lay-interpretable language for patient-accessible EHR information
- Incorporation of patient-generated data, including patient preferences
- Inclusion of core data elements that facilitate use of EHR data for clinical research.
- Strategy for seamless access to immunization history from immunization registries
- Strategy for consistent identification of patients

STAGE 3: 2015+

Stage 3 of meaningful use is expected to expand on requirements from stages 1 and 2, with more direct emphasis on improved patient outcomes through sharpened focus on quality, safety, efficiency, population health, and interoperability. Following are items, in addition to those noted above for stage 2, underscored in IOM discussions as being of particular and immediate importance to the impact of stage 3 enhancements on progress toward the Digital Infrastructure for the Learning Health System:

- Ability to access comprehensive, longitudinal patient record at point of care
- Incorporation of patient editing ability
- Demonstration of baseline semantic interoperability and exchange capacity among IT systems
- Integration of nonmedical, health-related information
- Seamless clinician–public health agency exchange on case-level information and alerts

semantic interoperability and exchange capacity among systems, the ability to access comprehensive patient records at the point of care, and seamless exchange of cases and alerts between clinicians and public health agencies. Participants also suggested strategies for including additional types of data—including nonmedical, health-related data—as well as providing patients with an annotated editing ability over their own records.

Stakeholder Responsibilities and Opportunities

Throughout each workshop, frequent reference was made to leadership responsibilities that fell naturally to individual stakeholders, or groups of stakeholders, to advance progress in the development of the digital infrastructure for the learning health system. In many cases, this involves leveraging ongoing efforts or building upon them with an orientation toward a continuous learning system. Summarized below are some of those most often noted.

Federal Government

Even though participants noted the decentralized manner in which localized innovation is likely to contribute to system progress, many of the central strategy elements and priority action targets discussed require strong leadership from federal agencies. Since a clear lead responsibility was given to ONC and the Secretary of HHS by the HITECH statute, many participants pointed to ONC as the natural leadership locus for activities needing coordination at the national level. Opportunities to build on the foundation laid by the HITECH requirements for work on standards, requirements, and certification criteria in meaningful use of EHRs include cooperation with other federal agencies in the development of a strategic plan for national HIT efforts; establishment of a governance mechanism for the NWHIN; accelerating, in cooperation with the National Institute for Standards and Technology, work on standards for exchange and interoperability; and work with FCC, FDA, and CMS to identify standards and reconcile regulations to facilitate wireless transmission of medical information. Participants noted that as the HITECH funds are used, the coordinating capacity of ONC will take on even greater importance, as coalitions will be needed to harmonize various key activities geared at developing the standards, policies, governance, and research projects necessary for effective progress toward a learning health system.

With respect to technical innovation, as the leading federal agency for funding computer science and engineering research, NSF was noted as a logical locus to work with ONC and NIH in the development of test beds for the rapid deployment and evaluation of innovative technological approaches. This work would have the potential to transform the functionality and capacity of the digital health infrastructure, as well as to shepherd the establishment of collaborative vehicles for the ongoing partnerships between the HIT and computational science communities.

Similarly, it was noted that progress in the quality and knowledge generation dimensions of the digital platform will require leadership from federal health agencies. AHRQ, working with ONC, professional societies, and groups such as NQF and the National Committee for Quality Assurance, is a natural steward for initiatives that enhance the utility of the digital infrastructure for quality improvement and health services research.

The CDC's focus on population health places it at the center of extending the scope of the digital infrastructure beyond health care. This carries implications for almost all elements of the system, but will be especially important for the support of public health processes and research as well as public engagement. To these ends, participants suggested development of templates and protocols for the integration of nonmedical population health and demographic information into the system.

As the nation's largest healthcare financing organization, CMS currently serves as the principal vehicle for applying economic incentives and standards to accelerate application of the meaningful use requirements. Furthermore, much promise for future innovation in health IT to support a learning system resides in the CMMI which provides an opportunity for testing innovative approaches suggested by workshop participants. These approaches include test beds for ULS-associated programs and new approaches to integrating clinical decision support with care coordination and delivery models.

On the research front, both NIH and NSF have mandates and networks to develop and demonstrate methods of improving the functionality of the digital infrastructure for health research applications. NIH, VHA, DOD, FDA, and AHRQ all have active programs under way that can evolve into cooperative leadership efforts to expand the use of EHRs for research into the clinical effectiveness of health interventions.

To build support and engagement among patients and the general population, AHRQ, FDA, NIH, and ONC have each established links to patient communities that can serve as the building blocks for a collaborative initiative to better characterize and communicate the health and economic advantages of public involvement in a digital platform for health improvement.

Given this level of activity, and the number of central stakeholders, the importance of ONC's coordination mandate was often underscored. Similarly emphasized was the need to cultivate strong counterpart capacity outside of government to partner in coordination and governance responsibilities.

State and Local Government Leadership

Given the regional emphasis of many of the ongoing efforts related to the digital learning health system—such as the establishment of regional health information exchanges—state and local governments and health departments have experience establishing governance structures and developing programs for engaging local stakeholders. As a result, participants noted, state and local bodies can function as resources and foundation stones for broader efforts. By collaborating with ONC, CMS, HRSA, and other federal initiatives, best practices and lessons learned can be leveraged from state and local efforts. Additionally, it was suggested that some of the more advanced local initiatives could serve as test beds for some of the innovative ULS-associated approaches suggested by participants.

Initiatives Outside Government

Outside of government, the entrepreneurial capacity of the commercial sector will certainly be a major driver of progress. Similarly, the full potential of the learning health system can only be achieved through the full engagement of patients and the public. Workshop discussants frequently underscored the roles of patient and clinician groups to facilitate dialogue between stakeholders and mediate public engagement. In particular, by using case studies to demonstrate the value of the digital infrastructure, participants felt these organizations could help develop the shared learning culture and trust necessary for the learning system to function. Many patient and clinician groups—such as the American College of Physicians, the American College of Cardiology, the Society of Thoracic Surgeons, and the National Partnership for Women and Families—are already involved in this type of work. Participants noted that these existing activities could be expanded to include issues of particular importance to a learning system.

Delivery systems, particularly those integrated across healthcare components, have been at the cutting edge of innovative EHR use, quality improvement, clinical data stewardship, patient engagement, quality initiatives, and distributed research efforts. Workshop conversations often pointed to these efforts, such as those at Kaiser Permanente and Geisinger Health System, suggesting that continued coordination between these delivery systems and relevant federal government agencies would be important in growing the digital health infrastructure.

As the stewards of the largest stores of clinical and transactional information outside of the federal government, insurers, payers, and product developers have an essential role to play in development of the digital infrastructure. Their use of transactional health data to assess utilization patterns, effectiveness, and efficiency is a foundational block on which strategies for broader knowledge generation can build. Furthermore, companies such as UnitedHealthcare have begun engaging the public in the use of data in health. These efforts often were cited during discussions as crucial first steps in establishing a learning culture.

Research is a fundamental aspect of the learning health system. Consequently, participants noted the fundamental role researchers have in developing the infrastructure necessary for continuous knowledge generation and application. Formation of multidisciplinary research communities was often cited as a critical step in accelerating many of the strategies discussed. Funding for these communities was noted as a clear opportunity for collaboration between NSF and NIH. Additionally, discussions highlighted that much work remains to be done in order to maximize the knowledge generation capabilities of the digital infrastructure, and that clinical research and product development communities have an essential role in building this capacity.

As much of the progress to date is a result of initiatives from many independent organizations, their continued efforts as facilitators and innovators were noted as crucial to accelerating progress. Reference was often made to the importance of these organizations as the foundational elements for coordination and governance leadership from outside government.

Finally, and ultimately of paramount importance, is the global perspective. As highlighted during workshop discussions and presentations (see Chapter 8), meeting the goals of a learning health system will inevitably require drawing upon resources and leadership of similar efforts throughout the world. Some of this activity has begun in the limited arena of infectious disease surveillance and monitoring and offers a hint of the potential opportunities—and challenges—in developing a truly global clinical data utility for health progress.

Collectively, the discussions captured in this publication represent unprecedented promise for innovation and progress in health and health care. Yet, the discussions also underscored that without successful efforts to create the conditions necessary for seamless interoperability, to create the protocols for enhanced access and use of available information for knowledge generation, and to build the culture of engagement and support on behalf of the sort of information utility possible, the potential will go unmet. By thoroughly and candidly engaging in discussions on the vision, the current state of the system, the key priorities for future work, and the strategic elements for accelerating progress, participants have set in motion perspectives that can quicken the progress in building the digital infrastructure required for the continuously learning health system necessary—and possible—to ensure better health for all.

REFERENCES

Blumenthal, D., and M. Tavenner. 2010. The "meaningful use" regulation for electronic health records. *New England Journal of Medicine* 363(6):501-504.

CHCF (California HealthCare Foundation). 2010. *New national survey finds personal health records motivate consumers to improve their health.* http://www.chcf.org/media/press-releases/2010/new-national-survey-finds-personal-health-records-motivate-consumers-to-improve-their-health#ixzz12kT8FU00 (accessed October 18, 2010).

DesRoches, C. M., E. G. Campbell, S. R. Rao, K. Donelan, T. G. Ferris, A. Jha, R. Kaushal, D. E. Levy, S. Rosenbaum, A. E. Shields, and D. Blumenthal. 2008. Electronic health records in ambulatory care—a national survey of physicians. *New England Journal of Medicine* 359(1):50-60.

Fox, S. 2010. *E-patients, cyberchondriacs, and why we should stop calling names.* http://www.pewinternet.org/Commentary/2010/August/Epatients-Cyberchondriacs.aspx (accessed October 19, 2010).

IOM (Institute of Medicine). 2001. *Crossing the quality chasm: A new health system for the 21st century.* Washington, DC: National Academy Press.

_____. 2007. *The Learning Healthcare System: Workshop Summary.* Washington, DC: The National Academies Press.

Jha, A. K., C. M. DesRoches, P. D. Kralovec, and M. S. Joshi. 2010. A progress report on electronic health records in U.S. hospitals. *Health Affairs (Millwood)* 29(10):1951-1957.

Northrop, L., P. H. Feiler, B. Pollak, and D. Pipitone. 2006. *Ultra-large-scale systems: The software challenge of the future.* Pittsburgh, PA: Software Engineering Institute, Carnegie Mellon University.

PCAST (President's Council of Advisors on Science and Technology). 2010. *Realizing the full potential of health information technology to improve healthcare for Americans: The path forward.* http://www.whitehouse.gov/sites/default/files/microsites/ostp/pcast-health-it-report.pdf (accessed December 12, 2010).

Smith, A. 2010. *Mobile access 2010.* http://www.pewinternet.org/Reports/2010/Mobile-Access-2010.aspx (accessed October 19, 2010).

1

Introduction

Health and health care are going digital. As multiple intersecting platforms evolve to form a novel operational foundation for health and health care—the nation's digital health utility—the stage is set for fundamental and unprecedented transformation. Most changes will occur virtually out of sight, and the pace and profile of the transformation will be determined by stewardship that fosters alignment of technology, science, and culture in support of a continuously learning health system. In the context of growing concerns about the quality and costs of care, the nation's health and economic security are interdependently linked to the success of that stewardship.

Progress in computational science, information technology, and biomedical and health research methods have made it possible to foresee the emergence of a learning health system that enables both the seamless and efficient delivery of best care practices and the real-time generation and application of new knowledge. Increases in the complexity and costs of care compel such a system. With rapid advances in approaches to diagnosis and treatment, and new genetics insights into individual variation, clinicians and patients must sort through exponentially increasing numbers of issues with each clinical decision. At the same time, healthcare costs are draining the purchasing power of consumers and handicapping the competitiveness of U.S. businesses, yet health outcomes are falling far short of the possible.

Against this backdrop of opportunity and urgency, the Institute of Medicine (IOM) of the National Academies, sponsored by the Office of the National Coordinator for Health Information Technology (ONC), convened a series of expert meetings to explore strategies for accelerating the development of the digital infrastructure for the learning health system. Major elements of those discussions are summarized in this publication, *Digital Infrastructure for the Learning Health System: The Foundation for Continuous Improvement in Health and Health Care.*

THE LEARNING HEALTH SYSTEM

In 2001, the IOM report *Crossing the Quality Chasm* called national attention to untenable deficiencies in health care, noting that every patient should expect care that is *safe, effective, patient-centered, timely, efficient, and equitable* (IOM, 2001). Based on the determination that health care is a complex adaptive system—one in which progress on its central purpose is shaped by tenets that are few, simple, and basic—the report identified several rules to guide health care. In particular, these rules underscore the importance of issues related to the locus of decisions, patient perspectives, evidence, transparency, and waste reduction. The report envisioned, in effect, engaging patients, providers, and policy makers alike to ensure that every healthcare decision is guided by timely, accurate, and comprehensive health information provided in real time to ensure constantly improving delivery of the right care to the right person for the right price.

The release of the IOM *Chasm* report stimulated broad activities related to clinical quality improvement and the effectiveness of health care, including the creation by the IOM of the Roundtable on Value & Science-Driven Health Care. Begun in 2006 as the IOM Roundtable on Evidence-Based Medicine, it has explored ways to improve the evidence base for medical decisions and sought the development of a learning health system "designed to generate and apply the best evidence for collaborative health choices of each patient and provider; to drive the process of discovery as a natural outgrowth of patient care; and to ensure innovation, quality, safety, and value in health care." From its inception, the Roundtable has conducted *The Learning Health System Series* of public meetings in an effort to outline components of the conceptual foundation of the learning health system. Since 2006 the IOM has conducted 15 workshops in the *Learning Health System Series*, with 10 reports published and in production:

- *The Learning Healthcare System*
- *Leadership Commitments to Improve Value in Health Care: Finding Common Ground*
- *Evidence-Based Medicine and the Changing Nature of Health Care*
- *Redesigning the Clinical Effectiveness Research Paradigm: Innovation and Practice-Based Approaches*
- *Clinical Data as the Basic Staple of Healthcare Learning: Creating and Protecting a Public Good*

- *Engineering a Learning Healthcare System: A Look at the Future*
- *Learning What Works: Infrastructure Required for Comparative Effectiveness Research*
- *Value in Health Care: Accounting for Cost, Quality, Safety, Outcomes, and Innovation*
- *The Healthcare Imperative: Lowering Costs and Improving Outcomes*
- *Patients Charting the Course: Citizen Engagement and the Learning Health System*

As the most recent contribution to this series, this publication considers what has been variously described as the system's nerve center, its circulation system, or the engine to drive the progress envisioned in the *Learning Health System Series*: the digital infrastructure.

As it has been laid out by the work of the Roundtable, in a learning health system patients and providers will have access to timely, accurate, and comprehensive health information that can be used to deliver services effectively and efficiently. Characteristics of such a system are noted in Box 1-1 and in matrix form in Appendix A.

Because information technology serves as the functional engine for the continuous learning system, this ONC-commissioned exploration was broadly conceived to consider the issues and strategies required for the emergence of a digital infrastructure that allows data collected during activities in various settings—clinical, research, and public health—to be integrated, analyzed, and broadly applied ("collect once, use for multiple purposes") to inform and improve clinical care decisions, promote patient education and self-management, design public health strategies, and support research and knowledge development efforts in a timely manner.

THE DIGITAL HEALTH INFRASTRUCTURE

The digital infrastructure for the learning health system will not solely be the result of features designed and built *de novo*; there is a growing body of existing initiatives and resources actively in play at multiple levels. These include expanding adoption of technologies such as electronic health records (EHRs), personal health records (PHRs), telehealth, health information portals, electronic monitoring devices, mobile health applications, and advances in molecular diagnostics. Also in play are collections of health information, such as biobanks, and health information databases maintained by large health systems, private insurers, and regulatory agencies. Each adds important capacity for clinical care, clinical and health services research, public health surveillance and intervention, patient education and self-management, and safety and cost monitoring.

Still, these capacities are relatively early in their development and as

> **BOX 1-1**
> **Learning Health System Characteristics**
>
> *Culture*: participatory, team-based, transparent, improving
>
> *Design and processes*: patient-anchored and tested
>
> *Patients and public*: fully and actively engaged
>
> *Decisions*: informed, facilitated, shared, and coordinated
>
> *Care*: starting with the best practice, every time
>
> *Outcomes and costs*: transparent and constantly assessed
>
> *Knowledge*: ongoing, seamless product of services and research
>
> *Digital technology*: the engine for continuous improvement
>
> *Health information*: a reliable, secure, and reusable resource
>
> *The Data utility*: data stewarded and used for the common good
>
> *Trust fabric*: strong, protected, and actively nurtured
>
> *Leadership*: multi-focal, networked, and dynamic
>
> SOURCE: Adapted from *The Learning Healthcare System* (IOM, 2007).

they continue to unfold, progress toward a digital health infrastructure depends on continuous improvement. Challenges include the fact that as of 2009, only about 12% of hospitals and 6% of clinician offices had an EHR in place (DesRoches et al., 2008; Jha et al., 2010) and only about 1 in 14 Americans had electronic access to any patient-oriented version of their health record (CHCF, 2010). On the other hand, since 2000, the number of Americans who have access to the Internet has jumped from 46% to 74%, and the number of American adults who have looked online for health information has jumped from 25% to 61% (Fox, 2010), suggesting a change in the way people access health information. Wireless technology is quickening the pace of change. With 6 in 10 American adults using wireless capability with a laptop or mobile device (Smith, 2010), mobile applications are rapidly developing for remote site access to health information, as well as diagnostic and even treatment services.

The striking progress in the capacity and influence of information technology on society over the past three decades is a blended product of interrelated initiatives arising from within the commercial, independent, and public sectors. Leaps in the speed and power of information processing, the efficiency of the operations, the development of the Internet and World Wide Web, and its use to facilitate near-universally available real-time access to information have spawned a new economy and new vehicles for progress.

Health information vendors, large and small, have emerged to meet the growing demand for capacity to manage the retrieval, storage, and delivery of information for agencies, institutions, professionals, and individuals in virtually every aspect of health and health care. The range of newly digitalized services—and the growth of vendors to provide them—is startling. Through technologies developed by companies such as Google, Microsoft, and Yahoo, the rapidly expanding amounts of health-related information available on the Internet have become increasingly easy to access and query. The amount of web-based health information accessed daily by individuals and clinicians, and the frequency with which they turn to the Internet for this information, is already transforming the care process.

Care Management Resources

Beyond publicly available digital resources, a vast array of specialized care management products have emerged to support a broad range of activities. A wide array of companies have emerged to support the various facets of clinical recordkeeping and information management needed to support clinical processes. Many of these, such as individual patient charting, are served through EHRs. Vendors include EPIC, Cerner, Greenway Medical, General Electric, and Allscripts, as well as newer companies that provide web-based services such as Practice Fusion. Most of these are comprehensive EHR products that integrate support of administrative processes such as scheduling, billing, claims processing, payment, and even supply and equipment inventory maintenance. Other products supporting health information management are PHRs—records maintained by individual consumers—that provide patients a format for contributing and managing their health information electronically. Microsoft HealthVault and Google Health are two of the leading efforts in this area, as well as Dossia, an employer-led, open source effort. Prescribing is another component of the clinical care continuum moving to the digital platform. Led by companies such as Surescripts—with an expansive network and increasing capabilities—e-prescribing is, in many ways, leading the way in current health information exchange.

EHRs, PHRs, and their associated functions represent a wealth of potential in the support of clinical decisions and as sources of information for research, surveillance, public health reporting, and patient–clinician communication. This is accomplished through portals for more regular, direct communication between patients and their providers; clinical research protocol processes; postmarket product monitoring; safety and hazard exposure monitoring; disease and intervention registries; and data aggregation, analysis, and modeling. Increased use of digital technology also includes remote examination and diagnosis through telehealth technologies, such as those used by the military and in rural locations. Furthermore, the use of monitoring sensors to follow patients remotely and collect information in real time is growing in use, especially among the chronically ill. Several organizations are actively involved in employing these technologies at their full potential, and some of these are highlighted in the case studies presented in Appendix B and discussed below.

Healthcare Delivery Organizations

Various large academic health centers and healthcare delivery organizations—Veterans Health Administration (VHA), Kaiser Permanente (see summary in Box 1-2, and the full written description in Appendix B), Geisinger Health System, Vanderbilt, MD Anderson, Palo Alto Medical Foundation, Group Health Cooperative, several Harvard facilities, Children's Hospital of Philadelphia, Virginia Mason, and the Mayo Clinic, to name a few—have invested substantially in the creation of advanced digital resources for administrative, patient care, and research functions. For example, the VHA established one of the first EHR systems, Veterans Health Information Systems and Technology Architecture (VISTA), and has been a pioneer in its use of health information technology (HIT) for quality improvement. More recently, VHA launched the 'My HealtheVet' program, a PHR system that allows veterans to track their clinical visits, tests, and prescriptions, while also having access to relevant health information and patient support communities. Other important HIT applications employed by these organizations include: clinical decision support technologies integrated within their EHR systems and data mining for adverse event surveillance and identification of populations at risk or in need of directed follow-up. Nonetheless, the diversity and limited compatibility of the products, coupled with the lack of economic incentives for their use, has, to date, restrained the uptake, application, and functional utility of these capacities across the broader system.

Independent Sector

A number of public, private, and independent sector initiatives have emerged to accelerate stakeholder action on various dimensions important

INTRODUCTION

> **BOX 1-2**
> **Case: Kaiser Permanente**
>
> In 2003, Kaiser Permanente (KP) launched a $4 billion health information system called KP HealthConnect that links its facilities and clinicians throughout their delivery system and represents the largest civilian installation of electronic health records (EHRs) in the United States. The EHR at the heart of KP HealthConnect provides a reliably accessible longitudinal record of member encounters across clinical settings including laboratory, medication, and imaging data; as well as supporting
>
> - Electronic prescribing and test ordering (computerized physician-order entry) with standard order sets to promote evidence-based care
> - Population and patient-panel management tools such as disease registries to track patients with chronic conditions
> - Decision support tools such as medication-safety alerts, preventive-care reminders, and online clinical guidelines
> - Electronic referrals that directly schedule patient appointments with specialty care physicians
> - Personal health records providing patients with the ability to view their personal clinical information including lab results, plus linkage with pharmacy, physician scheduling, and secure and confidential e-mail messaging with clinicians.
> - Performance monitoring and reporting capabilities
> - Patient registration and billing functions
>
> Physician leaders report that access to the EHR in the exam room is helping to promote compliance with evidence-based guidelines and treatment protocols, eliminate duplicate tests, and enable physicians to handle multiple complaints more efficiently within one visit. Ongoing evaluation by Kaiser indicates that patient satisfaction with outpatient physician encounters has increased and that the combination of computerized physician-order entry, medication bar coding, and electronic documentation tools is helping to reduce medication administration errors in hospital care.
>
> Overall, Kaiser's experience suggests that use of the EHR and online portal to support care management and new modes of patient encounters is having positive effects on utilization of services and patient engagement. For example, three-quarters or more of online users surveyed agreed that the portal enables them to manage their health care effectively and that it makes interacting with the healthcare team more convenient.

to progress. To supplement the relatively limited pre-2009 public investments, independent sector leadership has come from foundations such as the Markle Foundation, the Robert Wood Johnson Foundation (RWJF), and the California HealthCare Foundation (CHCF). For example, the

Markle Foundation has played a leading role in facilitating conversations in the areas of privacy and security in order to ensure that the patient is the ultimate beneficiary of a digitally–supported learning health system. Their Common Framework for sharing and protecting health information has been fundamental in identifying principles and approaches for safe health information exchange. Among many other activities, RWJF has led the way in stimulating innovation in PHRs through its Project HealthDesign, and CHCF has funded a number of projects to explore the use of HIT to improve the care of patients with chronic conditions.

As a result of the increased activity in the area, a number of facilitative stakeholder groups have emerged. A portion of these have taken the shape of capacity-building resources such as the Health Information Exchanges, which serve to work with clinicians and institutions to facilitate the exchange of health information between systems, often within a defined geographic area. Other groups include the Clinical Data Interchange Standards Consortium (CDISC) an organization involved in developing standards to enable aggregation of health information across datasets and methodologies to support its use for research, and Integrating the Healthcare Enterprise (IHE), which promotes coordinated use of established standards to improve health information interoperability. An example of the coordinative potential of these groups is found in the development of integration profiles by IHE and CDISC to support the use of EHRs for clinical research, quality and public health, and the testing and demonstration of these profiles by several vendors including Cerner, Allscripts, Greenway Medical, and GE Healthcare. Additionally, there are a number of organizations working to promote the use of information and information technology to improve health and health care. Notable among them are the eHealth Initiative, the National eHealth Collaborative, and the Healthcare Information and Management Systems Society. Finally, on the professional advancement dimension, the American Medical Informatics Association has emerged as a growing resource for the contributions of biomedical and health informaticians working in activities to organize, manage, analyze, and use information in health care.

Examples from Outside Health Care

The developing potential presents opportunities and challenges for stewardship. Issues related to interoperability, governance, engagement of patients and the general population, and privacy and security concerns resulting from the collection and use of health information will need to be better addressed for successful progress toward a learning health system. Given these challenges, workshop proceedings included the consideration of a number of different cases studies of innovative approaches from both within and outside the healthcare space to inform participants' considerations of the challenges ahead. These case studies are included in their entirety in Appendix B and summarized in boxes in several places throughout this introductory chapter. Two of those cases drawn from outside health care were VISA and Consumer Energy.

VISA was introduced as an example of an innovative approach to the governance of a highly decentralized network of service providers. Through the leadership of Dee Hock, a system based on a minimal set of core standards that maximized peripheral autonomy was created. The principles of this approach—which include maximizing human ingenuity, shared clarity on the purpose and principles of the group, pushing all possible operations to the periphery, and fostering and tolerating evolution—were specifically highlighted as important for consideration.

Consumer Energy's work in the Smart Grid Initiative was used to illustrate a systematic approach to implementation of a complex systems development project of nationwide scale. This approach, based on the ultra-large-scale (ULS) system principles, includes applying an engineering approach to accommodate and network a wide variety of legacy nodes while allowing for continuous expansion and evolution without the use of a comprehensive internal design or rigid standardization. The Smart Grid case is summarized in Box 1-3 and the full written description is included in Appendix B.

Regardless of the model, a key rationale for workshop discussions was the reality that effective and efficient progress in the growth and development of our national and global digital health infrastructure requires active cooperation, collaboration, and role delineation among many organizations, companies, and agencies—private and public—at the cutting edge of using HIT for improving health and health care.

Federal and State Governments

At the national level, stewardship of the digital health infrastructure has fallen primarily to the federal government. ONC was created in 2004 in the U.S. Department of Health and Human Services (HHS) to stimulate progress in the field by providing leadership, policy coordination, strategic planning, and infrastructure development for the adoption of HIT. Since 2009, with the enactment of the Health Information Technology for Economic and Clinical Health Act (HITECH) as part of the American Recovery and Reinvestment Act, the federal government leadership profile has become especially prominent. The principal goals of HITECH are to build approval for HIT adoption and meaningful use; increase patient and provider participation in electronic health information exchange; educate the public about the uses of personal health information and privacy and

> **BOX 1-3**
> **Case: The Smart Grid**
>
> The Smart Grid is a long-term, complex systems development project using an engineering approach to accommodate a wide variety of legacy nodes that are organic—constantly growing and evolving, much like a biological system. This continuous evolution allows the Smart Grid's architecture to preserve and encourage the capacity of each node to innovate locally and deal with complexity in a way that suits local and grid needs. As conceived, the Smart Grid will
>
> - Enable active participation by consumers
> - Accommodate all generation and storage options
> - Enable new products, services, and markets
> - Provide power equality for the digital economy
> - Optimize asset utilization and operate efficiently
> - Anticipate and respond to system disturbances (self-heal)
> - Operate resiliently against attack and natural disaster
>
> Because there is no need for consensus among the nodes on how they should operate within local boundaries, the Smart Grid development methodology is not based on comprehensive internal design and operating standards for each node on the Grid to follow. Instead, the approach accommodates highly diverse nodes connecting to the Smart Grid using open data translation protocols that standardize information management, rather than using the internal workings of each node. The Grid becomes a communications bus to which each node must be able to write, and from which each node must be able to read. This architecture preserves capacities for local operating autonomy and innovation throughout the Smart Grid. It also manages a standardized communications capacity among complex, and otherwise noninteroperable, legacy nodes on the Grid. These features are all characteristics of ultra-large-scale software-intensive systems.

security protections available to them; and use a comprehensive, integrated approach to successfully communicate about privacy, security, and meaningful use to target audiences. Meeting these goals has come with the commitment of unprecedented resources administered through the leadership of ONC. Implementation of HITECH by ONC has been done with the aid of two federal advisory committees made up of representatives from across all HIT stakeholder areas, the HIT Policy Committee and the HIT Standards Committee. The committees have guided ONC's work on meaningful use, certification and adoption, information exchange, strategic planning, privacy and security, and enrollment.

Under HITECH, ONC was granted $2 billion to facilitate the adoption and meaningful use of HIT. In addition, an estimated $27 billion was designated for the Centers for Medicare & Medicaid Services (CMS) to be distributed as incentive payments for physicians and hospitals to become meaningful users of HIT. Designed as a set of staged requirements to qualify for CMS incentive payments, the first-stage elements of "meaningful use" were released by CMS on July 13, 2010. These established a core set of requirements for eligible professionals and hospitals, as well as a menu of additional choices, from which five are to be chosen. The stage 1 meaningful use target elements are listed in summary fashion in Box 1-4, and details are contained in Appendix D. The subsequent stages of meaningful use are currently under development and are presented in Chapter 10, along with an indication of related issues flagged in workshop discussions.

In addition to the meaningful use requirements, ONC has funded a series of grant programs through HITECH such as the Beacon Community grants (aimed at demonstrating community-wide digital infrastructure capacity and use for health improvement) and the Strategic Health Information Technology Advanced Research Projects Program (aimed at fostering the capture of technological advances to improve system performance). At the broader level, ONC is pursuing a series of initiatives to foster health information exchange among stakeholders under the Nationwide Health Information Network.

Several additional HHS agencies have activities important to the development of the digital infrastructure for the learning health system. CMS has had primary responsibility for establishing rules for meaningful use and requirements for uniform condition identifiers central to healthcare payment and research. Additionally, the passage of the Affordable Care Act (ACA) created the $10 billion Center for Medicare and Medicaid Innovation (CMMI). CMMI will test innovative payment and program service delivery methods, many of which will rely on robust information technology systems.

Within the National Institutes of Health (NIH), the National Library of Medicine (NLM) serves as the central coordinating body for clinical terminology standards. In addition, NLM also supports a number of HIT system development tools—in areas such as language and knowledge processing—and offers grant programs in HIT education and training. The NIH Clinical and Translational Science Awards Program provides funding for a consortium of organizations to facilitate collaborative research and speed the adoption of clinical research results in the clinic including supporting the development and use of innovative technologies by individual grantee organizations. Additionally, the National Cancer Institute has a number of initiatives that serve as key contributors to building the capacity to derive scientific discovery from patient care. Among these are the Enterprise Vocabulary Services which provide controlled terminology and ontology services for use by researchers, and the cancer Biomedical Informatics Grid (caBIG®) which is designed to improve care and accelerate scientific discoveries by enabling the collection and analysis of large amounts of

> **BOX 1-4**
> **Meaningful Use Requirement Categories**
>
> Core structured personal data (age, sex, ethnicity, smoking status)
>
> Core list of active problems and diagnoses
>
> Core structured clinical data (vital signs, meds, [labs])
>
> Outpatient medications electronically prescribed
>
> Automated medication safeguard/reconciliation
>
> Clinical decision support
>
> Care coordination support/interoperability
>
> Visit-specific information to patients
>
> Automated patient reminders
>
> e-Record patient access (copy or patient portal)
>
> Embedded measures for clinical quality reporting
>
> Security safeguards
>
> Examples of optional elements:
> Advance directives for ages >65
> Condition-specific data retrieval capacity
> Public health reporting (reportable conditions)
>
> SOURCE: Adapted from Blumenthal and Tavenner (2010). See Appendix D for details.

biological and clinical information (see Box 1-5 and Appendix B for additional information).

Through its National Resource Center for Health IT and initiatives on patient registries, the Agency for Healthcare Research and Quality (AHRQ) supports a number of programs to advance the digital utility for healthcare quality and safety. Currently these programs are focused on the areas of support for HIT program management, guidance, assessment, and planning; HIT technical assistance, content development, and program-related projects and studies; HIT dissemination, communication, and marketing; and HIT portal infrastructure management and website design and usability

> **BOX 1-5**
> **Case: The National Cancer Institute's caBIG® Initiative**
>
> The National Cancer Institute of the National Institutes of Health has developed an informatics program designed to improve patient care and accelerate scientific discoveries by enabling the collection and analysis of large amounts of biological and clinical information and facilitating connectivity and collaboration among biomedical researchers and organizations. More than 700 different organizations are actively engaged in caBIG®, including basic and clinical researchers, consumers, physicians, advocates, software architects and developers, bioinformatics specialists and executives from academe, medical centers, government, and commercial software, pharmaceutical, and biotechnology companies from the United States and in 15+ countries around the globe.
>   At the heart of the caBIG® program is caGrid, a model-driven, service-oriented architecture that provides standards-based core "services," tools, and interfaces so the community can connect to share data and analyses efficiently and securely. More than 120 organizations are connected to caGrid. In partnership with the American Society of Clincal Oncology, caBIG® is developing specifications and services to support oncology-extended EHRs that are being deployed in community practice and hospital settings. caBIG® tools and technology are also being used by researchers working on cardiovascular health, arthritis, and AIDS. In addition, pilot projects have successfully connected caGrid to other networks, including the Nationwide Health Information Network, the CardioVascular Research Grid, and the computational network TeraGrid.

support. AHRQ also supports the National Guideline Clearinghouse which provides healthcare institutions, providers, and researchers access to objective, detailed information on clinical practice guidelines.

At the Food and Drug Administration (FDA), the Sentinel Initiative (see Box 1-6 and Appendix B) has been designed to build and implement a national electronic system for postmarket surveillance of approved drugs and other medical products. A smaller working pilot of the Sentinel system has been developed, under contract from the FDA, by Harvard Pilgrim Health Care to test epidemiological and statistical methodologies on distributed data sources.

As the federal focal point for programs in public health, the Centers for Disease Control and Prevention have supported several major HIT-anchored programs including the surveillance programs BioSense, EPI-X, and the National Healthcare Safety Network. The Health Resources and Services Administration, as the primary federal agency for improving access to healthcare services for the uninsured, isolated, or medically vulnerable, supports a portfolio of HIT programs aimed at improving care access and coordination for underserved populations and those in rural areas.

> **BOX 1-6**
> **Case: The FDA's Sentinel Initiative**
>
> In 2008, the Department of Health and Human Services and the Food and Drug Administration (FDA) announced the launch of FDA's Sentinel Initiative, a long-term program designed to build and implement a national electronic system—the Sentinel System—for monitoring the safety of FDA-approved drugs and other medical products. Data partners in the Sentinel System will include organizations such as academic medical centers, healthcare systems, and health insurance companies. As currently envisioned, participating data partners will access, maintain, and protect their respective data, functioning as part of a "distributed system."
>
> In a related pilot activity, FDA is working with Harvard Pilgrim Health Care, Inc. to develop a smaller working version of the future Sentinel System, dubbed "Mini-Sentinel." Through this pilot, FDA will learn more about some of the barriers and challenges, both internal and external, to establishing a Sentinel System for medical product safety monitoring. The Mini-Sentinel Coordinating Center (MSCC) represents a consortium of more than 20 collaborating institutions, working with participating data partners to use a common data model as the basis for their approach. Data partners transform their data into a standardized format, based upon which the MSCC will write a single analytical software program for a given safety question and provide it to each of the data partners. Each partner will conduct analyses behind its existing, secure firewall, and send only summary results to the MSCC for aggregation and further evaluation.
>
> As this pilot is being implemented, a governance structure is being developed to ensure that the activity encourages broad collaboration within appropriate guidelines for the conduct of public health surveillance activities. In order to accomplish that, the MSCC is developing a Statement of Principles and Policies that will include descriptions of the organizational structure and policies related to communication, privacy, confidentiality, data usage, conflicts of interest, and intellectual property.

Efforts to promote the development, implementation, and widespread adoption of HIT also build on a wide array of digital learning leadership efforts by other federal agencies. In particular, important contributions stem from responsibilities and activities of the VHA and the Department of Defense (DOD). The Telemedicine and Advanced Technology Research Center is a joint program between DOD and the VHA to promote research and applications in health informatics, telemedicine, and mobile health monitoring systems. Additionally, the DOD and VHA are working together to create a Virtual Lifetime Electronic Record to allow for seamless availability of healthcare, benefits, and services information for service members from enlistment to death. Additional efforts include defining a plan for HIT in the Federal Communications Commission's National Broadband Plan, and the National Science Foundation's Smart Health and Wellbeing initiative. Because of the deep and broad set of capabilities and initiatives collectively sponsored by federal agencies, their coordination and interface with private sector activities offer a vital strategic opportunity to accelerate the learning health system's development.

Testament to the compelling priority of the prospects, in December 2010 the President's Council of Advisors on Science and Technology (PCAST) issued its report, *Realizing the Full Potential of Health Information Technology to Improve Healthcare for Americans: The Path Forward* (PCAST, 2010). The PCAST report examines the opportunities and needs for the use of HIT to improve healthcare quality and reduce cost, as well as the activities and alignments of current federal programs with relevant responsibilities. It sets out a series of recommendations intended to facilitate private, entrepreneurial initiatives through governmental action to speed development of a "universal exchange language" for health information, the application of which would maximize the ability to use existing and developing electronic record systems. Specifically, it recommends action by the federal government—especially ONC and CMS—accelerate the identification of standards required for health information exchange using metadata-tagged data elements, map various existing semantic taxonomies onto the tagged elements, develop incentives for product use of tagged elements; foster use of metadata for security and safety protocols, bring federal program capacity and policy leverage to bear in implementing and guiding the efforts, and develop metrics to assess progress. The PCAST recommendations are included in Appendix E.

ABOUT THE DIGITAL INFRASTRUCTURE MEETINGS

As indicated by the title of this report, the primary intent of the meetings was to identify and explore strategic opportunities for accelerating the evolution of a digital infrastructure necessary to support and drive continuous assessment, learning, and improvement in health and health care. Three meetings were held in the summer and fall of 2010, bringing together researchers, computer scientists, privacy experts, clinicians, healthcare administrators, HIT professionals, representatives of patient advocacy groups, healthcare policy makers, and other stakeholders.

A planning committee,[1] composed of leading authorities on various aspects of the digital health learning process, established the main objectives for the workshop series. The series began by fostering a shared understand-

---

[1] Institute of Medicine planning committees are solely responsible for organizing the workshop, identifying topics, and choosing speakers. The responsibility for the published workshop summary rests with the workshop rapporteurs and the institution.

ing of the vision for the digital infrastructure for continuous learning and quality-driven health and healthcare programs by building on the existing foundations of HIT. Following the establishment of a vision, participants explored the current capacity, approaches, incentives, and policies and identified key technological, organizational, policy, and implementation priorities for the development of the digital infrastructure. Finally, participants considered strategy elements and priorities for accelerating progress on building a more seamless learning enterprise that will improve the health and health care of Americans.

Several contextual considerations informed the Committee's development of the agenda. These included rapid developments in information technology that promise to facilitate exponentially the potential of health data for knowledge generation and care improvement—these developments include federated and distributed research approaches that allow data to remain local while enabling querying and virtual pooling across systems, as well as ongoing innovation in search technologies with the potential to accelerate use of available data from multiple sources for new insights. Accordingly, considerations included developing standards that will facilitate distributed access to large datasets for comparative effectiveness research, biomarker validation, disease modeling, and improving research processes. This technological promise, coupled with policy initiatives like HITECH and the ACA that encourage the digital capture and storage of health data, provide starting points, incentives, and guidance, while encouraging innovation. Additionally, the committee considered the coevolving requirement for governance policies that foster strengthening the data utility as a core resource to advance the common good; in particular by cultivating the trust fabric among stakeholders and accelerating collaborative progress. Hand in hand with these were practical considerations including the increasing appreciation of the need to limit the burden of health data collection to the issues most important to patient care and knowledge generation.

The three workshops in the series progressed from a broad exploration of the state of play and various stakeholder perspectives on a learning health system, to a more specific identification of strategic approaches to components of the challenge, and concluded with detailed discussions of strategic elements, stakeholder responsibilities, and key crosscutting challenges. To maximize the identification and sharing of perspectives, expert presentations were followed by open discussion among participants and separate small group discussion sessions were incorporated in all of the workshops.

The first workshop, "Opportunities, Challenges, Priorities," considered the overall vision of the digital infrastructure for the learning health system as well as some of the prominent issues and opportunities related to technical progress, ensuring commitment to population and patient needs, development of the necessary trust fabric, stewardship and governance, and the implications of a global character of the health data trust. These presentations are captured in the speaker-authored manuscripts in Chapters 2 through 8. The second meeting, "The System After Next," went deeper into three cross cutting areas identified during the first workshop: engaging the patient and population, promoting technical advances, and fostering stewardship and governance structures. The third and final meeting of the series, "Strategy Scenarios," reviewed the common themes and information from the previous workshops and extended into deeper consideration of strategy elements, opportunities, responsibilities, and next steps for progress on four key focus areas: technical progress, knowledge generation and use, patient and population engagement, and governance. An integrated summary of the discussions during the second and third meetings is captured in Chapters 9 and 10.

Collectively, the discussions captured in this publication represent unprecedented promise for innovation and progress in health and health care. Yet, the discussions also underscored that without successful efforts to create the conditions necessary for seamless interoperability, to build the protocols for enhanced access and use of available information for knowledge generation, and to nurture a culture of engagement and support on behalf of the sort of information utility possible, the potential will go unmet. By thoroughly and candidly engaging in discussions on the vision, the current state of the system, the key priorities for future work, and the strategic elements for accelerating progress, participants have set in motion perspectives that can quicken the progress in building the digital infrastructure required for the continuously learning health system necessary to ensure better health for all.

REFERENCES

Blumenthal, D., and M. Tavenner. 2010. The "meaningful use" regulation for electronic health records. *New England Journal of Medicine* 363(6):501-504.

CHCF (California HealthCare Foundation). 2010. *New national survey finds personal health records motivate consumers to improve their health.* http://www.chcf.org/media/press-releases/2010/new-national-survey-finds-personal-health-records-motivate-consumers-to-improve-their-health#ixzz12kT8FU00 (accessed October 18, 2010).

DesRoches, C. M., E. G. Campbell, S. R. Rao, K. Donelan, T. G. Ferris, A. Jha, R. Kaushal, D. E. Levy, S. Rosenbaum, A. E. Shields, and D. Blumenthal. 2008. Electronic health records in ambulatory care—a national survey of physicians. *New England Journal of Medicine* 359(1):50-60.

Fox, S. 2010. *E-patients, cyberchondriacs, and why we should stop calling names.* http://www.pewinternet.org/Commentary/2010/August/Epatients-Cyberchondriacs.aspx (accessed October 19, 2010).

IOM (Institute of Medicine). 2001. *Crossing the quality chasm: A new health system for the 21st century.* Washington, DC: National Academy Press.

———. 2007. *The learning healthcare system: Workshop summary.* Washington, DC: The National Academies Press.

Jha, A. K., C. M. DesRoches, P. D. Kralovec, and M. S. Joshi. 2010. A progress report on electronic health records in U.S. hospitals. *Health Affairs (Millwood)* 29(10):1951-1957.

Smith, A. 2010. *Mobile access 2010.* http://www.pewinternet.org/Reports/2010/Mobile-Access-2010.aspx (accessed October 19, 2010).

2

Visioning Perspectives on the Digital Health Utility

INTRODUCTION

Building an effective learning health system requires a shared vision among a wide array of stakeholders with sometimes highly varied perspectives. Chapter 2 captures several of these perspectives, including those of the patient, the healthcare team, the quality and safety community, clinical researchers, and the population health community. The included manuscripts explore the current state of the digital infrastructure from their corresponding perspective, articulate their views of the potential for a learning health system supported by an integrated digital infrastructure, and identify sector-specific needs and priorities for progress.

Adam Clark, formerly of the Lance Armstrong Foundation (now FasterCures), shares his vision of a learning health system characterized by bidirectional exchange of health information (individuals are both donors and consumers). He describes the need to develop appropriate interfaces to encourage and facilitate participation in order to support this vision. This includes not only providing the most appropriate information to consumers in a format that is accessible to them, but accommodating the participation of family members and caregivers. Dr. Clark highlights the value of including consumers as information donors in the learning health system, pointing to their ability to contribute types of information—such as accounts of fatigue or depression—and provide a level of context that would otherwise not be captured. He cites data from the Lance Armstrong Foundation indicating that individuals want to share this information as long as their privacy concerns are addressed. Dr. Clark observes that the escalating complexity of medicine demands new kinds of relationships between patients, clinicians, and researchers, and that the digital infrastructure can serve as a platform for this going forward.

The perspective of the healthcare team is explored by Jim Walker of Geisinger Health System. He defines a learning health system as one of goal-oriented feedforward and feedback loops that create actionable information. Dr. Walker describes his experiences with health information technology (HIT) implementation at Geisinger and highlights the complex, sociotechnical nature of the challenge—requiring as much attention to the social aspects as is currently being given to technical capacity. Citing examples of healthcare system learning needs—such as the proper second-line treatment for diabetes—Walker lays out the potential for a learning system to address these questions and feed that information back to healthcare team members. He concludes by noting that this goal will require fundamental HIT systems redesign in order to support healthcare team decision making.

Janet Corrigan from the National Quality Forum (NQF) observes that little progress had been made to improve quality and safety since the publication of the *Quality Chasm* report (IOM, 2001), and that value has concurrently decreased. She states that increases in safety, quality, and effectiveness of health care will require investments in a digital infrastructure capable of collecting information across the longitudinal "patient-focused episode," and feeding back performance results along with clinical decision support for patients and clinicians. Dr. Corrigan describes the framework used by NQF to develop measures for reporting and value-based purchasing, and explores how a digital infrastructure could support capturing the relevant data. Finally, she states that achieving better health outcomes will require collecting information from, and enabling communication with, individuals both within and outside of traditional healthcare settings.

The growing information intensity of modern medicine and biomedical research, coupled with advances in computing capabilities, define the clinical research perspective as articulated by Christopher Chute from the Mayo Clinic. He observes that given these concurrent conditions, the technical requirements for information and knowledge management in health should be high-priority issues. Drawing from examples of "big science" disciplines such as astronomy and physics, he suggests that the future of biology and medicine will be characterized by collaborative efforts and shared data and knowledge. As such, he points to the need for standardization in order to allow for comparability and consistency in health information. Reviewing the historical state of standards uptake and development efforts, he suggests that meaningful use may be a transformative effort that moves health care in this direction.

Martin LaVenture, Sripriya Rajamani, and Jennifer Fritz from the Minnesota State Department of Health share their account of the opportunities and challenges surrounding a digital platform that supports population health activities. Acknowledging that the learning health system holds great promise for the improvement of health at the population level, they describe the need to improve the capacity and capabilities of population health services in order to realize this potential. The principal challenge, they note, is the lack of an integrated, modernized digital health infrastructure that is used by a trained workforce and stewarded by public health leaders who understand the potential benefits for population health. Accordingly, they articulate the need for a more unified vision of a digital infrastructure for population health, including development of a population health approach to data standards; aggregation and infrastructure; and intelligent, bidirectional messaging for patients and consumers.

INFORMED AND EMPOWERED PATIENTS: MOVING BEYOND A BYSTANDER IN CARE

Adam M. Clark, Ph.D.
Lance Armstrong Foundation (former)
FasterCures

The concept of a "learning health system" is one in which knowledge generation occurs as a natural outgrowth of healthcare delivery leading to improvements in innovation, quality, safety, and value in care while being inclusive of both patient and provider preferences (IOM, 2007). Fundamental and essential to the success of this concept are the two roles individuals will play in a bidirectional exchange as consumers and donators of health information. As consumers of healthcare information and utilities, a learning health system should provide individuals with information that is understandable, is pertinent to their health at the appropriate time, and is information they can act upon. The semantic content of the information will vary depending on where the individual is in the care continuum and whether the individual is acting as a patient, a caregiver, or a loved one. This will become increasingly important with the shift toward personalized medicine where prevention, screening, treatment, and care decisions become tailored to the individual.

As health information technology (HIT) continues to mature, individuals will increasingly participate in the meaningful exchange of health data. Understanding the needs of individuals as consumers and developing the appropriate interfaces with the individual and patient communities will allow the public to participate in their care and contribute to a research environment that improves both individual and population health. These interfaces could include applications such as personal health management programs, clinical advisory systems, treatment outcomes databases, clinical trials matching services, caregiver management resources, and molecular profiling tools. Provider interfaces will allow medical information exchange among the various members of the patient's clinical team and improve coordinated care. Individual interfaces to personal health records will would provide resources for individual health management, and could provide individuals with the control to donate and distribute their medical information as they see fit.

Individuals as Consumers of Health Information

The goal of patient-centered health care is to allow patients to play an active role in their healthcare decision making by working with healthcare providers to identify tools and knowledge appropriate for their health. Supporting the achievement of this goal will be an integrated health informatics infrastructure that allows appropriate information exchange among researchers, clinicians, and patients regarding treatment options, clinical outcomes, research engagement, and continuing care services.

Therefore, in a learning health system, individuals will be able to navigate through vast amounts of information to find that which is relevant to their needs. For example, a testicular cancer diagnosis touches a broad range of issues including finding oncologists in the area who have treated testicular cancer, treatment options, fertility issues, and counseling information to help address anxiety and emotional issues. In parallel, family members and loved ones who go through the cancer experience with the patient may also need information on caring for someone undergoing chemotherapy, emotional coping, appointment scheduling, and managing finances.

As consumers of health care, individuals enter the healthcare ecosystem searching for specific information that is relevant to their particular situation. In many cases the individual entering the healthcare system is not the patient, but still is searching for information related to care, understanding the disease, or identifying resources to help with practical matters. The Lance Armstrong Foundation supports a phone and online navigation program called LIVESTRONG Survivor*Care*[1] which provides free, confidential, one-on-one support, in English and Spanish, for anyone affected by cancer. LIVESTRONG Survivor*Care* provides resources and information on a range of issues including cancer diagnosis and treatment, clinical trials, counseling, financial concerns, insurance and employment concerns, and fertility preservation. Of those individuals contacting Survivor*Care* in 2009, approximately half of the individuals were not the patient diagnosed

---

[1] See http://www.livestrong.org/Get-Help/Get-One-On-One-Support (accessed August 8, 2010).

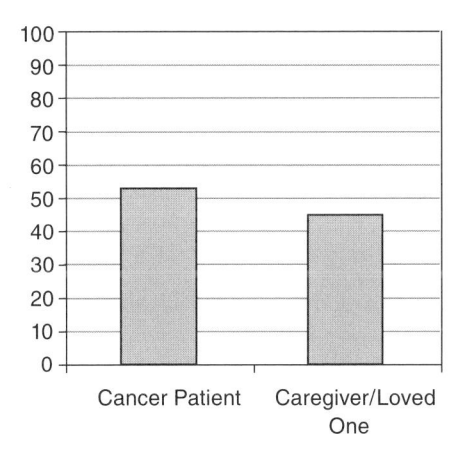

[Bar chart: Cancer Patient ~52, Caregiver/Loved One ~45]

FIGURE 2-1 The Lance Armstrong Foundation's LIVESTRONG Survivor*Care* program offers a navigation resource for anyone affected by cancer. Nearly half of the individuals contacting LIVESTRONG Survivor*Care* identify themselves as a caregiver or loved one of someone who has cancer.

with cancer (Figure 2-1). Thus, while individuals may be reaching out for information related to a particular disease, the personal context of their search varies.

A learning health system should account for this context, driving semantic content and resources useful to the individual. By linking patients' health information with an integrated electronic health information exchange, a knowledge environment can be built to connect clinical care, research, policy, and coverage that supports the best application of medical technologies for an individual patient's needs.

Individuals as Information Donors

The healthcare ecosystem is composed of a host of interconnected players: patients, doctors, regulatory agencies, insurance companies, and drug developers. In a learning health system, citizens will be equal contributors to building a learning environment, sharing their health data through HIT. In its current state, most information exchange tends to be one-directional, utilized for activities such as recordkeeping, physician reimbursement, and prescription orders. However, this model is shifting toward a bidirectional exchange as individuals adopt tools to help them participate in health management and personal health care.

There is growing evidence on the ability of electronic patient-reported outcomes (e.g., pain, sexual dysfunction, or psychological distress) to in-

TABLE 2-1 Results from the 2010 LIVESTRONG Electronic Health Information Survey

	Agree (%)	Disagree (%)	No Opinion (%)
EHRs should provide patients a way to share their medical information with scientists doing research—as long as the information cannot be linked back to them personally	86	10	4
EHRs should allow patients to enter information about their physical health for healthcare providers to review (e.g., pain, fatigue)	91	6	3
EHRs should allow patients to enter information about their emotional or mental health needs and concerns for healthcare providers to review (e.g., sadness, worry).	86	10	4

form clinicians on symptom management and direct medical interventions to improve patient quality of life (Abernethy et al., 2010a). These data are also valuable to researchers, as they provide information regarding the efficacy and/or toxicity of treatments from the perspective of the patient, particularly with respect to quality of life (FDA, 2009; Willke et al., 2004). Individuals can provide a wealth of information by linking clinically annotated data held in an electronic health record (EHR) to personal information such as pain, fatigue, or depression. This health information can be used to populate knowledge environments for analysis in health delivery services, comparative effectiveness research, and population health.

A LIVESTRONG survey[2] conducted in the spring of 2010 on electronic health information exchange discovered overwhelming support among the respondents for using electronic exchange to supply personal health information to providers as well as share clinically annotated information from their health records with researchers (Table 2-1). This suggests that individuals want to participate in the research environment, but they want to be in control of when and how they may participate. Additionally, the survey demonstrates that individuals recognize that electronic health exchange

---

[2] The LIVESTRONG Electronic Health Information Survey was conducted at the Lance Armstrong Foundation by Ruth Rechis, Ph.D., and Stephanie Nutt. Data not published. Survey publicly released April 7, 2010. Survey available at http://www.surveymonkey.com/s/healthinformationsurvey (accessed August 27, 2010).

is an appropriate tool to communicate with their providers on matters of personal health with 86% agreeing that EHRs can help share information about emotional/mental health needs and 91% agreeing EHRs can help share information about physical health needs.

Personalized Medicine and Personalized Care

Advances in biomedical research are revolutionizing our understanding of the molecular underpinnings of diseases as well as the ability to store, share, and compare large volumes of data in real time with integrated informatics platforms. In coming years, the role of the patient in research will expand, becoming a critical component in transforming the research environment. It is the hope that by 2014 the majority of Americans' health care will be supported through EHRs. In this same time frame, genetic technologies should have advanced to allow individual genome sequencing as a standard clinical analysis. The combination of these approaches will change our approach to diagnosing and treating complex diseases like cancer, drive molecularly informed comparative effectiveness research, aid in developing targeted treatments and personalized medicine, and improve care through federated health information exchanges.

The convergence of electronic personal health information, clinically annotated EHRs, and molecular medicine in an interconnected framework will help to realize the promise of both personalized medicine and personalized care (Abernethy et al., 2010b; Nadler and Downing, 2010). Patients, caregivers, doctors, and researchers will all have a participating role in a system that connects the laboratory bench, the clinical bedside, and the patient's home. In terms of treatment, as molecular understanding of disease improves, doctors will be able to make informed decisions about targeted drugs and predict patient response, enabling personalized treatment strategies. Similarly, patients will be able to provide valuable information to clinical staff regarding personal health and quality of life, and caregivers will have ready access to information and resources to improve care management.

Expansion and integration of health information exchange efforts can make it possible to aggregate millions of medical encounters in searchable data environments. This will allow for research hypothesis generation and enable researchers and clinicians to model the impact of care interventions. This will provide more detailed profiles to patients and help improve decision making. Additionally, this environment will support information for healthcare policy issues such as electronic information flow, drug/diagnostic approval for patient subpopulations, and reimbursement for targeted therapeutics. This new system relies on a new relationship among patients, doctors, and researchers whereby individuals and patients are all substantive consumers of HIT. However, in order to succeed, the system must ensure privacy, security, and individual control of personal health information for the patient, while allowing the patient to be both a donor and a recipient of information.

BUILDING A LEARNING HEALTH SYSTEM CLINICIANS WILL USE

James Walker, M.D.
Geisinger Health System

A learning health system will provide all of the healthcare team—patients, caregivers, and all different care providers—with up-to-date, care-process-integrated decision support that is based on the validated benefits and risks of potential interventions. This decision support will be developed through a learning system composed of multiple feedforward and feedback loops, connecting the relevant members of the healthcare team. When we execute this it will lead to marked improvement in population health; at least 100% improvement in delivery of patient-approved, evidence-based care; and at least a 30% reduction in the cost of evidence-based health care delivered (I am not promising decreased overall healthcare costs).

What is a learning system? My definition is a system of goal-directed, feedforward and feedback loops that creates usable and useful—which is to say actionable—information. All of the best data suggest that technology adoption is a function of usability and usefulness. If technology helps users achieve a goal they value and is usable, it will fly off the shelf. If it doesn't meet those two criteria, it is like most of our health information technology (HIT), and will sit on the shelf. An effective learning health system will need to be useful and usable to all healthcare team members: patients, caregivers, clinicians, public health workers, researchers, and policy makers.

In developing a learning health system, it will be important to consider the sociotechnical context. To systems engineers and increasingly to healthcare designers, it is obvious that any technology intervention is a sociotechnical phenomenon. While technology implementation and optimization are critical (and remarkably difficult), getting the social aspects of a system right is even more important (and more difficult). These social aspects include policies, mutually agreed roles, trust, standardization, resource allocation, mores, and conflict resolution. On the technical side, our existing infrastructure is adequate to support at least an order of magnitude more more shared, actionable learning than we currently achieve. For example, a relatively high-performance electronic health record (EHR) is available to serve well over 80 million Americans. On the social side, however, we miss more opportunities for cooperation than we act on. This lack of action is one significant reason that it has been difficult to demonstrate benefits of the technical infrastructure.

Building a Learning Health System

The first step in building a learning health system will be to identify the systems learning needs. In terms of clinical decision support, this could be questions like what is the best second-line therapy for type-2 diabetes (rosiglitazone or pioglitazone) or what is the cancer risk associated with antinogensin receptor blockers (ARBs). Other questions include: How are we going to use genomics to improve patient care? Do we need to send every doctor back to medical school? If faced with a public health emergency, can we give clinicians the questions to ask and clinical predictions that will help them to stratify patients for appropriate care? Can we build it into their EHRs? How rapidly?

After identifying the question, the next requirement for a learning system is to identify the information needed to answer the question and the best (most accurate, most efficient, most feasible) way to collect that information. In the case of questions impacting population health, agencies such as the Centers for Disease Control and Prevention and the Food and Drug Administration (FDA) are the logical actors to define the questions and commission user-centered development of the electronic tools that will make data collection efficient enough to be used in everyday care. The EHR infrastructure for collecting and reporting these data from tens of millions of Americans and their clinicians in near-real time is in everyday use today. So for questions like we're discussing, public health workers will find that if they design their questions to be asked and answered in HIT that clinicians and patients and their caregivers already use—and provide standard-of-care recommendations through that same HIT—they will be able to learn about emerging issues and guide care in days rather than months or years.

One of the most important ways for public health to reward information collection and submission is to feed back relevant information (e.g., trends in ARB adverse effects, patient outcomes on Avandia and other diabetes drugs and drug combinations) to clinicians and the public rapidly. Regarding new drugs for which safety information may emerge over the first years of use, FDA has the potential to make its guidance to care delivery organizations more usable by classifying drugs into one of four groups: (1) drugs that have been proven safe and effective; (2) drugs whose safety is under review and for which an indication for use should be documented and any of the FDA's standard list of potential adverse effects reported; (3) drugs like Avandia (rosiglitazone) for which significant adverse effects potentially in excess of benefits have been documented (documentation of the indication for use, patient's formal consent to treatment, and any adverse effects would be required to be reported; and (4) drugs that have been removed from the market.

In the end, what clinicians get is a set of tools—designed by the appropriate public health agency, developed by the HIT vendor, and implemented by their local HIT team—that would enable them to provide information on the benefits and adverse effects of different interventions and therapies without being distracted from their usual (and critically important) work.

Lessons from Geisinger

What have we at Geisinger learned so far? First, sociotechnical infrastructure development requires highly skilled care-process design teams and technical IT teams. Second, even when those teams work in an organization committed to change, it has taken us over 10 years to make organization-wide changes in 30–40% of our core clinical processes. It may be possible to accelerate this process, but the particularly isolated character of the delivery organizations that need to be integrated going forward make the optimal methods for HIT-supported process redesign a critical topic for research and development as well as careful monitoring. That said, once the infrastructure is in place, the rate at which an organization can make change becomes genuinely breathtaking. Geisinger can now run 5–10 major HIT-supported quality improvement initiatives simultaneously without overtaxing the organization—largely because the infrastructure dramatically decreases the administrative costs of process redesign and management. Finally, existing HIT systems need fundamental redesign to integrate feed-forward and feedback information loops into usable care processes. This is unsurprising, considering how preliminary our understanding of care processes and their information needs still is, but adds significant costs to process redesign and management. For example, Geisinger employs 176 people solely to support the EHR and networked personal health record.

Conclusions

First, we have enough HIT infrastructure in place now to create a much more effective learning health system. Second, our ability to agree among public health professionals, clinicians, HIT developers, patients, and others on the questions that are worth answering and the required information needs substantial development. Third, to optimize the learning system, HIT products and services need fundamental redesign based on actual and potential future needs. Finally, we must consider what will motivate delivery organizations to participate in such a learning system? Providing substantial reimbursement for participation is unlikely to be feasible, and sanctions for failure to participate are unlikely to be feasible or enforceable.

Alternatively, if participation is made optimally easy and enables delivery organizations to meet explicit societal standards of care reliably and cost-effectively, it will likely provide adequate incentive for participation.

IMPROVING QUALITY AND SAFETY
Janet M. Corrigan, Ph.D., M.B.A.
National Quality Forum

It has been 10 years since the Institute of Medicine issued its landmark reports, *To Err Is Human* and *Crossing the Quality Chasm*, focusing national attention on the need to improve health care quality and safety (IOM, 2000, 2001). Since that time, there have been some very important accomplishments, but overall, progress has been slow. Per capita expenditures in the United States far exceed those of all other industrialized countries, while quality and safety remain uneven (Fisher et al., 2003; IOM, 2010; Murray and Frenk, 2010).

Although there have been many very successful, localized quality improvement initiatives demonstrating that it is possible to close the quality gap, we have yet to take these innovations to scale. In our current health system, quality measurement and improvement are labor- and time-intensive activities. Measuring quality often involves abstracting information from paper charts or relying on administrative data sources that lack clinical richness. Clinicians may receive performance reports based on data that are a year old or more, and performance results (e.g., mammography rate) may not be accompanied by the necessary information to improve care (e.g., detailed listing of patients who should have received a mammogram but did not).

Our measurement and improvement efforts have also been hampered by the fragmented and siloed nature of the health system. Most quality improvement activities have been focused on aspects of the care process for which some data are captured, namely hospital care and ambulatory visits. Yet many serious safety and quality concerns arise from care transitions (e.g., discharge from the hospital to the community or referral from a primary care provider to a specialist).

In spite of the fact that health care consumes over 16% of U.S. gross domestic product, there is currently no system in place to measure patient outcomes (IOM, 2010). Currently, most available data are recorded by clinicians during health encounters. The health system lacks mechanisms to capture patient-derived data on health functioning, symptoms (e.g., fatigue, pain), health behaviors (e.g., exercise, diet, smoking), and adherence to treatment plans (e.g., medications).

Achieving higher levels of safety, quality, and efficiency requires investment in an electronic data platform capable of capturing the necessary longitudinal data *from* clinicians and patients, and providing real-time feedback and clinical decision support *to* clinicians and patients. With the passage of the Patient Protection and Affordable Care Act (ACA) of 2010, the stakes are now higher than ever before. ACA seeks to encourage and reward higher levels of performance and penalize those who fail to measure up through three key provisions:

- *Transparency*: expansion of public reporting websites pertaining to virtually all types of providers and clinicians to include safety, quality, and cost information.
- *Payment alignment*: creation of payment programs tied to performance, including paying more for higher value care and nonpayment for healthcare-acquired conditions.
- *Clinically-integrated delivery systems*: more favorable payment programs for health care homes and accountable care organizations capable of providing patient-centered, team-based care.

A digital infrastructure that can support robust performance measurement and improvement systems is a necessary prerequisite to succeed in this new environment.

Framework for Performance Measurement

A two-dimensional framework is guiding the development of performance measures and performance measurement requirements for public reporting and value-based purchasing:

- *Crosscutting areas*: The National Priorities Partnership convened by NQF has identified six crosscutting areas that impact most if not all persons/patients, including population health, safety, care coordination, patient/family engagement, palliative care, and overuse (National Priorities Partnership, 2008). Within each priority area, there are specific aspects of care that will be the focus of intense monitoring and improvement because these areas currently exhibit large quality, safety, and efficiency gaps (Box 2-1).
- *Clinical conditions*: A limited number of clinical conditions account for a sizable share of healthcare services and health burden (NQF, 2010). By focusing attention on these conditions, it should be possible to positively impact the lives of many patients while also removing waste from the system.

Figure 2-2 provides an example of this two-dimensional performance measurement framework applied to patients with acute myocardial infarc-

> **BOX 2-1**
> **National Priorities Partnership**
> **Key Cross-Cutting Areas and Goals**
>
> **Population health**
> - Key preventive services
> - Healthy lifestyle behaviors
>
> **Safety**
> - Hospital-level mortality rates
> - Serious adverse events
> - Healthcare-acquired Infections
>
> **Care coordination**
> - Medication reconciliation
> - Preventable hospital readmissions
> - Preventable emergency department visits
>
> **Patient/family engagement**
> - Informed decision making
> - Patient experience of care
> - Patient self-management
>
> **Palliative care**
> - Relief of physical symptoms
> - Help with psychological, social, and spiritual needs
> - Communication on treatment options, prognosis
> - Access to palliative care services
>
> **Overuse**
> - Nine major areas
>
> SOURCE: National Priorities Partnership (2008).

tion (AMI). To assess whether the health system is taking appropriate steps to prevent AMIs, information must be captured on the health status and risk behaviors of the entire population and the services provided to mitigate risk (e.g., programs to lower cholesterol levels through diet, exercise, and medication). Once an AMI occurs, information must be captured on the quality and safety of the emergency response system (including community-based and hospital services) and on how well the patient is managed throughout their hospital episode. Upon hospital discharge, the patient will require follow-up care emphasizing secondary and tertiary prevention and to ascertain whether expected outcomes have been achieved. The six cross-cutting areas also are relevant to AMI patients. For example, care coordination (e.g., transfer of treatment plan from hospital to rehabilitation provider with acknowledgement of receipt).

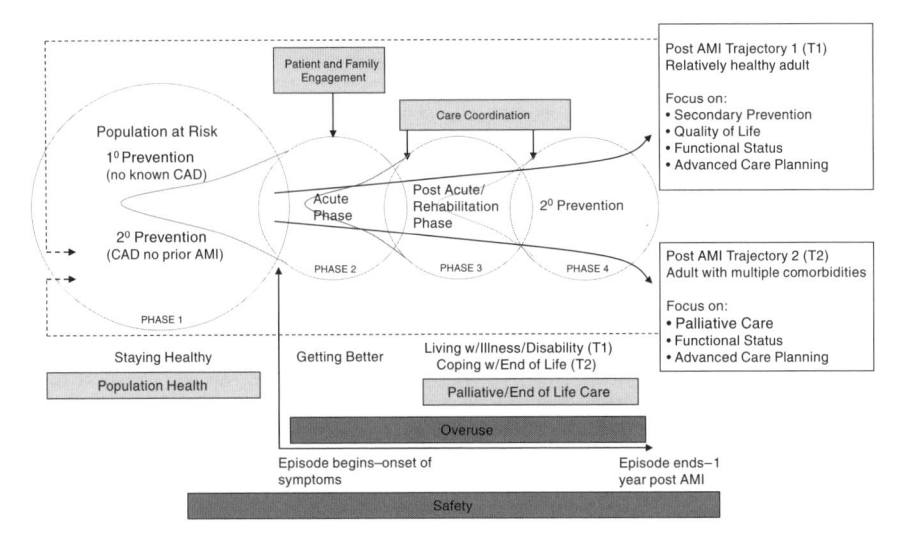

84   DIGITAL INFRASTRUCTURE FOR THE LEARNING HEALTH SYSTEM

FIGURE 2-2 Two-dimensional measurement framework applied to acute myocardial infarction.

Implications for the Digital Infrastructure

A patient-centered approach to designing the digital infrastructure will be needed to support quality measurement and improvement. The digital infrastructure must be capable of capturing the relevant data from clinicians and patients across the entire longitudinal, "patient-focused episode" to assess both cross-cutting and condition-specific aspects of quality. To achieve the greatest gains in improvement, there should be immediate feedback of performance results accompanied by clinical decision support to both clinicians and patients.

In general, the types of information that must be captured for a patient-focused episode fall into the following domains:

- Patient-level outcomes (better health)
  - morbidity and mortality
  - functional status
  - health-related quality of life
  - patient experience of care
- Processes of care (better care)
  - technical quality of care
  - care coordination and transitions
  - alignment with patients' preferences

- Cost and resource use (affordable care)
  o total cost of care across the episode
  o indirect costs

For some of these data—functional status, alignment with patient preferences—patients and family caregivers are the most reliable sources, so the digital infrastructure must provide for personal health records or other vehicles for incorporating a "patient voice."

Over time, it will also be important for the digital infrastructure to move beyond the traditional boundaries of the personal healthcare system. Achieving the best outcomes for patients and populations requires the ability to capture information from, and enable communication with, all residents of a community regardless of whether they use healthcare services. It will also be important to capture "context information," such as race, ethnicity, language, socioeconomic status, and employment, all of which influence adherence to treatment plans and patient outcomes, and are needed to inform policy.

CLINICAL RESEARCH IN THE INFORMATION AGE

Christopher G. Chute, Ph.D., Dr.P.H.
Mayo Clinic College of Medicine

The London Bills of Mortality were initiated by Henry the VIII of England during an onset of the Black Death in an effort to tabulate who was dying of what, mostly so that the nobility could know which areas were plague-infested and avoid them. An unexpected consequence was the publication over a century later of John of Graunt's seminal work, "Natural and Political Observations . . . Upon the London Bills of Mortality," first published in 1662. Through his systematic analyses of these data, public health was transformed into a quantitative science, replete with the introduction of endemic and epidemic patterns, small area analyses of mortality, and the foundation of epidemiological and biostatistical principles (Glass et al., 1963). As with all such seminal work, it was largely ignored for 200 years, but it was probably the first work to show that the systematic collection of mortality statistics could inform the world about much more than where not to travel to avoid the plague.

The Information-Intensive Nature of Modern Health Care

The distinguishing characteristic of modern medicine is the information-intensive nature of its practice. Modern health care comprises two things: managing information and procedural interventions. Virtually everything done clinically—from gathering a history and a physical, to working through differential diagnoses, managing preventive measures, and most importantly, accessing the wealth of extant medical knowledge—involves information. Humans have been adept at processing clinical information for generations. However, in the midst of the continuously escalating rate of biomedical discovery and knowledge generation, even the most adept among us are overwhelmed. Requirements for computational assistance in the clinical process are apparent.

Equivalently, the formalized improvement of care inevitably involves the definition of numerators and denominators corresponding to clinical phenotypes. Patients are classified into these strata, a process that increasingly cannot rely on human abstraction and judgment. Comparisons among strata are computed, often involving sophisticated numerical or machine learning methods, and inferences made with respect to quality of care, technology assessment, best evidence discovery, or comparative effectiveness. Thus, most of our science associated with care improvement is inexorably linked to information processes.

If we accept that biomedical advancement and clinical practice have become unified as an information-intensive domain, then the technical requirements for information and knowledge management are now high-profile and high-priority issues.

The Transformation of Information Processing

In parallel with the explosion of biomedical knowledge has evolved the transformative change in our capacity to manage and interpret information. Moore's Law (for Intel founder Gordon Moore), postulated in 1965, asserts that integrated circuit density would double every 2 years. The well-known corollary is that computation power would double every 18 months (the acceleration being due to processor design improvements). Both laws have proven uncannily accurate. Computing capacity has increased on the order of 10^{12}-fold over the past 60 years. The supercomputing power that nations would have sacrificed the lives of spies to secure as recently as 20 years ago are now under Christmas trees as game platforms for children.

However, raw computation power is not the only dimension over which we can meaningfully measure information processing capability. Network performance has experienced dramatic increases in bandwidth from 110-baud teletypes to 100-Gb backbones—an increase of 10^9 over 50 years. Furthermore, the raw number of high-bandwidth connections around the globe has successfully saturated four generations of IP protocols—another 10^9 increase. Correspondingly, local memory stores on machines have grown from handfuls of vacuum tubes to 100-Gb RAM configurations not uncommon on intermediate server platforms today—an approximate 10^{11}-fold increase in capacity. Not to be forgotten are data storage capabilities, exploding from paper-tape holes (where one could reassuringly see those bits) to petabyte drive assemblies—at least a 10^{15}-fold increase.

All these measures of computational capability are gross underestimates in the face of emerging cloud computing and data storage resources, which are arbitrarily scalable to sizes that make these comparisons ultimately irrelevant. Nevertheless, if we add the exponents above—which is really multiplying, since we are in exponential space—humanity has achieved a 10^{56}-fold increase in our capacity to manage and manipulate information during my lifetime. This is a conservative estimate, and a vast, genuinely astronomical number by most measures. Despite its frail arithmetical basis, the conclusion persists that we have experienced a profound increase in our ability to manage information. This must have a profound impact on domains that are information intensive. We are only in the opening chapters of a massive social and cultural transformation of biomedicine. It is without precedent.

These conclusions are concordant with predictions emerging from the genomics community and consistent with our everyday experience with unprecedented access to most anything we could want to know on the Internet. Our Google-aided society can research topics with a speed and depth unimaginable a generation ago. So, too, will our capabilities in biomedical discovery and clinical practice evolve.

The Emergence of "Big Science"

The lessons of astronomy and physics are informative as we consider the future of biology and medicine. These disciplines have evolved into a "big science" paradigm, where the work of collective groups and the amassed knowledge and data resources of the field dominate over the contributions of independent investigators. Gone are the days when a Galileo could gaze into the skies from his porch and make seminal discoveries in astronomy. Similarly, the tabletop experiments of Rutherford, while profound, cannot be matched in the present era in terms of scientific impact or advancement. Both fields today depend on large teams of interdisciplinary scientists, who draw from and contribute to a vast commons of shared data and imputed knowledge.

The duality of biology and medicine having become information-intensive domains, coupled with our vast capacities to manage and manipulate information, make it inevitable that a similar "commons" of biomedical information will form a hub from and to which investigators and practitioners will draw and contribute. A foreshadowing of this reality is already evident in the genomic community, with the myriad of publicly accessible databases that surround the original Genbank suite of resources.

If clinical medicine is to truly become "big science," we must recognize that this implies that we can learn from the historical experience of patients, study their outcomes, and learn what interventions help or hurt for particular characterizations of patients, diseases, comorbidity, risk factors, genomic traits, and social or patient preferences. While randomized clinical trials remain the gold standard of biomedical evidence, we can and will learn more from empirical studies of patient outcomes. Presently, the meticulous surveys, chart abstractions, quality studies, or comparative effectiveness efforts have yet to coalesce into anything like a scientific commons for large-scale analyses and understanding. Clinical evidence, together with the healthcare delivery infrastructure, remain trapped in a cottage industry–level effort, fraught with noncomparable information and profound barriers to data sharing and access. Medicine, from a knowledge management perspective, remains in a pre-Grauntian state. We are unable to tabulate our fate using 16th century data spreadsheets or other quantitative means for lack of consistent and comparable information about what we do clinically or what happens to patients.

Comparability and Consistency in Healthcare Information

What then would correspond to a present-day London Bills that could sustain the analyses of the intellectual descendents of Graunt and improve our understanding, practice, and outcomes in clinical care? A widely shared vision is the notion of a repository of patient experience, where electronic records were made available under supervised and consented conditions to epidemiologists, health services researchers, biostatisticians, and others to scalably discover best evidence for care, and ultimately a mechanism that would predict best therapies or preventions for specific categories of people. While presently many obstacles—including privacy, confidentiality, and intellectual property concerns—make this vision impractical, one critical path issue remains the reality. Most health information is neither comparable nor consistent among providers, record systems, or researchers. We lack standards for representing patient findings, events, or interventions in a comparable or consistent way. This obviates any scalable analyses without expensive and typically humanly intensive abstraction and harmonization of the data.

The absence of standards is not due to technical obstacles or an absence of specification. Among the cottages of healthcare delivery have emerged what may be characterized as wanton idiosyncrasies. There is no good technical reason why every hospital and clinic feels compelled to create de novo codes and identifiers for clinical laboratory measures; the foundation of the publicly accessible and free-for-use LOINC codes for laboratories could solve this one problem overnight. Furthermore, most electronic medical record systems developers have been slow to contribute to or adopt clinical information standards; that those who have invested the least in health information technology (HIT) standards development appear to be the most successful in the marketplace suggests there are misaligned incentives operating in the healthcare marketplace—not a new observation, to be sure.

William Farr, a great 19th century English leader of public health, asserted in 1839 that "nomenclature is of as much importance in [medicine], as weights and measures in the physical sciences, and should be settled without delay" (Langmuir, 1976). The metaphor is apt with our big science analogies. How could we conduct astronomy or physics without notions of a meter, second, or gram? We seem as a society not to have heeded Farr's admonition about nomenclature, since even something as relatively uncontroversial as a serum sodium measure has virtually no adoption of standard nomenclature or code system.

The U.S. Standards Experiments

If we accept that health care is information intensive, that computational capacity has transformed our ability to manage and understand information, that comparable and consistent representation of clinical data using HIT standards is on our critical path to improved healthcare efficacy and efficiency, why have we not fully developed and adopted HIT standards?

There has been no lack of efforts to establish consensus forums in the United States and globally for the specification of HIT standards. The overused quip that "the nice thing about standards is that there are so many to choose from" might apply equivalently to HIT standards bodies and consensus forums. Beginning with the Health Information Standards Planning Panel in the early 1990s, and moving through the American National Standards Institute's Healthcare Informatics Standards Board, the Health Information Portability and Accountability Act, the Healthcare Information Technology Standards Panel, and the Office of the National Coordinator for HIT (ONC) HIT Standards Committee, there have been significant resources expended on this problem. Few have lasted more than a few years, and most have had minimal impact on clinical practice or biomedical discovery.

"Meaningful use" may be a transformative effort, where the likelihood of broadly based adoption—premised on the suite of incentives and penalties under the Health Information Technology for Economic and Clinical Health Act—may be substantial. If so, then for the first time the United States will have a basis for comparable and consistent representation of clinical data beyond billing codes. The implications of this for future science, enabling the establishment of federated repositories of patient data that can sustain inference and discovery, are profound.

INTEGRATING THE PUBLIC HEALTH PERSPECTIVE

Martin LaVenture, Ph.D., M.P.H., Sripriya Rajamani, Ph.D., M.P.H., and Jennifer Fritz, M.P.H.
Office of Health Information Technology,
Minnesota Department of Health

Achieving the vision for a *Digital Infrastructure for the Learning Health System* will make profound improvements in the health of individuals, communities, and the entire population. Successfully achieving this vision requires improving the capability and capacity of population health services provided by governmental public health organizations at the local, state, and federal levels; close integration with clinical stakeholders; and fully engaging the general public.

Background

The Health Information Technology for Economic and Clinical Health (HITECH) Act and the Patient Protection and Affordable Care Act (ACA) have provided the nation with an unprecedented opportunity to accelerate the pace for improving healthcare quality, increasing patient safety, reducing healthcare costs, and enabling individuals and communities to make the best possible health decisions. Coordination and training were identified as key issues for the national public health informatics agenda at a meeting of stakeholders almost a decade ago (Yasnoff et al., 2001). These issues are currently being addressed at the national level through initiatives that focus on adoption and use of electronic health records (EHRs) through incentives, technical assistance, training, and support for health information technology (HIT) innovation (Blumenthal, 2010). The extensive policy, governance, and technical foundation established locally to date needs to be leveraged and integrated closely with national efforts facilitated through the Office of the National Coordinator for HIT.

A digital infrastructure for the learning health system can offer immense opportunities for population health improvement in public health surveillance and response, population-based research and policy, coordination and quality improvement, and health education and communication. Challenges to achieving this vision include a lack of a sound electronic public health infrastructure, the need to advance workforce skills, polices that force categorical use of funds and short budget cycles, and uneven understanding among programmatic leaders about public health benefits of HIT. A shared vision and commitment to a clear path are critical, with emphasis on addressing the needs identified above.

Population Health Opportunities of Digital Infrastructure

The meaning of population health varies, but working definitions used by the Minnesota e-Health Initiative are as follows (Minnesota e-Health Initiative, 2010; Westera et al., 2010):

Population health: a conceptual approach to measure the aggregate health of a community or jurisdictional region with a collective goal of improving those measurements and reducing health inequities among population groups. Stepping beyond the individual-level focus of mainstream medicine, population health acknowledges and addresses a broad range of social determinant factors that impact health. Emphasizing environment, social structure, and resource distribution, population health is less focused on the relatively minor impact that medicine and healthcare have on improving health overall. (Koo et al., 2001)

Governmental public health: a core infrastructural entity that is legislatively authorized to protect the public. Public health organizations provide the backbone to the infrastructure for population health improvements. It depends on other sectors (e.g., health care system, academia, business community) to improve the overall health of a community based on population health analysis. (Minnesota e-Health Initiative, 2008)

The digital infrastructure for the learning health system can offer immense opportunities for population health improvement and, more importantly, can serve as a conduit for bringing the domains of population health together. Table 2-2 identifies five areas of population health services and

TABLE 2-2 Types of Population Health Activities and Opportunities for Provider Engagement

Population Health Area	Opportunity for Provider Engagement
Surveillance and response	Identify sentinel events, emerging illness, and injury trends. Access to cross-sectional and longitudinal data to identify patterns, trends, and support response actions
Health status/disease measurement	Leverage resources available to optimize health status and outcome measurement
Health education/communication	Use new medical information for targeted knowledge/recommendations
Population-based health care	Clinic-based profiles of patients informing decision-support programs to assist members in developing/improving self-care skills
Population-based research	Applied research to improve care for individuals/the community

example opportunities for provider engagement in each domain. Achieving a healthier population requires that federal, state, and local organizations be fully engaged. Given the challenges described above, the capacity and capability of public health information systems need to be modernized. Box 2-2 identifies some of the benefits of an integrated, modernized electronic infrastructure that enables secure, authorized bidirectional communications with governmental public health agencies and other organizations providing population health services. All of these activities seek to improve the health of individuals and communities.

Current State of Play

Achieving the population health improvements possible in a learning health system requires significant improvement in the digital infrastructure. This cannot be achieved on a national scale by simply adding some population health fields onto an EHR. We need to achieve a much broader understanding of how we are going to collect, analyze, distribute, and use information to better provide care coordination and other activities at the community level.

Table 2-3 identifies three levels of public health infrastructure in the United States and their general areas of responsibility. Infrastructure varies significantly across these agencies. The systems they employ vary in functional capability as well as capacity. Improvements in individual and organization skills in informatics and information technology are needed. Most agencies are currently experiencing significant budget challenges. Additionally, system capability and capacity as well as workforce informatics skills needs remain barriers to achieving a broader vision.

Figure 2-3 presents an example from Minnesota where plans for HIT incorporate a strategic model that is designed to integrate across the continuum of care, including public health. As a result, the integration of public health into this plan is a core element for achieving a broader population health vision.

Challenges

Many challenges face public health organizations as they seek to modernize and maintain an infrastructure that can support a learning environment. In general, key needs fall into several categories: modernize technical infrastructure, advance the skills of the workforce, commit to development of common business processes across jurisdictions, modify policies that force categorical use of funds and short budget cycles, address the uneven understanding among programmatic leaders about how HIT benefits public health needs; and improve understanding of public health's role in care coordination.

BOX 2-2
Bidirectional Benefits of Public Health Participation in a Learning Health System

Public health contributions
- Knowledge and skills on population health measurement
- Intervention expertise to health reform/quality improvement efforts
- Leadership on community-focused population health efforts that increase utilization of primary prevention services
- Improvements in care coordination especially for chronic diseases (e.g., diabetes, asthma, hypertension)
- Can provide data based on select characteristics (summary-level data, epidemiological data)
- Can provide "evidenced-based practice" as well as "practice-based evidence"
- Collaborative efforts to implement clinical decision support systems
- Leadership on efforts to measure and monitor the health of the community by applying data analysis competence
- Capability to execute large population health/community-level changes through recommendations, guidelines, and public policies
- Ability to translate impact of interventions to public health problems
- Optimize systems for disease surveillance, analysis, and alerting
- Coordinate efforts to implement clinical decision support systems that better integrate decision support across multiple diseases/conditions to improve disease management

Benefits to public health
- Ability to use outcomes data from electronic health records and other HIT to supplement existing surveillance methodologies and information
- Ability to optimize systems for disease surveillance, analysis, and alerting based on lessons learned
- Gain new knowledge to improve care coordination and outcomes, especially for chronic diseases
- Quicker translation of insights gained from clinical environment to potential interventions to possible public health recommendations
- Coordination of services and research with academic and learning community
- Creation of a framework where the trend of new and existing acute and chronic conditions are correlated with select population-level metrics (e.g., demographics, socioeconomic status, prevalence of other comorbidities, community characteristics)

SOURCE: Adapted from Improving Population Health and the Minnesota e-Health Initiative fact sheet. http://www.health.state.mn.us/e-health/phphin/index.html (accessed February 22, 2011).

TABLE 2-3 Governmental Public Health Agencies

Governmental Entity	Number and Scale of the Agencies
Cities and counties	~3,000 health departments
State/territory	50 state health departments, 6 territories
Federal	Centers for Disease Control and Prevention as the lead agency Centers for Medicare & Medicaid Services Health Resources and Services Administration Office of the National Coordinator for Health IT Agency for Healthcare Research and Quality

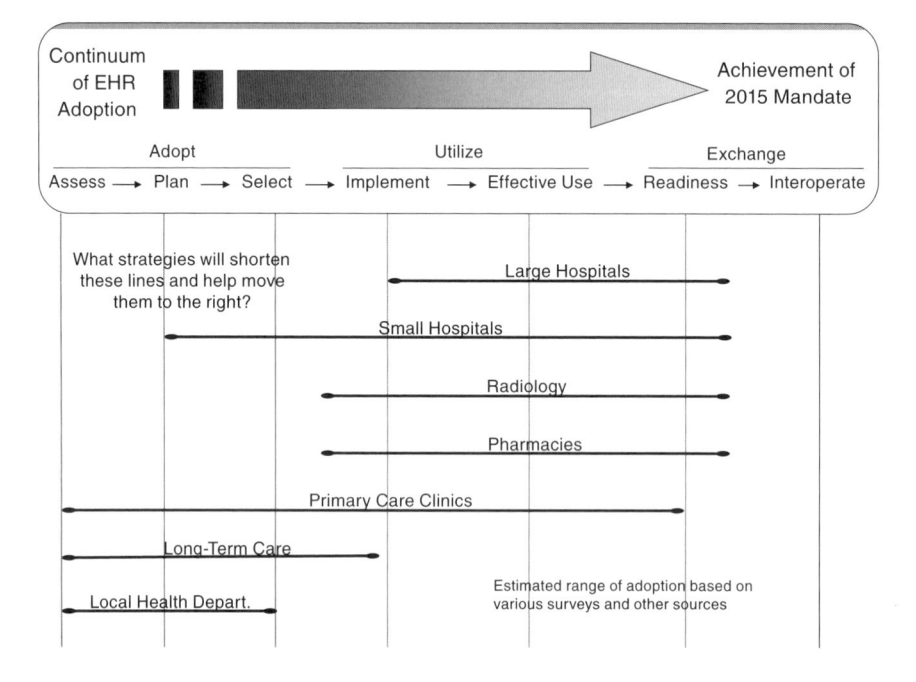

FIGURE 2-3 Minnesota example of public health infrastructure relative to other systems.

Recommendations

Establish a *shared vision and action plan for population health and a clear path to success*. The lack of coordination of efforts in the past has proven to be a barrier and must be addressed in order to realize the opportunities before us today. The Minnesota e-Health Initiative[3] provides an example of one state's shared vision and how it was incorporated into the statewide plan for e-health to ensure success. The critical components to ensure success include

- A commitment to the development of common business requirements and processes across jurisdictions, starting with local health departments.
- Improved standards, specifications, and certification criteria for interoperability of public health–focused data on individuals and population aggregate information.
- A commitment to modernizing infrastructure using a coordinated and integrated approach.
- A commitment to close the gap in core and advanced informatics skills of the workforce.
- A transition to policies that encourage integrated approaches to programs supporting the larger vision.
- A cohesive message to advance common understanding of how EHRs/HIT benefit public health.

Adopt specific approaches to data standards, aggregation, and/or infrastructure that will help achieve better population health outcomes

- Improve federal and state leadership and coordination on identification and use of standards for interoperability including technical, semantic, and process interoperability.
- Establish the framework for tools that can present population health data in ways that can profile the health status and disease burdens of communities. This should include the ability to analyze patterns of injury and illness in relationship to health status and risk in the community. What gets measured is better understood and often gets done.
- Utilize existing tools to create an informatics profile for public health agencies and expand and adapt the tool to meet evolving needs (Fritz et al., 2009).
- Implement population health dashboard applications that provide community health profile in near-real time. Establishing a population health dashboard will empower individuals and providers with data they need to support the learning health system.

---

[3] More information on Minnesota's Statewide Plan for e-Health can be accessed at www.health.state.mn.us/ehealth (accessed September 30, 2010).

- Adopt the standards for the full set of transactions for meaningful use requirements. For example, expand immunization transactions beyond submission to include request, return of history, and the options for forecasting using decision support.
- Adopt standards for all transactions associated with reportable conditions including alerting function capability.
- Certifications of public health software applications are vital. Pursue "orphan" software classification if needed to obtain vendor participation.
- Build upon national standards and large-scale models for implementation strategies. Avoid duplication of population health–only infrastructures.

Implement intelligent, bidirectional public health messaging for providers and consumers. The potential for effective health communication and key messages to the public to modify beliefs and influence behavior has been recognized by the public health community for many years. In order to drive effective messaging, public health agencies and others responsible for population health improvement should fully engage consumers by presenting health information in effective formats that drive improved outcomes and also extend reach through utilization of emerging venues of communication such as social networks and other new media mechanisms. Consumers must be fully engaged and messages based on trusted information sources should

- Articulate the value public health information can bring to them—in terms of quality, cost, and convenience.
- Explain how patient privacy is protected both by law and through the use of appropriate security measures.

Conclusion

A learning health system provides the opportunity to improve the health of the population in profound ways. Significant improvements are needed to modernize information systems, improve needed functional capability, and achieve better trained workforce. "Informatics savvy" organizations are a vital component to achieve the goal of improved population health.

REFERENCES

Abernethy, A. P., A. Ahmad, S. Y. Zafar, J. L. Wheeler, J. B. Reese, and H. K. Lyerly. 2010a. Electronic patient-reported data capture as a foundation of rapid learning cancer care. *Medical Care* 48(6 Suppl):S32-S38.

Abernethy, A. P., L. M. Etheredge, P. A. Ganz, P. Wallace, R. R. German, C. Neti, P. B. Bach, and S. B. Murphy. 2010b. Rapid-learning system for cancer care. *Journal of Clinical Oncology*.

Blumenthal, D. 2010. Launching HITECH. *New England Journal of Medicine* 362(5):382-385.

FDA (Food and Drug Administration). 2009. *Guidance for industry patient-reported outcome measures: Use in medical product development to support labeling claims*. http://www.fda.gov/downloads/Drugs/GuidanceComplianceRegulatoryInformation/Guidances/UCM193282.pdf (accessed September 10, 2010).

Fisher, E., D. Wennberg, T. Stukel, D. Gottlieb, F. Lucas, and Ã. Pinder. 2003. The implications of regional variations in Medicare spending. Part 1: The content, quality, and accessibility of care. *Annals of Internal Medicine* 138(4):273-287.

Fritz, J. E., P. Rajamani, and M. LaVenture. 2009. *Developing a public health informatics profile: A toolkit for state and local health departments to assess their informatics capacity*. http://www.phii.org/resources/doc/MN%20PHIP%20Toolkit%20FINAL.pdf (accessed September 30, 2010).

Glass, D. V., M. E. Ogborn, and I. Sutherland. 1963. John Graunt and his natural and political observations [and discussion]. *Proceedings of the Royal Society of London. Series B, Biological Sciences* 159(974):2-37.

IOM (Institute of Medicine). 2000. *To err is human: Building a safer health system*. Washington, DC: National Academy Press.

———. 2001. *Crossing the quality chasm: A new health system for the 21st century*. Washington, DC: National Academy Press.

———. 2007. *The learning healthcare system: Workshop summary*. Washington, DC: The National Academies Press.

———. 2010. *Healthcare imperative: Lowering costs and improving outcomes: Workshop series summary*. Washington, DC: The National Academies Press.

Koo, D., P. O'Carroll, and M. LaVenture. 2001. Public Health 101 for informaticians. *Journal of the American Medical Informatics Association* 8(6):585-597.

Langmuir, A. D. 1976. William Farr: Founder of modern concepts of surveillance. *International Journal of Epidemiology* 5(1):13-18.

Minnesota e-Health Initiative. 2010. *Minnesota e-health Initiative: Vision*. http://www.health.state.mn.us/e-health/abouthome.html (accessed September 30, 2010).

———. 2008. *Population health and health information technology framework: Definitions, conceptual model, and principles*. http://www.health.state.mn.us/e-health/phphin/phmodel2008.pdf (accessed September 30, 2010).

Murray, C. J. L., and J. Frenk. 2010. Ranking 37th—measuring the performance of the U.S. health care system. *New England Journal of Medicine* 362(2):98-99.

Nadler, J. J., and G. J. Downing. 2010. Liberating health data for clinical research applications. *Science Translational Medicine* 2(18):18cm16.

National Priorities Partnership. 2008. *National priorities and goals: Aligning our efforts to transform America's healthcare*. Washington, DC: National Quality Forum.

NQF (National Quality Forum). 2010. *Prioritization of high-impact Medicare conditions and measure gaps*. http://www.qualityforum.org/projects/prioritization.aspx?section=MeasurePrioritizationAdvisoryCommitteeReport2010-05-24 (accessed February 23, 2011).

Westera, B., M. LaVenture, B. Wills, and S. Rajamani. 2010. Case study 14d. Minnesota e-health Initiative. In *Nursing and informatics for the 21st century: An international look at practice, education and EHR trends*, edited by C. A. Weaver, C. W. Delaney, P. Weber, and R. L. Carr. Chicago, IL: Healthcare Information and Management Systems Society and American Medical Informatics Association. pp. 312-322.

Willke, R. J., L. B. Burke, and P. Erickson. 2004. Measuring treatment impact: A review of patient-reported outcomes and other efficacy endpoints in approved product labels. *Controlled Clinical Trials* 25(6):535-552.

Yasnoff, W. A., J. M. Overhage, B. L. Humphreys, M. LaVenture, K. W. Goodman, L. Gatewood, D. A. Ross, J. Reid, W. E. Hammond, D. Dwyer, S. M. Huff, I. Gotham, R. Kukafka, J. W. Loonsk, and M. M. Wagner. 2001. A national agenda for public health informatics. *Journal of Public Health Management and Practice* 7(6):1-21.

3

Technical Issues for the Digital Health Infrastructure

INTRODUCTION

Information technology drives the digital learning health system, and technological innovation in several key areas will be crucial in meeting future needs for security, healthcare quality, and clinical and public health applications. These issues include building off of the foundation laid by the implementation of the American Recovery and Reinvestment Act initiatives, working toward systems interoperability, ensuring secure data liquidity, maximizing computing potential, and finding strategies to harmonize data from diverse sources. This chapter explores these issues with a vision for leveraging current technologies and identifying priorities for innovation in order to ensure that data collected in one system can be utilized across many others for a variety of different uses—for example, quality, research, public health—all of which will improve health and health care.

Douglas Fridsma from the Office of the National Coordinator for Health IT provides an update on the current standards and interoperability framework being developed. He reviews several lessons learned by past standards development efforts currently informing their approach, such as the notion that standards must be adopted not imposed, and not to let perfection be the enemy of the good. Dr. Fridsma describes the priorities shaping the work of the Office of Standards and Interoperability, highlighting the need to manage the life cycle of standards and interoperability activities by providing mechanisms for continuous refinement. He details the model being used in the development of the standards and interoperability framework which consists of interplay between community engagement, harmonization of core concepts with other exchange models, development of implementation specifications, reference implementation, and incorporation into certification and testing initiatives. Dr. Fridsma emphasizes the need to leverage existing work, coordinate capacity, and integrate successful initiatives into the framework.

Rebecca Kush from the Clinical Data Interchange Standards Consortium shared the Institute of Electrical and Electronics Engineers' definition of interoperability—"the ability of two or more systems or components to exchange information and to use the information that has been exchanged" (IEEE, 1990). Building on this, she suggests that one approach to defining interoperability within the digital infrastructure of the learning health system might be the exchange and aggregation of information upon which trustworthy healthcare decisions can be made. Dr. Kush cites existing enablers that will contribute to this goal, including the Coalition Against Major Diseases's Alzheimer's initiative to share and pool clinical trial data across pharmaceutical companies. Furthermore, she posits that a standardized core dataset of electronic health record information that could be repurposed for research, safety monitoring, quality reporting, and population health would help facilitate an interoperable digital health infrastructure. Dr. Kush shares several examples of existing standards initiatives that could be leveraged as a foundation for the learning health system, for example, increasing adverse drug event (ADE) reporting through the implementation of the ADE Spontaneous Triggered Events Recording trial.

Echoing the notion of health care as a complex adaptive system, Jonathan Silverstein, formerly of the University of Chicago (now at NorthShore University Health System), asserts that current technological failures of the healthcare system are a result of incompatibility between the technology employed and the nature of the system. He suggests that what is needed is secure data liquidity supported by a functional architecture that enables ever-expanding secure uses of health data. Dr. Silverstein proposes that this can be achieved by employing provable electronic policy enforcement in regard to access, provenance, and logging, as well through scalable data transport mechanisms and transformations that make data unambiguous and computable. He predicts that the increasing scale and complexity of medicine and biology will lead to more collaborative endeavors and sharing of resources—both data and technical. Consequently, approaches to sharing technical resources through federated hosted services such as grids and clouds—which provide scalable ways to leverage existing distributed data, transport standards, and individual expertise—promise to be a crucial part of the digital infrastructure.

Drawing on his experiences with the Indiana Network for Patient Care, Shaun Grannis of the Regenstrief Institute shares his thoughts on what will be needed to mitigate data heterogeneity in a learning health system.

Because information needed to support the functions of a learning health system must be compiled from a number of diverse data sources, integration of these data is a major barrier to learning. Dr. Grannis suggests that efforts to specify standards for vocabularies, messaging, and data transactions through interoperability specifications, standards, and use cases have not been sufficient to address this issue and new approaches are needed. He suggests that new strategies to deal with patient and provider identity management, vocabulary standardization, and value set maintenance by addressing elements including patient- and provider-level aggregation, and health system metadata, and value set maintenance should be prioritized.

BUILDING A STANDARDS AND INTEROPERABILITY FRAMEWORK

Douglas Fridsma, M.D., Ph.D.
Office of the National Coordinator for Health Information Technology

The Office of Interoperability and Standards, a division within the Office of the National Coordinator for Health Information Technology (ONC), provides leadership and direction to support the secure and seamless exchange of health information in alignment with the national health information technology (HIT) agenda. Responsibilities of the office include advancing the development, adoption, and implementation of HIT standards; promoting the development of performance measures related to the adoption of these standards; and working with various federal agencies to evaluate mechanisms for harmonizing security and privacy practices in an interoperable HIT architecture. One of the office's principal projects is the development of a standards and interoperability (S&I) framework—an open government initiative that uses integrated processes, tools, and resources with the goal of developing and supporting specifications guided by the healthcare and technology industry. This paper presents some background on the project and proposes a preliminary version of the framework.[1]

Lessons from Previous Efforts

There is a large body of existing work that can be used to inform ONC's development of the S&I framework. Specifically, the Healthcare Information Technology Standards Panel (HITSP)—a cooperative partnership between public and private sectors—has already worked on several

---

[1] The S&I framework was officially launched on January 7, 2011. More information can be found at http://jira.siframework.org/wiki/pages/viewpage.action?pageId=4194700 (accessed March 8, 2011).

of the key issues surrounding HIT standards and interoperability, and has accumulated important lessons and best practices that can be applied to the S&I Framework:

- *Standards are not imposed, they are adopted.* Widespread adoption of standards will be more effective if individuals are drawn in because of their utility, not because they are forced to by the federal government. In order to be useful, standards must address real problems, not abstract ones. This is where learning from problems encountered in previous efforts can be extremely helpful. Furthermore, engaging the community in the development of standards fosters a feeling of ownership. When stakeholders have a sense that they contributed to the development of standards they are more likely to adopt them.
- *Standards should be harmonized and commissioned based on clearly articulated priorities.* Without unlimited resources, there must be some degree of coordination in the development of standards. This will entail prioritizing what issues to work on and will require a governance strategy to oversee the coordination and prioritization process.
- *Adoption of standards is accelerated by tools.* Creating tools such as vocabulary and terminology registries will facilitate adoption. Furthermore, it is necessary to make implementation specifications easy to use. It must be clear to users that when they implement standards and engage with the system, the environment is in place so that an exchange of information is going to happen readily.
- *Keep it as simple as possible but no simpler.* This is the parsimony principle. Care must be taken not to "boil the ocean" but instead focus on the real problems that stand in the way of adoption.
- *Perfection can be the enemy of the good.* Developing standards that are perfect would take at least 5 or 10 years at which point they would no longer meet contemporary needs. It is far more useful to accelerate the development and implementation of standards so that they can be integrated into real-world settings. Once implemented, the standards can continue to be refined and improved in an iterative fashion.

Building on Existing Efforts

One of the responsibilities of the Office of Interoperability and Standards is to remain cognizant of these lessons when developing an S&I framework. Past experiences have indicated that the following priorities are crucial when moving forward:

- *Move toward more "computational" implementation specifications.* Developing implementation specifications that are explicit—and therefore less subject to interpretation—will increase the efficiency of development and maintenance. For example, rather than using a Word document that describes standards and how to implement them, producing an .xml file that can be implemented and customized will be much more useful and not as subject to interpretation by the user.
- *Link use cases and standards from inception to certification.* Certification needs to be tightly linked to the process of developing standards and implementation specifications. ONC is working to develop certification criteria and a certification process that makes it possible to test whether people are following suggested standards and specifications. Coming up with an implementation specification that cannot be tested or certified against will introduce enormous challenges down the road.
- *Integrate multiple service delivery organizations with different expertise across the process.* It is important that, when working to solve problems around meaningful use and other issues, ONC remain cognizant of the need to integrate across a whole host of organizations that have existing standards. For example, an electronic prescribing use case requires vocabularies and terminologies from different organizations, different transportation packages, and different standards.
- *Managing the life cycle.* There needs to be a controlled way to manage all of the activities within the standards and interoperability realm, from identification of a needed capability to implementation and operations. This will help to ensure that the standards developed are not static, but change as new technologies are developed and the practice of medicine evolves. A framework must serve as a mechanism for continuous refinement.
- *Reuse.* Standards development and harmonization efforts need to accommodate multiple stakeholders and business scenarios to ensure reuse across many communities. Within the federal government alone, there are a tremendous number of silos of excellence, all of which are creating wonderful standards but are not sharing. It will be necessary to leverage descriptions of standards and services that are being provided across different silos.
- *Semantic discipline.* Work products need to be developed in a way that ensures machine and human readability and traceability throughout the entire life cycle. This allows for the uniformity of concept definition that is needed to solve challenging healthcare problems where understanding of terms is critical.
- *Human consensus.* Achieving human consensus is a prerequisite

for computable interoperability. If stakeholders cannot agree on what a term or a concept is (or means), it will be impossible for a computer to do so.

Bottom-Up Innovation

The Office of Standards and Interoperability has in the past been perceived as employing a governance strategy that is both "command and control" as well as "1,000 flowers blooming." The goal of the S&I framework is to find the "sweet spot" between the two—called focused collaboration (see Figure 3-1). Focused collaboration engages a broad array of stakeholders in the development process, but manages their work properly to ensure efficiency and efficacy. This avoids the pitfalls inherent in both a high degree of focus (top-down, heavy-handed, government-driven process) with little participation from outside stakeholders as well as a highly participatory

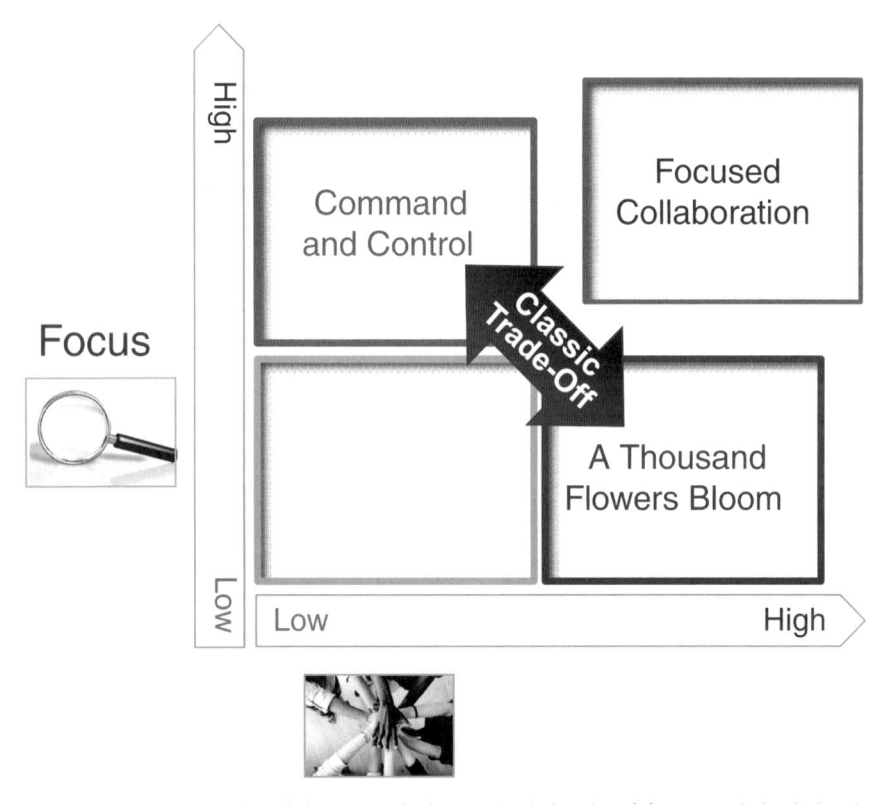

FIGURE 3-1 Focused collaboration balances high levels of focus with high levels of participation.

process with no strong focus that generates many good ideas, but no results. This creates an environment that is results oriented but at the same time is inclusive and fosters "bottom-up innovation."

Process Overview of the S&I Framework

The S&I framework being developed by ONC is an attempt to leverage the work of HITSP and other previous standards development efforts, while designing a new process to embrace the lessons learned and best practices of prior efforts. This process is not something that will be built *de novo*, but will leverage and harmonize past activity. The framework (Figure 3-2) is broken down into a series of functions that are intended to guide healthcare interoperability initiatives. The first is *use case and functional requirements*—ONC's outward-focused activity aimed at engaging the healthcare community by developing business scenarios to help make the case for adoption.

The next function in this model is the *harmonization of core concepts*. This function includes usage and adoption of the National Information Exchange Model (NIEM), and is a process that has been developed that focuses on taking use cases developed by the healthcare community and harmonizing existing standards in support. This allows for two important functions: (1) describing the data needed for information exchange and (2) describing the behaviors, functions, and services and how the information exchange supports them. The first function focuses on specifying the data that are important to be exchanged, and the second function specifies what can be done with it. Along with a policy and trust framework, this function defines what is needed to successfully exchange information.

Successfully harmonizing core concepts is a necessary step in developing *implementation specifications*. In many ways, developing successful imple-

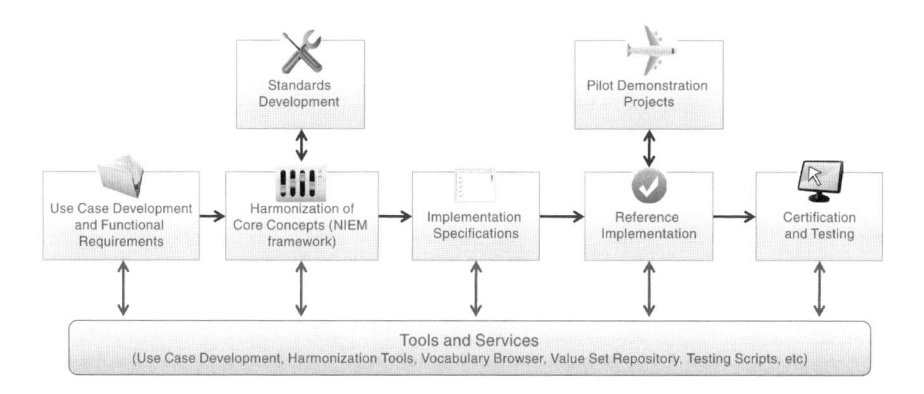

FIGURE 3-2 Preliminary schematic of the S&I framework.

mentation specifications is the way interoperability is achieved—taking all of the standards and services (ingredients) and combining them in a way that serves a particular purpose (recipe). That recipe is the implementation specification, and the S&I framework is also focused on making sure the "recipe" is understandable and "easy to bake." Once an implementation specification has been defined, the next functions in the framework are focused on developing a *reference implementation*, which is a fully functioning version of the defined implementation specification, and *certification and testing*, which ensures that the implementation is certified against a set of requirements and fully tested. As part of these functions, *pilot environments* are also created so that ONC and its partners in the private and public healthcare sectors can test and evaluate how the reference implementations work.

Without reference implementations it is not possible to test whether or not implementation specifications that have been developed are usable without unforeseen problems. ONC works with the National Institute of Standards and Technology to develop the certification and testing requirements needed to test reference implementations.

It is important to note that not all of the components that are outputs of the S&I framework will be built within ONC. The vision of the framework is that, in its coordinating capacity, ONC will take the best examples and work products currently available and integrate them into a common framework, so that best-of-breed solutions come to the forefront.

Situating in the Broader Context

The S&I framework is designed to map to NIEM and its foundational structure, based on the Information Exchange Package Documentation (IEPD). (Figure 3-3). The NIEM IEPD lays out a series of artifacts that define what is needed for interoperability, and when combined with the outputs of the framework, it is expected that S&I Framework interoperability initiatives will produce the logical and foundational artifacts needed to enable health information exchange. As indicated in the figure, the S&I Framework also augments NIEM with additional features. One is a description of services, known as service specifications. While the NIEM IEPD defines exchange, it does not describe services explicitly. Additionally, the S&I framework adds implementation, testing, and certification to the NIEM model, so that information exchanges are not just developed, but tested and certified to promote adoption. These additional features are examples of how ONC is working to integrate existing initiatives such as NIEM into a broader standardization and interoperability framework for health care.

It is important to remember that the S&I framework is not designed to operate in a vacuum, as noted in (Figure 3-4). The Health Information Technology Policy Committee (HITPC) will be providing use cases and pri-

TECHNICAL ISSUES FOR THE DIGITAL HEALTH INFRASTRUCTURE   107

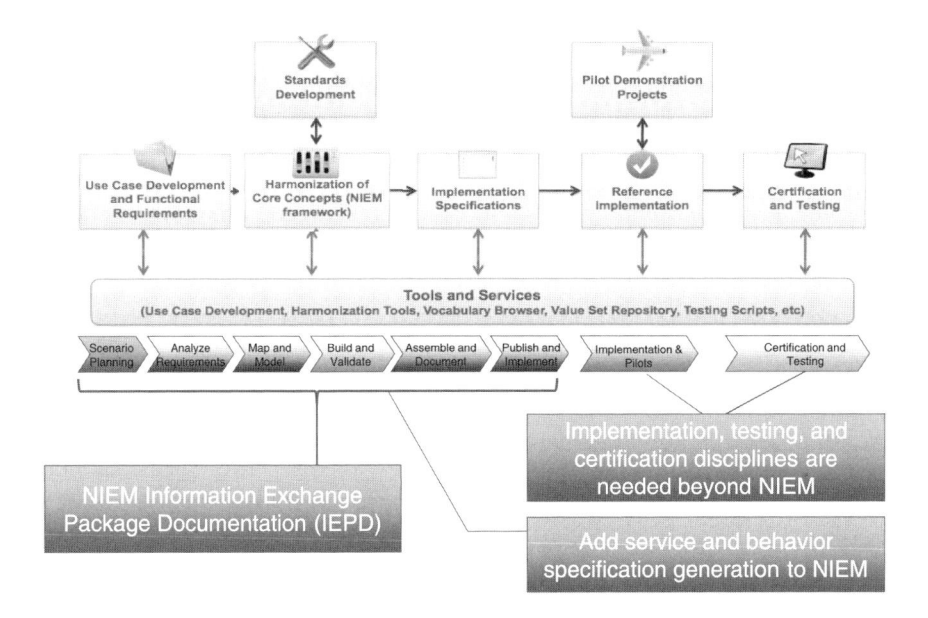

FIGURE 3-3 Mapping the S&I framework to NIEM processes.

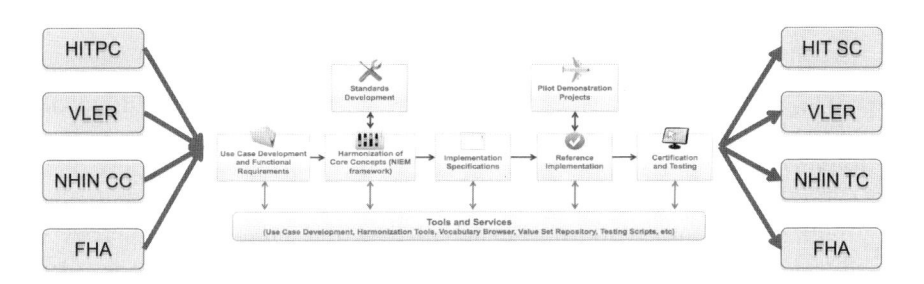

FIGURE 3-4 The S&I framework will enable stakeholder coordination throughout the standards and interoperability development life cycle.

orities to the framework and will serve as the primary source for interoperability initiatives. The Health Information Technology Standards Committee evaluates the work completed through the S&I framework process and may propose additional standards that need to be incorporated. Other programs are also integrated into the framework as important stakeholders, including the joint Department of Defense–Department of Veterans' Affairs Virtual Lifetime Electronic Record (VLER) project, the Nationwide Health Information Network (NWHIN) Coordinating Committee (CC) and Technical Committees (TCs), and the Federal Health Architecture (FHA). This level of broad participation and integration ensures that S&I framework functions are always aligned to the needs of the broader healthcare community.

INTEROPERABILITY FOR THE LEARNING HEALTH SYSTEM

Rebecca D. Kush, Ph.D.
Clinical Data Interchange Standards Consortium

The digital infrastructure for a learning health system must be based upon information possessing integrity and quality such that users can trust in the system and important medical decisions can be made based upon accurate information and knowledge. While search engines, signal detection, natural language processing, and other state-of-the-art techniques can potentially surface indicators and interesting information, the knowledge held in these search results is only as good as the underlying research data available. To optimize the quality of patient care, rigorous scientific methods with adequate sample sizes and comparable data should be the basis for the evidence upon which medical decisions are made. Unfortunately, the time frame cited today for bringing research results into clinical care decisions is purportedly on the order of 17 years (Lamont, 2005). Recent government incentives in the United States have provided a new opportunity to change the current "ignorant" system into a true learning system by creating an appropriate electronic digital infrastructure as electronic health records (EHRs) are adopted across the nation. Interoperability to enable data sharing and the ability to aggregate adequate, analyzable information upon which to base scientific conclusions are at the heart of this infrastructure.

Interoperability has been defined by the Institute of Electrical and Electronics Engineers as "the ability of two or more systems or components to exchange information and to use the information that has been exchanged" (IEEE, 1990). To be more specific, one can differentiate between syntactic and semantic interoperability. *Syntactic interoperability* occurs if two or more systems are capable of communicating and exchanging data. Fundamental to this type of communication are specified data formats or communication protocols (such as SQL, XML, or even ASCII). Syntactic interoperability is a requirement for any further attempts at interoperability. *Semantic interoperability,* which goes beyond simply exchanging information, is the ability to automatically interpret the information exchanged meaningfully and accurately in order to produce useful results. Semantic interoperability requires a common information exchange reference model to ensure that what is sent is understood by the recipient.

In the cycle of an informed healthcare system, medical research is based upon healthcare information and, in turn, clinical decisions are based upon research results. Medical research or clinical research are terms used broadly in this context. They include the understanding of diseases, discovery and testing of new therapies, comparative effectiveness research (CER), understanding responses to therapies (e.g., personalized health care, biomarkers, and genomics), safety monitoring, biosurveillance, and evaluating quality. For the purpose of defining a digital infrastructure and understanding the essential role of interoperability, one aspect of the definition of a learning health system could be *efficient exchange (and aggregation) of sufficient high quality, meaningful information upon which trustworthy decisions can be leveraged to improve health care for all of us, as patients.*

The path to interoperability, in an *ideal situation* would rely on both a common information exchange reference model as well as controlled terminology. However, the *real situation* is that we are faced with competing terminologies and repositories; mapping, legacy data conversion, and normalization; and we have competing models and "mini-models" such as clinical data elements, detailed clinical models, archetypes, and clinical element models. Approaches to deal with this reality are surfacing solutions such as service-oriented architecture and Services-Aware Interoperability Framework. These issues will need to be addressed in terms of the digital infrastructure to turn an inefficient and ignorant system into a learning health system.

Valuable Enablers to a Learning Healthcare System

The Critical Path Institute[2] has brought the Food and Drug Administration (FDA), the European Medicines Agency (EMA), the National Institutes of Health, and biopharmaceutical companies together to form the Coalition Against Major Diseases (CAMD). CAMD—a unique public–private partnership tasked with better understanding neuro-degenerative diseases—has now produced a new database of information on more than 4,000 Alzheimer's disease patients who have participated in 11 industry-sponsored clinical trials. This is the first database of combined clinical trials to be openly shared by pharmaceutical companies and made available to qualified researchers around the world. Disease modeling, biomarker validation, and the gleaning of knowledge from failed therapies and placebo patient data for Alzheimer's disease are techniques anticipated to enable an improved process of therapy development and evaluation.

The aggregation of sufficient information from these patients required a "common model" for which CAMD selected the Study Data Tabulation

---

[2] See http://www.c-path.org/CAMD.cfm (accessed September 13, 2010).

Model (SDTM). SDTM was developed through a global, open consensus-based standards development process led by the Clinical Data Interchange Standards Consortium (CDISC). Unfortunately, since the original clinical trials were conducted using proprietary standards, or no standards at all, the data had to be mapped into the SDTM format before the database could be developed. Also, standard formats for the Alzheimer's-specific efficacy data were necessary to augment the existing SDTM standard safety data domains. Now that these are available, future research studies on Alzheimer's patients can be designed to collect the data in the standard format "up front," which will facilitate ready aggregation into the database in the future.

This will also accelerate study start-up. A business case conducted with Gartner indicated that the use of CDISC standards at the beginning of the medical research process (study startup) can reduce startup (cycle time) by 70–90% (Rozwell et al., 2007). In other words, a study can be initiated faster and with significantly fewer resources (time and personnel) if standards are employed. In addition to these objective savings, the use of the standards resulted in higher data quality and integrity, improved communication among stakeholders/project teams, and flexibility in selecting technologies that work together. The standards enable ready data aggregation and semantic interoperability among proprietary or unique technologies as long as these technologies inherently support the research standards.

One key enabler of a learning health system would be to have a core dataset (with common value sets and terminology) that is "standard" as a base to support multiple purposes. Ideally, these data would be collected once in an EHR and the be repurposed for multiple different uses, including but not limited to medical research, CER, safety monitoring, quality reporting, public and population health, and other uses.

This is not feasible today since we cannot even all agree, for example, on whether a patient's sex (or gender) is collected as male/female, M/F, 2/1, 1/2, or even if there are 2, 4, or 15 options in the value set for gender (or is it sex?). Automated teller machines and credit cards work today because there is a core set of information that has been agreed upon and standardized across banks/card issuers—that is, codes for credit card type, cardholder type, 16-digit card number, expiration data, 3-digit code on the back. Such electronic data interchange standards allow access to personal banking and funds around the world.

Dr. John Halamka, in his blog comments[3] on ONC's HIT Standards Committee Testimony, listed a set of "Gold Star Ideas." The following three stand out:

---

[3] See http://geekdoctor.blogspot.com/2009_10_01_archive.html (accessed February 23, 2011).

1. We've learned from other industries that starting with simple standards works well.
2. Keep the standards as minimal as possible to support the business goal.
3. Start immediately rather than waiting for the perfect standard.

This begs the question of what is available that could be used now as a foundation upon which a learning healthcare system can build. It is critically important to start now to ensure convergence of the current "meaningful use" criteria with future efforts to enable a healthcare system that can take rapid advantage of scientific findings.

Leveraging Existing Enablers

Following are existing enablers that could be leveraged now to provide a foundation for a learning healthcare system.

eSource Data Interchange (eSDI) Initiative

The purpose of this initiative (a collaboration between CDISC and FDA) was to facilitate the use of electronic technology in the context of existing regulations for the collection of eSource data in clinical research. The term eSource pertains to collecting data electronically initially through such technologies as e-diaries, e-patient-reported outcomes, e-data collection instruments, and EHRs. The overarching goals of this initiative were to make it easier for physicians to conduct clinical research, to collect data only once in a global research standard format for multiple downstream uses, and to improve data quality and patient safety. The product is the eSDI Document,[4] which contains 12 requirements for eSource that comply with existing regulations for electronic record retention good clinical practices. This document and the 12 requirements, specifically, are cited by the EMA for their field auditors.[5]

Workflow Integration

The eSDI Initiative formed the basis for the *Retrieve Form for Data Capture (RFD) Integration Profile*,[6] which was collaboratively developed

---

[4] See http://www.cdisc.org/eSDI/eSDI.pdf (accessed September 14, 2010).
[5] See http://www.ema.europa.eu/ema/index.jsp?curl=pages/regulation/document_listing/document_listing_000136.jsp&jsenabled=true (accessed September 14, 2010).
[6] See http://wiki.ihe.net/index.php?title=Retrieve_Form_for_Data_Capture (accessed September 14, 2010).

by CDISC and Integrating the Healthcare Enterprise (IHE). This is an extremely powerful workflow integration profile that streamlines the use of an EHR for a variety of purposes. It is easily implemented, which has led to its endorsement by the EHR Association.[7]

Global Clinical Research Standards and BRIDG

Through a global, consensus-based standards development process, a suite of open and freely available standards has been developed to support medical research from protocol through reporting. These are harmonized through the Biomedical Research Integrated Domain Group (BRIDG) model and have a common set of controlled terminology openly housed and curated through the National Cancer Institute (NCI) Enterprise Vocabulary Services (EVS). The BRIDG model was so named because it bridges research and health care in addition to bridging organizations and stakeholders. The harmonized global research standards are depicted in Figure 3-5. One particular standard that would pave the way for a learning health system is the Clinical Data Acquisition Standards Harmonization (CDASH),[8] which defines a core minimum research dataset.

Standards-Inspired Innovation

The mission of CDISC is *to develop and support global, platform-independent data standards that enable information system interoperability to improve medical research and related areas of health care.* To this end, a concerted effort has been made to ensure interoperability between research and health care. In addition to the BRIDG model, through the development of the CDISC IHE RFD integration profile the eSDI work has been leveraged to streamline the workflow from EHRs/clinicians who wish to conduct research or support other enhanced uses of clinical information. CDASH, in particular, was developed collaboratively through the FDA's Critical Path Initiative. CDASH is a case report form/data collection standard that represents a core minimum dataset to support 18 domains for any clinical research study. CDASH has been "mapped" to the CCD (or the Continuity of Care Document) such that EHRs can produce a core research dataset (the CDASH clinical research data elements). Together the CCD, the IHE RFD integration profile, and CDASH constitute an interoperability specification that readily supports the conduct of clinical research using EHRs, while adhering to existing regulations for research (Figure 3-6).

---

[7] See http://www.cdisc.org/stuff/contentmgr/files/0/f5a0121d251a348a87466028e156d3c3/miscdocs/ehra_cdisc_endorsement_letter_100908.pdf (accessed September 14, 2010).

[8] See http://www.cdisc.org/cdash (accessed September 14, 2010).

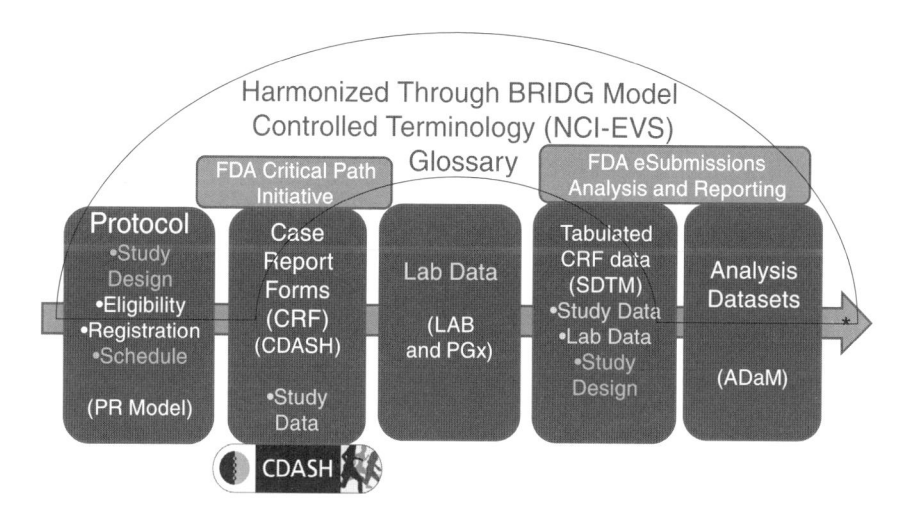

TECHNICAL ISSUES FOR THE DIGITAL HEALTH INFRASTRUCTURE   113

FIGURE 3-5 CDISC global content standards for clinical research.

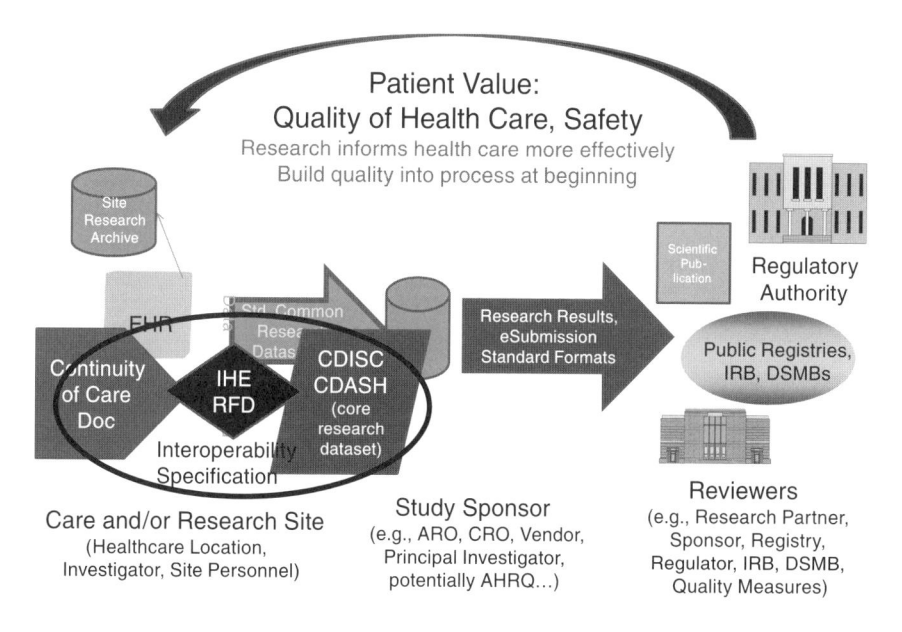

FIGURE 3-6 Schematic depicting a sample interoperability specification involving the CCD, the IHE RFD integration profile, and CDASH.

Unfortunately, standards are frequently misperceived as stifling creativity in research. However, they have been known to inspire innovation in other industries. In the aforementioned interoperability specification, standards are, in reality, enablers of workflow and efficiencies in the processes associated with a learning health system. A number of implementations are now in place around the world to leverage enablers. For example, the Adverse Drug Event Spontaneous Triggered Event Recording study has brought safety reporting from >34 minutes (which meant that a busy clinician would not make such a report) to less than a minute (which increased reporting dramatically) (Neuer, 2009). Other use cases include outbreak reporting and clinical research studies, with the potential to harmonize with quality reporting measures. Currently in progress is a new integration profile (based on Business Process Execution Language) that will leverage the CDISC Protocol Representation Model to automate research subject identification, patient scheduling, and data collection by visit, thus making it far easier for physicians to conduct research or adhere to reporting requirements.

Standards-Inspired Innovation

A core dataset with standard value sets and terminology can dramatically reduce time and effort to report key information for safety, research, and public health; accommodate e-diaries and other patient-entered data; improve data quality; enable data aggregation and analysis or queries; be extensible and pave the way for more complex research and clinical genomics for personalized health care; and be readily implemented by EHR vendors.

While search engines and signal detection have their place in the learning health system, ensuring the integrity of the search results—and thus trust in the knowledge upon which clinical decisions are based—a learning health system must support rigorous scientific research. The current research process is antiquated and ripe for transformation. EHRs may provide the impetus for necessary changes.

PROMOTING SECURE DATA LIQUIDITY

Jonathan C. Silverstein, M.D., M.S.
The University of Chicago (formerly)
North Shore University Health System

Any healthcare system is made up of individual people and institutions. Whether focused on clinical care, population health, quality, or research, each entity is goal directed while being dependent upon the activities of others. In the current healthcare environment, these dependencies are often problematic due to misalignment of individual incentives, policy restrictions, and competition for control rather than competition for value (Porter and Teisberg, 2006). This is sufficiently obvious in the fact that it is acceptable to assert that the U.S. healthcare system is failing to systematically deliver measurable quality at acceptable cost.

Health Care Is a Complex Adaptive System

We do not assign the assertion that the system is failing as fault to any entity. In fact, there are exceptional institutions that can effectively deliver measurable quality at acceptable cost. Unfortunately, this cannot be demonstrated for the system as a whole. Rather, we assert that the failure at the system level is a result of not matching the technology required to enable a functioning system with the nature of the system itself. Health care and biomedicine in the United States exist as complex adaptive systems and needs the underpinning technology infrastructure to match.

A complex adaptive system is a collection of individual agents that have the freedom to act in ways that are not always predictable and whose actions are interconnected. (IOM, 2001). Ralph Stacey (1996) describes these essential characteristics of a complex adaptive system:

- Nonlinear and dynamic.
- Agents are independent and intelligent.
- Goals and behaviors often in conflict.
- Self-organization through adaptation and learning.
- No single point(s) of control.
- Hierarchical decomposition has limited value.

The Need for Secure Data Liquidity

If we accept that these characteristics of a complex adaptive system match the reality of the healthcare system, as we develop shared responsibility, policy, governance, and competition for value, we will need matching infrastructures that are driven from a systems-level perspective and that *scale*. Such infrastructures must enable integration, interoperation, and secured appropriate access to biomedical data on a national scale. Useful data will emerge from multiple sources and need to be distributed for multiple creative reuses to drive better understanding and decision making. This, in turn, drives the need for provably secure systems that work across organizations. In short, we need to develop and deploy systems for secure data liquidity.

Secure data liquidity is a catch phrase for a functional architecture that enables an explosion of new uses of healthcare data by making two things possible: provable electronic policy enforcement in regard to who is delivered precisely what data for what purpose (flexible, robust access control, provenance, and logging—or "secure data"); and scalable data pipelines and transformations that make data unambiguous and computable such that data from multiple sources can be used together in meaningful ways ("liquid data"). We need to break through from having data locked up and unlinked, to a situation where data flow for many purposes, with provable security in regard to who is permitted to use, and is, using, which data for what purpose ("secure data liquidity"). Too often the Health Insurance Portability and Accountability Act has been interpreted defensively, driving risk avoidance rather than motivating best practices for systems and data management. As a result, secure data liquidity has, to date, been undesirable by individual organizations and therefore unattainable. The limitations are not technical but sociotechnical.

As biology and medicine undergo their digital transformation, more and more collaborative endeavors among investigators and clinicians will emerge. Technical resources will be increasingly shared as well. Even the world's largest supercomputers—standing as silos, rather than connected—aren't enough to move, store, or analyze all of the available data. When multiple entities need to share, there are natural security concerns, resource utilization and scheduling problems, and the need for data movement across organizations. These cannot be satisfied in a single, monolithic system with the required multiorganizational security, flexibility, extensibility, redundancy, stability, robustness in multiple industries, openness, and lack of central ownership. These technical requirements underpinning multi-institutional resource sharing toward common goals are just beginning to be appreciated by the private sector and governments. As they begin to face the issues squarely, some technology will need to be deployed in order to harvest these socioeconomic benefits.

Federated, Hosted Services (e.g., Grids and Clouds)

Ian Foster described a federated framework of service-oriented science based in grid computing approaches in which individuals with varying expertise can *create services* (e.g., data services, algorithms, pipelines) which others *discover* and compose to create a new function, and then *publish* as a new service (Foster, 2005). In this model, each actor in the system does not have to become an expert in operating services and computer infrastructure. Instead, they depend upon "others" to host services and manage the underpinning security, reliability, and scalability. In this way, everyone is leveraged for their own expertise. Federation and hosting of services allows people, organizations, or institutions to "outsource the complex and mundane activities" to third parties. These enabling features map quite closely to the problems facing health and biomedical systems—that of multiple, often competing, and differentially motivated entities—that need to work together to care for patients, improve public health, and conduct research. Thus, effective use of federation and hosted technical approaches have great potential impact in enabling the learning healthcare system.

Grossly oversimplified, grid approaches can be thought of as federations toward data and computation sharing across assemblies of multiple organizations driven by complex multiorganizational functional requirements. The grid paradigm is a combination of philosophy and technology including principles and mechanisms for dynamic sets of individuals and/or institutions engaged in the controlled sharing of resources in pursuit of common goals (virtual organizations), leveraging service-oriented architecture, loose coupling of data and services, and open software and architecture (Foster, 2002; Foster et al., 2001). Grid is not a technology, but rather a set of approaches that have moved through several technological generations in the last 15 years. This approach remains robust, flexible, secure, and is increasingly deployed in the biomedical sciences.[9]

In contrast, clouds can be thought of as an approach toward data and computation hosting driven by business models leveraging outsourcing and economies of scale. This is most prototypically achieved technically by deploying on-the-fly multiple identical virtual machines—infrastructure-as-a-service. Amazon's Elastic Compute Cloud[10] is a prime example. Cloud approaches also provide scalable software-as-a-service (Salesforce.com[11]) and platform-as-as-service (Google's App Engine[12]).

These science-based approaches and business-based technical approaches need to converge to support the complex nature of biomedicine and promote the development of a learning health system. Both grids and clouds leverage core Internet protocols and services and are typically deployed in a services-oriented approach. Thus, combining characteristics of grids and clouds in a *hosted federation of services* is required for the digital infrastructure of the learning health system. At the same time we are learning to value crowd-sourced information, or information that is annotated and curated by individuals most familiar with the data.

---

[9] For examples of the grid approach, see http://www.opensciencegrid.org; http://www.birn-community.org; http://www.cagrid.org (accessed December 17, 2010).
[10] See http://aws.amazon.com/ec2/ (accessed December 17, 2010).
[11] See http://www.salesforce.com (accessed December 17, 2010).
[12] See http://code.google.com/appengine/ (accessed December 17, 2010).

Hosted Federations of Services Can Transform Health Care

Facing squarely the many sociotechnical issues in the health domain will drive deeper understanding among healthcare policy makers, health information managers, and lawyers. This in turn should drive individual organizational social behaviors away from risk avoidance and fear in regard to health information privacy, and toward good data management practices that effectively reduce risk.

Although health and medicine have their own custom set of requirements—particularly in regard to specific workflows and data standards—we need to leverage the existing distributed computing models and Internet standards as we address problems of scale instead of attempting to build new healthcare-specific infrastructures. This cannot occur in a monolithic system. Thus, there is an inevitable need for a distributed computing approach that will foster the generation of new knowledge and drive better care based on that knowledge. The convergence of grid and cloud systems can address the required enabling multiorganizational, scalable technical characteristics:

- Attribute-based authorization.
- Distributed identity management.
- End-to-end security.
- Data naming, linking, movement, and integration.
- Flexible, but enforceable policy/sociability.
- Extensibility.
- Redundancy.
- Robust in multiple industries/stability.
- Without central ownership/manageability.

Summary

The issues facing health and biomedical systems of multiple—often competing and differentially motivated—entities that need to work together to care for patients, improve population health, and conduct research can be addressed by federated (grid) approaches in combination with hosted (cloud) approaches. The general idea of infrastructure on demand drove both cloud and grid. Whereas cloud emerged from virtualization of machines, business models, and flexible capacity, grid evolved from virtualization of organizations, social models, flexible capabilities, security, and open services. Both head toward *hosted federation of services* which are promising paths to transforming healthcare into a high performing system.

INNOVATIVE APPROACHES TO INFORMATION DIVERSITY

Shaun Grannis, M.D., M.S.
Regenstrief Institute

Comprehensive clinical information stitched together from a diverse set of data sources supports many healthcare processes including direct patient care, population health management, quality improvement, and comparative effectiveness research (CER). However, these data are captured from many independent systems with complex relationships where information is stored as separate islands with different identifiers, names, and codes. Such heterogeneity impedes seamless integration of data by the healthcare system. Therefore, to effectively and efficiently support the informational needs of a variety of healthcare processes, approaches to managing system complexities and information heterogeneity are needed.

Adding to the challenge is that fundamental perspectives on the nature of complexity often differ. To illustrate, Alan Perlis, a computer science luminary, suggests that complexity can be abrogated when he said, "Fools ignore complexity. Pragmatists suffer with it. Some people can avoid it. Geniuses remove it" (Perlis, 1982). If simplicity can be taken as the opposite of complexity, Albert Einstein suggested that achieving maximal simplicity (and thus minimizing complexity) may be ill-advised with his exhortation to "make things as simple as possible, but no simpler."[13] With differing perspectives on the degree to which complexity can or should be mitigated, strategies designed to address the challenge may vary substantively.

The Challenge of Heterogeneous Data

These strategies are critical to the success of Health Information Exchanges (HIEs) because HIEs are an amalgamation of many healthcare data sources with data quality characteristics that vary both by data source and by time. Consequently, HIEs pose particularly illustrative data heterogeneity challenges. These challenges are driving HIEs to become emergent centers of innovation in health data management with core competencies that focus on standardizing and integrating clinical data to support the informational needs of myriad healthcare processes. Stated simply, addressing the complex task of managing information heterogeneity is an intrinsic HIE function.

As clinical data are captured from an increasing number of sources, heterogeneity of data threatens to impede progress toward meaningful use,

---

[13] See http://rescomp.stanford.edu/~cheshire/EinsteinQuotes.html (accessed February 23, 2011).

CER, and high-quality delivery of health care. Specifying standards for vocabularies, messages, and transactions will not be sufficient to mitigate substantial variations in data from different systems. New strategies will be required in the areas of patient and provider identity management, vocabulary standardization, and value set maintenance to facilitate quality reporting and disease surveillance in the future.

The fundamental premise of this paper is that while much energy has been spent on interoperability specifications, on standards, and on use cases, they are not sufficient. There are other necessary elements required to enable electronic sharing of semantically interoperable data. These elements include patient-level data aggregation, physician-level data aggregation, healthcare system metadata, and value set maintenance. In this paper I will draw on our experience with the Indiana Network for Patient Care (INPC), one of the nation's most comprehensive and longest-tenured HIEs, to highlight some of these additional elements.

Differing opinions on the degree to which healthcare system complexity can or should be mitigated leads to differing strategies for addressing the challenges. Some may disagree with our approaches. What I hope this paper does is put a pebble in your shoe. You might not agree with how we went about a certain operation—but hopefully this discomfort may motivate you to understand the reason why we are doing it.

The Indiana Network for Patient Care

The INPC contains more than 3.1 billion coded standardized clinical observations, and a global patient index that holds more than 20 million person:source entities that represent more than 12 million unique individuals. Since the mid-1990s, the INPC global patient identity resolution service resolves identities from real-time clinical data streams provided by myriad sources with widely varying data quality. Currently, the INPC global patient identity resolution service adjudicates identities for between 350,000 and 1 million transactions received daily from over 1,100 distinct participating HIE sources.

With data extending back over 30 years, the INPC connects over 80 hospitals, as well as numerous outpatient clinics, ancillary laboratory systems, and public health organizations (Figure 3-7). These data are used for population health, population and clinical decision support, quality reporting, and research—all supported using standards that existed in the late 1990s and early 2000s. Of the 500,000 to 1 million clinical transactions per day being added to the system, about 99% of the data are in HL7 version 2. Hospitals, clinics, and other sources submit their data to the system utilizing their own local code. There was an effort to have the participating organizations standardize their data sources before submit-

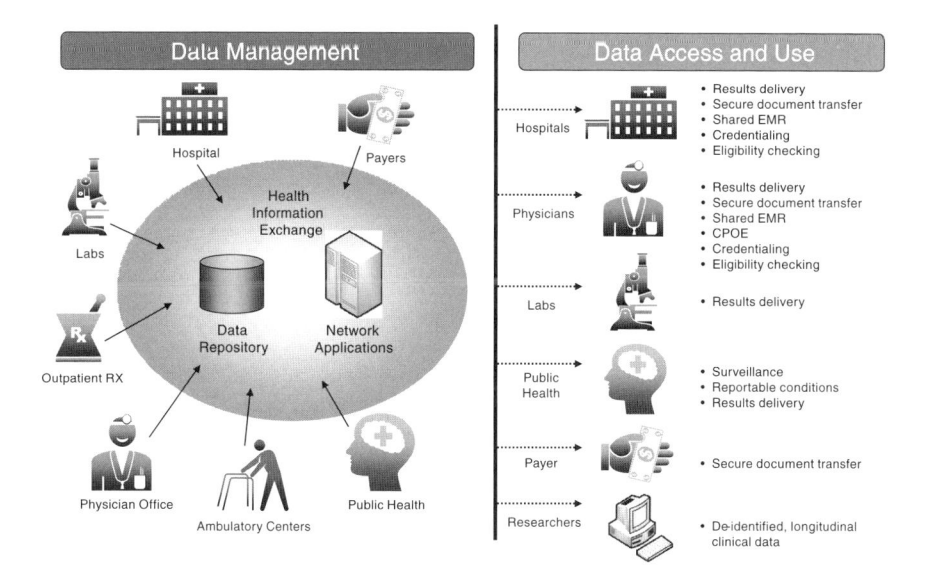

FIGURE 3-7 Schematic of the Indiana Network for Patient Care.

ting them to the system, but this did not last long. The administrators basically said that if there was value in having the data standardized then we would have do it ourselves. They did not see the value in this. Their priorities were taking care of patients, submitting bills, and the like. So, now we've hired five full-time employees whose entire job is mapping and clinical standardization.

All of the data for each provider or business entity go into a separate logical vault. We employ an entity-attribute-value data model, so as new terms are created and new vocabulary standards are produced, we are able to simply add new observation types to our database. Hence, the data model changes little over time. Although there are incremental changes, the core of the data model has been the same since the 1980s.

Domains of Data Standardization

The focus of our data standardization work falls into three main areas. First, patient data need to be standardized so that we can identify the same patient who is seen at many different parts of the healthcare system. We also need to standardize physician data since a single doctor can practice at multiple hospitals and be at multiple clinics throughout the week. Finally, we need to standardize metadata including business rules, knowledge basis, and so forth.

Patient-Level Aggregation

Many might assume that patient-level aggregation has been solved. But all of the studies to date on patient linking have been conducted using homogeneous data sources, not the kind of heterogeneous data that exist within most systems. Common errors in data input—a certain registration clerk at the local community hospital who always puts the date of birth in the wrong field or who always switches the last name and the first name—also present challenges. But these are the real-world issues that need to be addressed. What sort of matching methodologies would be needed to accommodate this kind of data heterogeneity?

A classic example of patient-level identification uncertainty is with newborns. When a baby is born, the first name is often not known and there is certainly not a social security number available. Yet, we still need to be able to link individual children from the newborn screening record to vital statistics. We also need to know if a patient has been screened for newborn diseases. In order to do that at INPC, we actually query the health department's newborn screening registry. When a patient is not in the newborn screening registry we send out an alert that a match needs to be found. The matching algorithms of the vast majority of commercial products, such as maximum likelihood estimators, fail in this population.

Our research has shown that there are ways to accommodate this kind of matching. However, until we actually start to look at the diverse data sources—and understand the different cohorts and pieces—we are not going to develop solutions. It is crucial that we look at the data as they exist today so that we can move from a diverse set of data to something more standard and interoperable. This work can only take place incrementally. We will not get all of the way there in 5, or even 10 years. In the meantime, however, we need to share strategies to understand the implications of data heterogeneity and begin to design solutions.

Physician-Level Aggregation

The second area for standardization research is physician-level aggregation. Despite the fact that a National Provider ID is mandated by Medicaid, there are many clinical transactions that lack a provider ID. Even on the billing side, Medicaid had to push back the deadline an entire year because hospitals were not ready to implement physician identifiers.

In addition, many clinical transactions do not contain sufficient physician data to generate quality reports for providers. As a result, the identifying information must be added manually by contacting the clinic to confirm which physician or provider was involved in a particular case. So, the national provider ID helps, but is not prevalent enough yet.

Healthcare System Metadata

At the level of healthcare system metadata, there are pieces of information that are important as we look at CER or quality reporting. This information includes which providers practice together, how different providers influence the quality of care, etc.

Another challenging area is patient-provider attribution that links a specific patient to the specific provider who performed the care. Knowing that information is critical to quality reporting so that outcomes can be assessed for providers and groups of providers. Other important information includes when new equipment, devices, and interventions were available for clinical use at specific locations and under which drug formulary a particular doctor was practicing? This information is crucial to understand healthcare outcomes.

Maintaining Value Sets

The final component to our research on data standardization and interoperability research is on maintaining value sets. A value set is a collection of concepts drawn from one or more controlled terminology systems and grouped together for a specific purpose—for example, ICD-9, SNOMED, and LOINC®. In addition to establishing specifications for individual value sets, the relationships between value sets needs to be maintained.

For example, INPC has an automated public health reporting system called the Notifiable Condition Detector. This system tracks hundreds of thousands of transactions every day and determines whether each transaction is a reportable event or not. To accomplish this, it uses a reference table called the Public Health Information Network Notifiable Condition Mapping Table (PHIN-NCMT), which was developed jointly by the Centers for Disease Control and Prevention (CDC), the Council of State and Territorial Epidemiologists, and the Regenstrief Institute to map standardized test codes to the conditions for which that test may be reportable.

Since the time of the initial PHIN-NCMT development, however, stakeholders at CDC and Regenstrief have maintained the reference table independently and the two tables have diverged considerably. There is currently no coordination among stakeholders when the disease list is changed or a new test added. Yet, if there is to be consistent reporting nationwide, these tables need to be maintained and synchronized.

Conclusion

As clinical data are collected from an increasing number of divergent systems, the prevalence of data heterogeneity will only increase. This variation impedes the aggregation of individual data across sources and hinders the use of these data in the delivery of care, public health reporting, clinical research, and related activities. Specifying standards is just one element of the solution to information heterogeneity. New strategies are also needed in the areas of patient matching, physician linkage, and value set maintenance to provide the most comprehensive health information for the benefit of individual and public health.

REFERENCES

Foster, I. 2002. The grid: A new infrastructure for 21st century science. *Physics Today* 55:42-47.
———. 2005. Service-oriented science. *Science* 308(5723):814-817.
Foster, I., C. Kesselman, and S. Tuecke. 2001. The anatomy of the grid: Enabling scalable virtual organizations. *International Journal of High Performance Computing* 15(3):200-222.
IEEE (Institute of Electrical and Electronics Engineers). 1990. *IEEE standard computer dictionary: A compilation of IEEE standard computer glossaries*. New York: IEEE.
IOM (Institute of Medicine). 2001. *Crossing the quality chasm: A new health system for the 21st century*. Washington, DC: National Academy Press.
Lamont, J. 2005. *How KM can help cure medical errors*. http://www.kmworld.com/Articles/Editorial/Feature/How-KM-can-help-cure-medical-errors-9606.aspx (accessed September 14, 2010).
Neuer, A. 2009. *ASTER study jumpstarts adverse event reporting*. http://www.ecliniqua.com/eCliniqua_article.aspx?id=93784 (accessed September 14, 2010).
Perlis, A. J. 1982. Special feature: Epigrams on programming. *Association for Computing Machinery SIGPLAN Notices* 17(9):7-13.
Porter, M. E., and E. O. Teisberg. 2006. *Redefining health care: Creating value-based competition on results*. Boston, MA: Harvard Business School Press.
Rozwell, C., R. Kush, and E. Helton. 2007. Saving time and money. *Applied Clinical Trials* 16(6):70-74.
Stacey, R. D. 1996. *Complexity and creativity in organizations*. San Francisco, CA: Berrett-Koehler.

4

Engaging Patient and Population Needs

INTRODUCTION

In order to truly improve health and health care, the digital infrastructure will require appreciation, support, enthusiasm, and active involvement from patients, providers, and the population as a whole. Papers included in this chapter highlight strategies for engaging of stakeholders and facilitating higher value care, including putting more relevant information under their control, leveraging health information to better coordinate care of chronically ill patients, and combating health disparities.

Mark McClellan from the Brookings Institution details the essential components of a digital infrastructure that can more closely align quality measurement and improvement in order to achieve high-value health care. He notes that patient-centered measures, repurposing data already being used to coordinate care for performance measurement, and alignment of these processes with other reform efforts—namely, value incentives—will be necessary to improve care and lower costs. Dr. McClellan uses diabetes care coordination to highlight ways in which information could be used to help providers improve care in a timely way, help patients obtain better care, and serve as the basis for driving value-based reforms. He notes that pilots such as accountable care organizations and Office of the National Coordinator for Health Information Technology (ONC)-funded Beacon Communities will be instrumental in helping identify best practices and aligning processes and incentives for systemwide change.

Addressing the issue of engaging individuals in population health monitoring, Kenneth Mandl from Children's Hospital Boston asserts that harnessing the knowledge possessed by populations through longitudinal studies of large, distributed, consenting populations, will be the focus of work in population health over the next decade. Based on his experience developing Indivo—a patient-centered health record that places patients in control of their own health information—coupled with federal incentive initiatives, he predicts a shift in the health information economy from institutional to individual or patient control. This shift will likely change population health research in a way already being seen through forums such as PatientsLikeMe. Finally, Dr. Mandl suggests that a critical outstanding research question is how to achieve sustained engagement of patients in research.

Sophia Chang from the California HealthCare Foundation states that a digital infrastructure provides important opportunities for informing and improving the care of patients with chronic disease. She discusses the potential to actively engage patients in management of their conditions, but notes that, currently, the locus of control lies solely with the healthcare providers and not the patient. Additionally, Dr. Chang points to the lack of common nomenclature, data formats, and protocols for incorporating patient-generated information as barriers to aggregating and translating health data into useful decision support. Pointing to Kaiser Permanente and the Veterans Health Administration as examples of institutions that have successfully used electronic health records (EHRs) for population health management, she notes that smaller institutions or individual physicians might have less opportunity for exposure, and therefore be less aware of their value. In order to maximize the value of EHRs, she asserts, research paradigms must shift to real-time knowledge development and feedback. Finally, Dr. Chang highlights several steps to move toward the goals of re-centering the system around the patient, such as providing useful support for chronic disease management, aligning EHR data elements with patient priorities, and developing better paradigms for learning from patient data.

M. Christopher Gibbons of the Johns Hopkins Urban Health Institute discusses opportunities for using a digitally supported learning health system to better comprehend and combat health disparities. Noting that understanding and treating health disparities requires integration of knowledge spanning many sources and disciplines, he points to several demographic trends that make this challenge ever more pressing—rising prevalence of chronic disease, an aging population, and the growing racial and ethnic diversity of the U.S. population. Dr. Gibbons introduces the terms "populomics" and "populovigilance" to describe the integrative, systems-oriented, and informatics-intensive approaches to understanding and monitoring the complex causes and manifestations of diseases and disparities. He suggests that as more and more data from diverse sources are collected and available for analysis, it will be important to adopt these new perspectives in order to enable advances in treatment, public health, and healthcare disparities.

ELECTRONIC HEALTH DATA FOR HIGH-VALUE HEALTH CARE
Mark McClellan, M.D., Ph.D.
The Brookings Institution

Achieving real healthcare reform requires aligning all five elements of the quality enterprise: measurement and data collection, payment reform, benefit reform, better evidence, and quality improvement support. Electronic data exchange is an essential tool to support these strategies. While all five of these elements are important, this paper will focus on the role of the data collection and reporting infrastructure in improving quality and lowering costs.

The essential features of the data collection infrastructure are implementing technically sound strategies to obtain patient-centered measures, utilizing electronic data that are already being used to coordinate care for performance measurement, and ensuring that this process is consistent with the implementation of other related reform efforts. The overarching goal for an improved data collection infrastructure is to be able to measure performance with the same data being collected during the routine delivery of care.

Improving the Data Collection Infrastructure

The focus of the improvements to the data collection infrastructure is on identifying scalable methods to coordinate the flow of information from existing sources. This approach is aligned with ongoing health information technology (HIT) reform efforts in the areas of meaningful use, value-based purchasing, pay-for-reporting, and others. It is also important to incorporate efforts from a wide array of stakeholders to facilitate coordination across the broad spectrum of initiatives in the public and private sectors.

Work in the area of improved data collection should build on existing progress and account for alternative sources in exchanging data and generating functionally equivalent performance information. Effort should also be made to identify nationally consistent methods and approaches through pilot projects prior to nationwide implementation. Finally, the resulting systems should effectively cover the vast majority of providers and patients in a timely fashion.

Healthcare reform is a complex undertaking, but at its core, reform is about how we can provide better care and value for patients. Patient care takes place within a complicated ecosystem composed of many stakeholders, from physicians and hospitals to labs and pharmacies. A tremendous amount of valuable health information is generated at each patient encounter along this continuum. With funding from the American Reinvestment and Recovery Act of 2009 to encourage the adoption and meaningful use of HIT, we can expect that more of this health information will be collected electronically and that it will be more easily exchanged to better coordinate care and to provide valuable feedback to healthcare providers. For example, registry functions, decision support tools, and medication alerts all have the potential to help healthcare providers deliver better, safer, high-value health care (Figure 4-1).

The contribution of claims data from public and private payers further enhances the value of the feedback and enables consistent performance measurement. Payment and service delivery are inextricably linked. The fragmented care that we currently have is, in large part, because of the fragmented way in which we pay for care. What this means for testing healthcare innovations is that we can expect changes in the payment to drive changes in service delivery. Those changes can be compared and evaluated to determine which payment models produce comparatively better quality at lower cost.

On the demand side of health care, performance information can also be provided to patients to enable them to select high-value healthcare providers, reinforcing broader health reform efforts that attempt to foster greater accountability for care. Patients can also make valuable contributions to healthcare information. Data they provide on their experience of care and their demographic backgrounds will help us improve patient satisfaction and track and reduce healthcare disparities. Additionally, patient

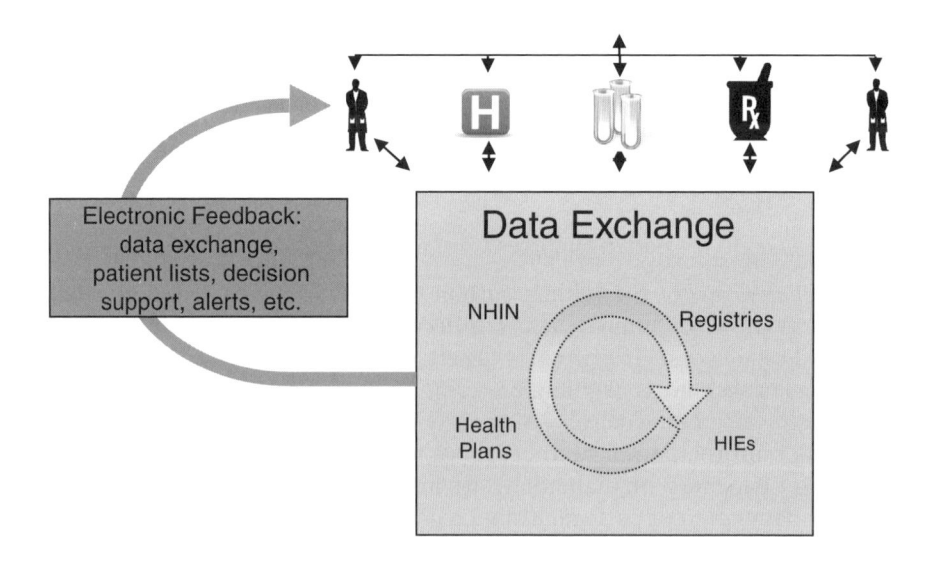

FIGURE 4-1 Basic data exchange infrastructure in a learning health system.

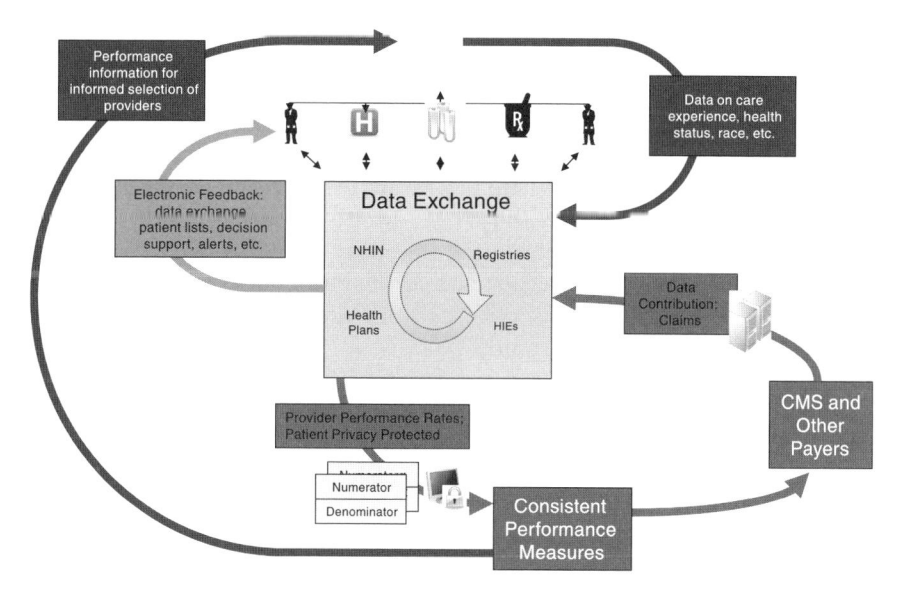

FIGURE 4-2 Electronic health data as the center of a model for better care at lower cost.

data on the quality of their healthcare experience can be used by other consumers in making future choices about healthcare providers.

Incorporating all of these elements—coordinating data exchange among healthcare providers, using payment models as levers to reform service delivery to improve quality and reduce costs, and involving the consumer in both data collection and use—can form the basis of a reform model to improve care and lower costs (Figure 4-2).

Better Diabetes Care at Lower Cost

Diabetes, one of the leading chronic diseases in the nation, highlights many ways in which improvements in electronic data exchange can enhance care and reduce costs (Figure 4-3). There is already electronic information exchange in such areas as filling prescriptions and managing laboratory results that is used in the delivery of care. With feedback from these electronic sources of information, it becomes more feasible to support improvements in care for patients with diabetes by driving evidence-based treatments for a defined population of patients from a registry who may be at risk from certain diabetic complications and also to measure costs. This does not require pooling all information. As long as the systems from different providers

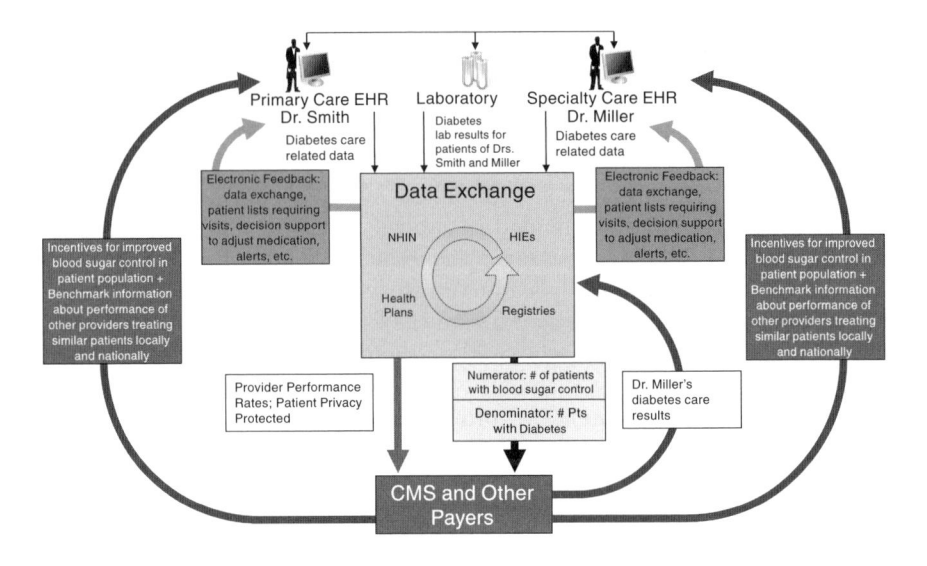

FIGURE 4-3 Schematic in Figure 4-2 applied to diabetes. The result: better care at lower cost.

and organizations are using consistent methodologies for constructing the measures, it is possible to get a more comprehensive picture of quality of care. The information can then be utilized in several areas: by providers to help them improve care in a timely way, by patients to help them identify ways to obtain better care, and as the basis for payment and benefit reform.

Accountable Care Organizations

Many of the lessons learned from how to utilize existing data to improve quality and reduce costs are being applied on launching performance measurement programs for five pilot accountable care organizations (ACOs) supported by the Brookings-Dartmouth Learning Network for Accountable Care Organizations. These pilot sites and their payer partners are attempting to implement changes in payments around value at the organizational level. These efforts typically begin with the information that they already have available in existing systems—such as claims—which in many cases, are the only data available.

Efforts to implement learning networks at ACOs could involve three stages. In the basic phase, ACOs utilize existing data from medical, pharmacy, and laboratory claims from payers. In the intermediate phase, ACOs incorporate specific clinical data, such as electronic laboratory results, as well as limited survey data. In the advanced phase, ACOs add more complete clinical data, such as electronic records and registries, and robust patient-generated data, such as health risk appraisals and functional status.

These incremental improvements in the utilization of available health data can have simultaneous impacts in several key areas including care effectiveness (in individual and public health), safety, patient engagement, and efficiency (reducing overuse). More detailed description of the measures within these categories is provided in Table 4-1.

Advances in HIT and quality measurement, along with coordination between efforts will ultimately lead to improved care and better quality and cost information. In the coming years, as the various aspects of quality measurement and HIT are each improved on their own, additional attention is needed to ensure that these elements work together to produce increasingly sophisticated, patient-centered information about quality, costs, and care experience (Figure 4-4).

The Path Forward

The focus for the next 3 years will be on identifying and expanding best practices, as well as developing and aligning incentives that support the quality reporting infrastructure. Recent successes that can be expanded include pilot projects to demonstrate the feasibility of integrating additional data to support more clinically sophisticated, person-centered measures over time.

Incentives will continue to play a central role in quality improvement efforts and it will be increasingly important to align measures between public and private sector payers to further promote effective incentives. Also required will be a clear plan for implementation of increasingly sophisticated patient-centered measures to encourage continuing progress in coordinating care.

Since different data sources and data collection methods may be used by different organizations, one specific area for work is on producing functionally equivalent performance results. Finally, the use of incentives will contribute to quality improvement efforts such as e-prescribing and HIT payments, quality reporting payments, shared savings, and other performance-based payments.

Using Pilot Programs to Improve Quality Reporting

Pilot programs, such as those funded by the Office of the National Coordinator (ONC) for Health Information Technology's Beacon Community Program, have the opportunity to drive movement toward nationally consistent methods in quality reporting. Some areas to be tested with future pilot programs include the use of consistent summary reporting methods,

TABLE 4-1 Incorporating Advanced Measures Through Accountable Care Organizations

Basic Phase—Claims-Based Measures ACOs have access to medical, pharmacy, and laboratory claims from payers	
ACO Impact	Quality Improvement Measure
Care effectiveness/ population health	Cancer care acreenings Diabetes care (LDL and A1c tests, eye exams, etc.) Coronary artery disease care (LDL test)
Safety	High-risk medication for the elderly Appropriate testing for patients using high-risk medications
Overuse/efficiency	Imaging for low back pain (in absence of "red flags") during first 30 days Inappropriate antibiotic prescribing Utilization rates of select services (e.g., C-section)
Intermediate Phase—Limited Clinical and Survey Measures ACOs use specific clinical data (e.g., electronic laboratory results) and limited survey data	
ACO Impact	Quality Improvement Measure
Care effectiveness/ population health	Immunization rates for children and adolescents Patients with diabetes whose blood sugar (A1c) are in control Patients with diabetes or ischemic vascular disease whose lipids are in control Patients with hypertension whose blood pressure is in control
Safety	"Never events" in hospitals
Patient engagement	Physician instructions understood (Consumer Assessment of Health Providers and Systems [CAHPS]) Care received when needed (CAHPS)
Overuse/efficiency	Episode-based resource use—linked to quality measures for common medical (e.g., diabetes, acute myocardial infarction [AMI]) and common surgical conditions (e.g., hip replacement)
Advanced Phase—Comprehensive Patient-Focused Measures More complete clinical and robust patient-generated data	
ACO Impact	Quality Improvement Measure
Care effectiveness/ population health	Comprehensive health risk summary score (body mass index, blood pressure, cholesterol, smoking, exercise, alcohol) Stage-specific quality of life and functional outcomes for common cancers Quality of life and functional outcomes for common conditions (e.g., AMI, hip replacement, diabetes)
Safety	Hospital infection and risk-adjusted mortality rates Outpatient medication errors

TABLE 4-1 Continued

Patient engagement	Care plans—patient activation and engagement in chronic/other conditions Preference-sensitive conditions—level of information communicated regarding patient choice (e.g., knee surgery) Patient preferences—adherence to design and execution of care plan (e.g., advanced directives)
Overuse/efficiency	Episode-based resource use—linked to quality of life, functional and patient engagement measures for common medical (e.g., diabetes, AMI) and surgical conditions (e.g., hip replacement)

methods to ensure complete reporting (representing all patients without double counting), mechanisms to generate provider feedback, and the ability to capture and use information on race, ethnicity, language, and other valuable patient data. Successful pilot programs in these and other areas will provide links to measurable improvements in patient outcomes, error reductions, and administrative burdens. They will also provide better evidence to identify best practices going forward. The overarching goal of such efforts is to assemble the electronic infrastructure with currently available data sources, while promoting pilot programs to improve methods.

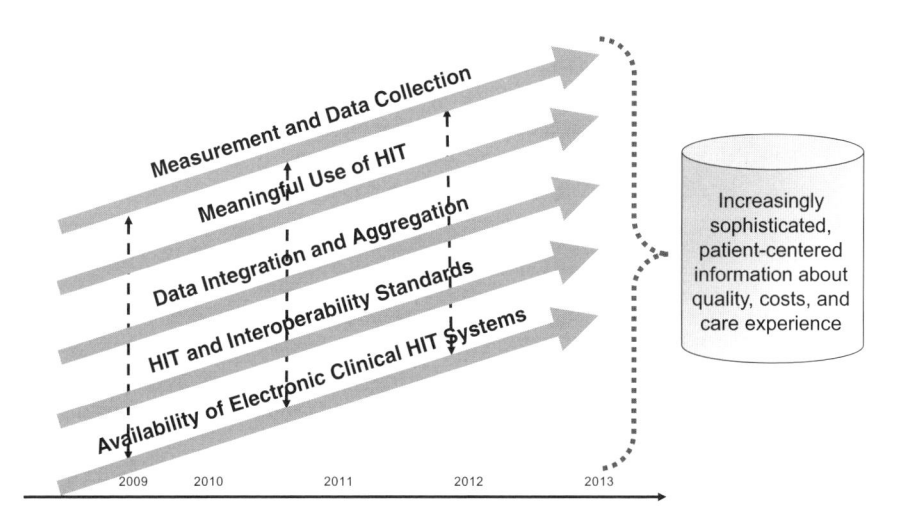

FIGURE 4-4 All aspects of quality improvement must work in concert to improve care.

Key Next Steps

Quality measurement and improvement will be crucial to healthcare delivery reform. All five elements—measurement and data collection, payment reform, benefit reform, better evidence, and quality improvement support—are important, but the focus in this paper has been on the data collection and reporting infrastructure and its role in improving quality and lowering costs. Some of the crucial areas for work in the near term are to identify best practices for quality reporting and payment reform, to expand successful pilots projects for measurement and payment reform, and to develop and pilot more advanced patient-focused measures. Ultimately, momentum in all of these areas will combine synergistically to yield more advanced patient-focused measures and more sophisticated delivery of care.

ENGAGING INDIVIDUALS IN POPULATION HEALTH MONITORING

Kenneth D. Mandl, M.D., M.P.H.
Children's Hospital Boston

The next major step in the evolution of population research is to engage large, distributed consenting populations in longitudinal study. By treating individuals as collaborators and not just subjects in research or cases in public health we will mine a largely untapped source of knowledge about health and disease—the patient. Emerging patient-oriented health information technologies will transform the research enterprise, helping to establish a learning health system.

Following are four near-term predictions all informed by our experiences in developing, evaluating, and diffusing the Indivo personally controlled health record (PCHR) to engage the patient in medicine, research, and public health (Mandl et al., 2007).

- Individuals will share their own data and observations for the public good.
- As data begin to flow into patient-controlled mechanisms (such as PCHRs), populations of individuals will control datasets that are larger and more complete than those traditionally used in population research.
- Present-day online social networks are a rudimentary version of a major pillar in an emerging health information technology (HIT) infrastructure.
- Engaging populations will require development of incentives and enticements as well as blurring the boundaries between clinical care and research.

The Personally Controlled Health Record

In 1998, structural and sociopolitical concerns motivated us to define a new approach to managing electronic health information. Though most health information at the time was stored on paper, we anticipated a time when it would be stored electronically. That time has been slow to arrive. Studies have shown that, even now, very few outpatient or inpatient settings have a complete electronic health record (EHR) (DesRoches et al., 2008; Jha et al., 2009). In the 1990s, the main problem was that the information stored in EHR systems was—and for the most part still is—generally stored locally at the site where it was recorded. As a result, EHR data were often unavailable at the point of care (Bourgeois et al., 2010). In response, we developed the PCHR—a subset of personal health records (PHRs)—which inverts the standard model and instead allows a patient to assemble, maintain, and manage a secure copy of their medical data. Originally called the Personal Internetworked Notary and Guardian, and created under funding from the National Library of Medicine, Indivo is an open source, open standards PCHR platform. Indivo, much like Quicken and MINT.com function for financial data, is a tool that enables patients to collect copies of their data longitudinally across sites of care. Similar to the iPhone and Apple's App Store, Indivo exposes those data (under patient control) to third-party applications across an open application programming interface (Mandl and Kohane, 2009). Hence, Indivo is designed to spawn an ecosystem of apps, providing functionality and promoting innovation (Figure 4-5). Reflecting on the promise of the PCHR model, Harvard Professor Clayton Christensen observes: "We cannot overstate how important PHRs are to the efficient functioning of a low-cost, high quality health-care system. . . . We think that the Indivo system, or something like it is a good place to start" (Christensen et al., 2009).

After diffusion of the PCHR model at two Harvard Medical School invitational conferences,[1] Indivo has become the reference model for subsequent PCHRs: Microsoft's HealthVault used Indivo software code; Google-Health implemented the model on its own servers with its own code; and the Dossia consortium contracted with the Indivo creators to create a version for deployment to populations of employees from organizations such as Wal-Mart, AT&T, and Intel.

The Next Stage

Uptake of PCHRs has been gradual primarily because PCHRs work best when they can readily obtain a copy of data from EHRs, and EHR vendors have been slow to allow data liquidity. Yet there is reason for

---
[1] See www.pchri2006.org and www.pchri2007.org (accessed February 24, 2011).

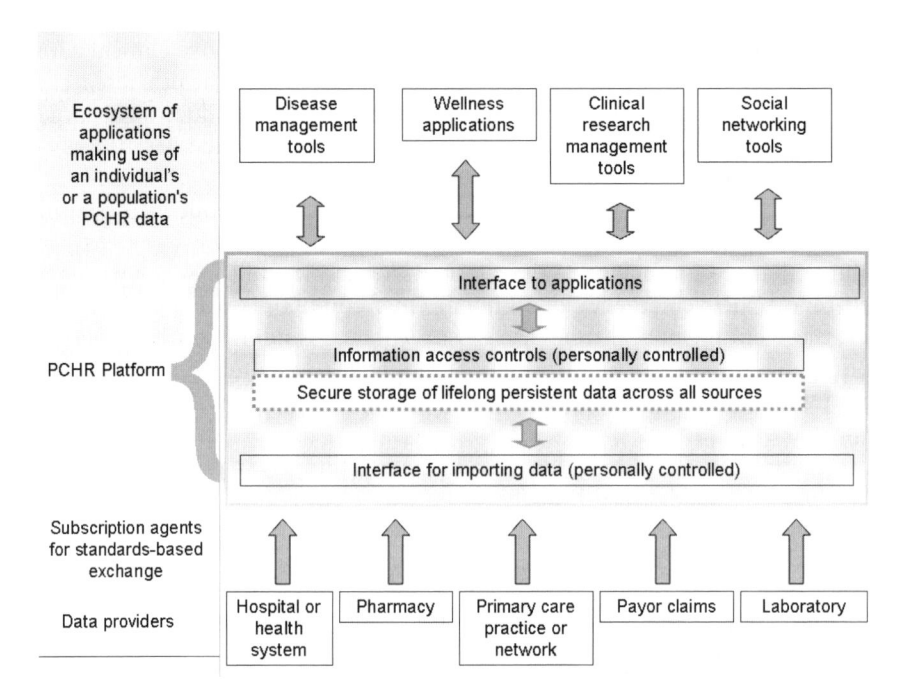

FIGURE 4-5 The personally controlled health record (PCHR) architecture.
SOURCE: Adapted from (Mandl and Kohane, 2008).

optimism. The Health Information Technology for Economic and Clinical Health Act provides that for covered entities using or maintaining an EHR, "the individual shall have a right to obtain from such covered entity a copy of such information in an electronic format." By 2013, this feature of EHRs will be required under the final rule for "meaningful use" of certified EHR technology. In preparation, early-stage efforts have arisen to promote this data liquidity, including the very well marketed "Blue Button" initiative (Chopra et al., 2010). Hence we can expect that even before 2013 a "tectonic shift in the health information economy" will begin, mediated by a change in the locus of control of health information from institutions to individuals (Mandl and Kohane, 2008). For this shift to happen, we must learn to entice populations of patients to share data for research and public health by engaging them on their own terms. The PCHR is a technology designed to do just that. PCHRs enable the patient to authorize access to information—views or even copies of the record—to intelligent software agents ("apps") or individuals including clinical providers, family members, healthcare proxies, and researchers.

While this shift will be largely driven by a need to improve clinical care processes, it will also have a deep impact on population health research. The ability to reach out to populations directly will produce very large cohorts of individuals who can share EHR data and provide detailed self-reported information about their care and health status.

Evidence suggests that patients are faithful reporters about their health. In fact, parents report more accurately on the past medical history of their infants than do physicians in the chart (Porter et al., 2000). When patients self-report their emergency department chief complaints using a brief survey, the accuracy of real-time disease surveillance systems greatly improves (Bourgeois et al., 2007). Furthermore, patient reports about adverse events are timelier and more concordant with their actual health status than those reported by clinicians (Basch, 2010).

There is also evidence that patients are willing to share data with researchers and public health professionals. In a population of patients that had used an early version of a PCHR for over a year, only 9% were unwilling to allow researchers or public health professionals access to an anonymized copy of those data. Patients were most willing to share when they were guaranteed anonymity and that the data would be used primarily for research. While altruism was clearly a motivator, willingness to share was increased if the subjects were offered compensation (Weitzman et al., 2010).

Recent studies also suggest that returning information about health, even in aggregate, to an online community is highly gratifying and promotes information altruism. The for-profit online social networking community PatientsLikeMe has demonstrated that individuals with a severe chronic disease are highly willing—even without compensation—to contribute data and observations to a patient community in order to accelerate learning about their disease (Frost and Massagli, 2008). Similarly, we recently ran a "data donation drive" in a nonprofit online social network of patients with diabetes,[2] rapidly recruiting a cohort of nearly 2,000 individuals sharing data under an implied consent model. What was returned to the community was a "riskscape" picture of glycemic control displayed to the community in aggregate form on maps and graphs. In this experiment, funded by the Centers for Disease Control and Prevention, over 95% of participating network members were willing to be recontacted about opportunities to participate in research.

Engaging Patients

A critical research question is how to engage individuals in *sustained* participation in research cohorts. Across multiple domains, the data col-

---

[2] See www.tudiabetes.org (accessed February 24, 2011).

lected in research are becoming increasingly relevant in clinical settings. For example, as genomic data acquired for research become more clinically pertinent to individuals, inventing creative mechanisms to manage this communication will become an imperative. There is a mounting consensus that participants in genomic research deserve to learn of findings pertinent to their health and well-being (Fabsitz et al., 2010). At Children's Hospital Boston's Gene Partnership Project,[3] we have begun to engage our patients as collaborators in research, developing ethically sound approaches to returning actionable results directly to patients (Kohane et al., 2007).

Focused study is needed to determine whether, and under what circumstances, it is research results, aggregate community-level views, information about "patients like me," financial incentives, pure altruism, or something else that most motivates individuals to share information in a sustained manner. Unlocking the knowledge possessed by populations of individuals is the work of the next decade.

OPTIMIZING CHRONIC DISEASE CARE AND CONTROL

Sophia W. Chang, M.D., M.P.H.
California HealthCare Foundation

Chronic disease care provides important opportunities for the use of electronic health information to inform care delivery. The prevalence of chronic disease in the United States continues to increase and 20% of the population currently accounts for 80% of healthcare costs (Anderson and Wilson, 2006). The opportunity for better quality and more cost-effective care lies in identifying and delivering useful interventions in a timely and nonduplicative manner. The prevalence of comorbid conditions (over 50% of those with a chronic condition) also raises important questions about better care management approaches (Anderson and Wilson, 2006). There is already indication that overemphasis on the close management of a single condition may cause harm—for example, in the setting of diabetes and cardiovascular disease (Skyler et al., 2009). Beyond the knowledge gained from randomized controlled trials, systematic review of population data may allow us to reap timely information about optimal therapies and approaches from clinical observation, experience, and documented patient outcomes.

Leveraging Patient Health Data

As the most powerful actors in care, actively engaging patients in the management of their chronic conditions is going to be vital to any system-

---
[3] See www.geneparnership.org (accessed February 24, 2011).

wide improvements in healthcare delivery. The need for increased and more timely use of electronic health data provides an opportunity to involve patients in providing, validating, and using their own health information, priming them to reap significant benefits in both health and quality of life. This requires a paradigm and culture shift from our present systems where shared data infrastructures are solely controlled by healthcare providers.

The existing healthcare data infrastructure has a number of limitations that make it difficult for healthcare professionals and patients to effectively use patient health data. Currently, there is a lack of commonly accepted standardized nomenclatures and data formats—and only limited use of what does exist—for items consistently included in medical documentation (e.g., chief complaints or symptoms, laboratory results, radiology and pathology interpretations). This lack of standardization limits the ability to aggregate meaningful information across providers and even within large institutions. These same limitations also prevent widespread decision rules and tools from being used effectively to support the consistent practice of evidence-based care (i.e., robust clinical decision support). Furthermore, opportunities to include quality of life, functional status, and self-management measures—all of which would be predominantly provided by patients—are also hindered by the lack of standardization and system functionality. Current patient portal approaches to sharing EHR information generally lack the ability for patients to extract and use their own structured electronic data. In addition, these records do not include the concrete information that often is most valuable for patients managing a chronic condition: how to make dietary changes, adhere to medications, manage side effects, incorporate exercise into their schedules, etc.

While we progress toward the paradigm of engaging patients in the management of their own electronic health data, an important stepping stone is the clear understanding that data within the record belong to the patient and not to either the provider or the institution (Ralston et al., 2010; Walker et al., 2009). Using EHR data as a mode of communication between patients and providers simultaneously validates data quality and engenders trust in its use for clinical care decisions. Although to date no organization has a truly interactive and shared patient record system, some have developed successful patient portals that may move in that direction.

Large enterprises like Kaiser Permanente and the Veterans Health Administration (VHA) have maintained population management systems in parallel to their transactional EHR systems (High Value Health Care Project, 2010). The VHA recently published their experience in managing a national data warehouse (disease registry) for the high-cost chronic conditions of HIV/AIDS and Hepatitis C. Focusing on data use for quality management, the VHA's approach uses a system that pulls data nationally from its EHR system and includes local clinicians at each medical center who systematically confirm patients in each population. A key enabler of adoption was providing local clinical support and query tools to help clinicians validate data elements and manage patient populations locally. Adoption and use are further supported through national-level reporting of quality measures, which are in turn tied to financial bonuses and incentives (Backus et al., 2009).

A similar example exists in the Health Maintenance Organization (HMO) Research Network (HMORN), an organization of HMO research programs. HMORN creates virtual data warehouses pulled from EHR systems across 16 provider organizations. It should be noted that each HMO in the network has been using its EHR system in the context of a robust quality improvement culture and infrastructure. That is, the review and use of EHR data for clinical management play a significant role in providing validated data for research purposes.

Challenges and Next Steps

Small physician offices not affiliated with a large system have, to date, had less opportunity to receive rapid-cycle quality improvement feedback and participate in clinical research. Recognizing the need for and value of aggregated population-level data, a growing number of regional health information exchanges are offering (or plan to offer) population reports to support improvements in disease management. Furthermore, it is hoped that federal investments in regional extension centers will support smaller practices in EHR adoption. Experience to date, however, has demonstrated that the EHR adoption effort is highly time- and resource-intensive and requires ongoing local management and feedback in order to reap improvements in clinical care (Nutting et al., 2009).

To maximize the value of EHRs—for both improved quality of care and increased patient satisfaction—existing research paradigms need to shift toward real-time feedback and knowledge development. Electronic data hold the promise of being able to provide more timely and extensive comparative effectiveness data. Especially in settings of comorbid conditions, it will be increasingly difficult to have a single evidence-based best practice. More likely, we will have a range of options, with associated potential risks and benefits, to support shared decision making between clinicians and patients on which chronic disease management course to take. The important next step is the ability to collect and aggregate those treatment regimens and outcomes to better inform current and future practice. To bring the patient back into the center, data about care processes, quality of life, and side-effect experiences will be increasingly valued, collected, and shared directly with patients.

To move toward these goals, some next steps should include

- *Wider adoption of standardized core data elements.* Current implementation efforts are time-consuming and expensive, and may be redundant without national requirements.
- *Better align what is important to patients with the data elements collected by EHRs.* This requires a move beyond portals toward new paradigms for patient-entered data and for data sharing, with sharing directed by patients to a range of providers and others who support them in the management of their health.
- *Learn how to incorporate patient experience into our knowledge base and data systems.* If we spend too much time, effort, and expense on the provider side, we are missing the biggest opportunities to improve chronic disease. The care experience goes well beyond what is documented in a health record, and a "learning system" must be able to understand, document, and improve care processes outside the clinical encounter.
- *Develop a better paradigm for learning from patient data.* Our expanding Health Insurance Portability and Accountability Act privacy framework is a start, but a clearer continuum for data use—quality improvement, system improvement, clinical effectiveness, and health services research—is needed. There is a blurring of the lines between real-time data feedback, measuring to improve care processes, and improving clinical outcomes when EHR data can be used to meet all these needs.
- *Better translate what we already "know" about population health into actionable information.* The potential to mine aggregated data to improve the health of populations gives us incredible power. Given the value of these potential data, how do we ensure that new knowledge is put into practice when we do a poor job of doing so already?

In the end, we must be wary of arguments about "primary" vs. "secondary" use of clinical data, and keep in mind that it is the patients who own their clinical information and live with their chronic conditions. It is incumbent upon us to ensure that the investments made in automating this vital information are brought to the service of patients who, in the end, will at some point be every single one of us.

TARGETING POPULATION HEALTH DISPARITIES

M. Christopher Gibbons, M.D., M.P.H.
Johns Hopkins Urban Health Institute

Traditionally, modern medicine has sought to understand health and disease largely through elucidating molecular, physiological, or psychological mechanisms and determinants. While this approach has yielded significant gains in individual longevity, achieving sustained population-wide gains has been much more elusive (NRC, 2001). This reality is perhaps most convincingly illustrated by the existence of healthcare disparities. Systematically reducing healthcare disparities is a vexing challenge that, to date, has yet to be accomplished. Part of the challenge lies in our understanding of the causes of these disparities. Disease causation in general, and health disparities in particular, results from complex interactions of many factors that simultaneously and often cooperatively act longitudinally across more than one level of influence (Gibbons et al., 2007). As such, a comprehensive understanding of disparities requires the integration of knowledge derived from the bench with that from sociobehavioral and population sciences. In a similar fashion, treating disease at the bedside and addressing healthcare disparities in the population will require an integrating health and social care systems with a focus on clinical, behavioral, and environmental determinants of health.

Demographic Trends and Challenges

Several national trends suggest the pressing need for this type of integrated approach to population health and health disparities. First, the high prevalence of chronic disease in our society represents a challenge for a healthcare system largely oriented to acute care episodes. Chronic diseases are the leading cause of illness, disability, and death with over 15% of the U.S. population suffering from activity limitations resulting from chronic diseases (IOM, 2001). Because individuals suffering from chronic disease often have these diseases for many years, yet only need acute clinical services for relatively short periods of time, most of the "care" they will receive will be provided by relatives and friends in the home or community (IOM, 2001). To complicate matters further, the United States is experiencing a burgeoning of the senior population. In 2000, 35.0 million people (12%) were over the age of 65 (Meyer, 2001). The proportion of seniors in the U.S. population (age ≥ 65) is expected to increase to approximately 20% in 2030 (71 million seniors). The number of persons age > 80 years is expected to increase from about 9 million in 2000 to 19 million in 2030. With 80% of all seniors burdened by a chronic condition, and 50% having two or more, these trends will challenge our ability to provide chronic disease care (CDC, 2003).

The United States is also becoming more racially and ethnically diverse. Between 2000 and 2050, the number of Asians is expected to increase by 22.7 million (213%), while the number in the "all other races" (which includes American Indians and Alaska Natives, Native Hawaiians and other Pacific Islanders, and individuals who identify with two or more races) category will increase by 15.3 million (217%). The population of Hispanic or Latino origin is projected to steadily increase as a percentage of the total U.S. population through 2050, rising from 12.6% in 2000 to 24.4% in 2050 (Shrestha, 2006). This increase is occurring even as the U.S. population overall is also expected to grow and reach approximately 420 million persons by year 2050.

These population-level increases come at a time when the physician and nurse workforces are rapidly aging (HRSA, 2003). This will inevitably result in greater patient reliance on family and informal caregivers to help meet healthcare management needs. The actions of these caregivers and patients will be influenced by cultural norms, attitudes, beliefs, and practices that could influence healthcare decision making and health outcomes. Taken together, these trends suggest a growing importance of "nonclinical" factors in the genesis and treatment of disease as well as the reduction of healthcare disparities.

Populomics

Elucidation of mechanisms of action and understanding disease pathogenesis in an integrated way will require the generation and synthesis of large, complex, and diverse datasets. In addition, treating disease from this perspective will require real-time synthesis and analysis of multilevel data at the point of care. As such, advances in health information technology (HIT), electronic health records (EHRs), and health information exchanges offer significant promise in bringing these needs into reality. The term populomics has emerged from the synthesis of the population sciences, medicine, and informatics to describe this integrative, systems-oriented perspective (Abrams, 2006; Gibbons, 2005). Populomics is focused on transdisciplinary, integrative disease/risk characterization, interdiction, and mitigation and relies heavily on innovations in computer and information technologies to characterize the interplay of sociobehavioral pathways, and biophysiological/molecular mechanisms that work across levels of existence to impact health at the individual and population levels (Gibbons, 2008).

Research paradigms like the sociobiologic integrative model provide a conceptual framework for populomics-oriented research and analysis (Gibbons et al., 2007). This model posits that individuals are constantly being exposed to many health-impacting factors in the environments in which they live. These are collectively called "inputs." Some of these inputs may be modified to increase or attenuate their effects via "other" environmental factors. These other factors are called indirect environmental inputs. Once an individual or population is exposed to a given factor or set of factors, these direct and indirect inputs are, in turn, acted upon by metabolic, digestive, and/or detoxification systems within the body. If inputs or their metabolic products overwhelm bodily defense or regulatory mechanisms, illness and disease will occur (Gibbons et al., 2007). Because inputs, biological processes, and outcomes exist on several levels, the model is conceived as operating on the cellular, individual, and population levels—temporally proceeding from input (exposure) to cellular-, individual-, or population-level outcomes. Within this context, disease will only occur if the magnitude of impact produced by inputs and metabolic processes is sufficient to overwhelm bodily reparative, restorative, or compensatory mechanisms and cause genotypic, phenotypic, or psychological abnormalities that ultimately result in a disease state or health deficit (Gibbons et al., 2007). If the resulting deficits manifest only at the cellular level, it may be detectable as a change in susceptibility or predisposition. If they manifest at the individual level, it would result in a disease or illness state. If they occur in a large number of people in a given population, it could be detected as an epidemic, pandemic, or disparity. Science must organize and define the inputs, biological processes, and outcomes that exist and the relationships between them that undergird disease at each level of exposure (Gibbons et al., 2007).

Populovigilance

Recent advances in information technology and computer science are making the capture, organization, and synthesis of large amounts of data possible. With the evolution of EHRs, personal health records, consumer health informatics, and social media, we are entering an era when this synthesis and analysis are possible at the bedside in real-time. In the future, working from this integrative perspective, we may find that understanding single etiologies or factors (bacteria, viruses, poverty, race, ethnicity) might be less important than knowing that a given group of factors work together, across levels of analysis (cellular, individual, and population), to collectively influence discreet biomolecular mechanisms and result in a given outcome. These groups of individual- and population-level factors that predictably coexist and act cooperatively to influence discrete health outcomes could then form the basis of so-called sociobehavioral disparities phenotypes. Further, scientists may be able to usher in a new generation of genome-wide association studies (GWAS) that actually start at the population level. Here, scientists would seek to define one or more sociobehavioral phenotypes across a given population of consumers or patients and then link them with underlying biophysiological, psychological, and molecular mechanisms, constructing "causal profiles."

Across a group of patients with a given disease or disparities, one or more causal profiles may exist. This suggests that across a population of patients, with a given disease (breast cancer) or disparity (elevated prostate cancer rates among African Americans), there exist multiple pathways to a given outcome. Because this form of analysis starts at the population level—by first elucidating those sociobehavioral phenotypes that actually exist across that population—this "PheGe" (phenotypic-genotypic) analysis may be more cost-effective than typical GWAS that attempt to first identify molecular pathways and then determine the prevalence of the identified pathway in a defined population. For similar reasons, these causal profiles could ultimately prove to have more predictive value than commonly used constructs like race, ethnicity, or any other single factor thought to be a "fundamental" cause of disparities.

Rather than debating "fundamental causes" as the only credible starting point for disparities research, it may be possible to think in terms of a disparities-oriented "populovigilance" where scientists work to collect, monitor, and evaluate data from defined populations, on the adverse effects of disparate care, environmental hazards, behavior, and policies. Implemented effectively, this could identify hazards and/or sentinel events associated with the existence of healthcare disparities as well as prevent harm to patients and individuals among the target subpopulations (disparities harm reduction research).

Clearly, many challenges must be overcome prior to accomplishing these tasks and realizing these goals. While the future is unknown, the potential of HIT to yield novel insights and enable new advances in treatment, public health, and healthcare disparities is certainly significant.

REFERENCES

Abrams, D. B. 2006. Applying transdisciplinary research strategies to understanding and eliminating health disparities. *Health Education and Behavior* 33(4):515-531.

Anderson, G. F., and K. B. Wilson. 2006. *Chronic disease in California: Facts and figures*. http://www.chcf.org/publications/2006/10/chronic-disease-in-california-facts-and-figures (accessed September 10, 2010).

Backus, L. I., S. Gavrilov, T. P. Loomis, J. P. Halloran, B. R. Phillips, P. S. Belperio, and L. A. Mole. 2009. Clinical case registries: Simultaneous local and national disease registries for population quality management. *Journal of the American Medical Informatics Association* 16(6):775-783.

Basch, E. 2010. The missing voice of patients in drug-safety reporting. *New England Journal of Medicine* 362(10):865-869.

Bourgeois, F. C., K. L. Olson, and K. D. Mandl. 2010. Patients treated at multiple acute health care facilities: Quantifying information fragmentation. *Archives of Internal Medicine* 170(22):1989-1995.

Bourgeois, F. T., S. C. Porter, C. Valim, T. Jackson, E. F. Cook, and K. D. Mandl. 2007. The value of patient self-report for disease surveillance. *Journal of the American Medical Informatics Association* 14(6):765-771.

CDC (Centers for Disease Control and Prevention). 2003. Trends in aging—United States and worldwide. *Morbidity & Mortality Weekly Report* 52(6):101.

Chopra, A., T. Park, and P. Levin. 2010. "Blue Button" provides access to downloadable personal health data. http://www.whitehouse.gov/blog/2010/10/07/blue-button-provides-access-downloadable-personal-health-data (accessed March 11, 2011).

Christensen, C., J. Grossman, and J. Hwang. 2009. *The innovator's prescription: A disruptive solution for health care.* New York: McGraw-Hill.

DesRoches, C. M., E. G. Campbell, S. R. Rao, K. Donelan, T. G. Ferris, A. Jha, R. Kaushal, D. E. Levy, S. Rosenbaum, A. E. Shields, and D. Blumenthal. 2008. Electronic health records in ambulatory care—a national survey of physicians. *New England Journal of Medicine* 359(1):50-60.

Fabsitz, R. R., A. McGuire, R. R. Sharp, M. Puggal, L. M. Beskow, L. G. Biesecker, E. Bookman, W. Burke, E. G. Burchard, G. Church, E. W. Clayton, J. H. Eckfeldt, C. V. Fernandez, R. Fisher, S. M. Fullerton, S. Gabriel, F. Gachupin, C. James, G. P. Jarvik, R. Kittles, J. R. Leib, C. O'Donnell, P. P. O'Rourke, L. L. Rodriguez, S. D. Schully, A. R. Shuldiner, R. K. Sze, J. V. Thakuria, S. M. Wolf, and G. L. Burke. 2010. Ethical and practical guidelines for reporting genetic research results to study participants: Updated guidelines from a national heart, lung, and blood institute working group. *Circulation: Cardiovascular Genetics* 3(6):574-580.

Frost, J. H., and M. P. Massagli. 2008. Social uses of personal health information within PatientsLikeMe, an online patient community: What can happen when patients have access to one another's data. *Journal of Medical Internet Research* 10(3):e15.

Gibbons, M. C. 2005. A historical overview of health disparities and the potential of eHealth solutions. *Journal of Medical Internet Research* 7(5):e50.

———. 2008. Populomics. *Studies in Health Technology and Informatics* 137:265-268.

Gibbons, M. C., M. Brock, A. J. Alberg, T. Glass, T. A. LaVeist, S. Baylin, D. Levine, and C. E. Fox. 2007. The sociobiologic integrative model (SBIM): Enhancing the integration of sociobehavioral, environmental, and biomolecular knowledge in urban health and disparities research. *Journal of Urban Health* 84(2):198-211.

High Value Health Care Project. 2010. *How registries can help performance measurement improve care.* http://www.rwjf.org/files/research/65448.pdf (accessed September 10, 2010).

HRSA (Health Resources and Services Administration). 2003. *Changing demographics: Implications for physicians, nurses, and other health workers* ftp://ftp.hrsa.gov/bhpr/nationalcenter/changedemo.pdf (accessed January 18, 2011).

IOM (Institute of Medicine). 2001. *Crossing the quality chasm: A new health system for the 21st century.* Washington, DC: National Academy Press.

Jha, A. K., C. M. DesRoches, E. G. Campbell, K. Donelan, S. R. Rao, T. G. Ferris, A. Shields, S. Rosenbaum, and D. Blumenthal. 2009. Use of electronic health records in U.S. hospitals. *New England Journal of Medicine* 360(16):1628-1638.

Kohane, I. S., K. D. Mandl, P. L. Taylor, I. A. Holm, D. J. Nigrin, and L. M. Kunkel. 2007. Medicine. Reestablishing the researcher-patient compact. *Science* 316(5826):836-837.

Mandl, K. D., and I. S. Kohane. 2008. Tectonic shifts in the health information economy. *New England Journal of Medicine* 358(16):1732-1737.

———. 2009. No small change for the health information economy. *New England Journal of Medicine* 360(13):1278-1281.

Mandl, K. D., W. W. Simons, W. C. Crawford, and J. M. Abbett. 2007. Indivo: A personally controlled health record for health information exchange and communication. *BMC Medical Informatics and Decision Making* 7:25.

Meyer, J. 2001. *Age 2000.* Washington, DC: U.S. Census Bureau.

NRC (National Research Council). 2001. *New horizons in health: An integrative approach.* Washington, DC: National Academy Press.

Nutting, P. A., W. L. Miller, B. F. Crabtree, C. R. Jaen, E. E. Stewart, and K. C. Stange. 2009. Initial lessons from the first national demonstration project on practice transformation to a patient-centered medical home. *Annals of Family Medicine* 7(3):254-260.

Porter, S. C., M. T. Silvia, G. R. Fleisher, I. S. Kohane, C. J. Homer, and K. D. Mandl. 2000. Parents as direct contributors to the medical record: Validation of their electronic input. *Annals of Emergency Medicine* 35(4):346-352.

Ralston, J. D., K. Coleman, R. J. Reid, M. R. Handley, and E. B. Larson. 2010. Patient experience should be part of meaningful-use criteria. *Health Affairs* 29:607-613.

Shrestha, L. B. 2006. *The changing demographic profile of the United States.* http://digital.library.unt.edu/ark:/67531/metacrs9276/ (accessed January 18, 2011).

Skyler, J. S., R. Bergenstal, R. O. Bonow, J. Buse, P. Deedwania, E. A. Gale, B. V. Howard, M. S. Kirkman, M. Kosiborod, P. Reaven, and R. S. Sherwin. 2009. Intensive glycemic control and the prevention of cardiovascular events: Implications of the ACCORD, ADVANCE, and VA diabetes trials: A position statement of the American Diabetes Association and a scientific statement of the American College of Cardiology Foundation and the American Heart Association. *Circulation* 119(2):351-357.

Walker, J., D. K. Ahern, L. X. Le, and T. Delbanco. 2009. Insights for internists: "I want the computer to know who I am." *Journal of General Internal Medicine* 24(6):727-732.

Weitzman, E. R., L. Kaci, and K. D. Mandl. 2010. Sharing medical data for health research: The early personal health record experience. *Journal of Medical Internet Research* 12(2):e14.

5

Weaving a Strong Trust Fabric

INTRODUCTION

Building trust among all stakeholders of the digital infrastructure—in particular the patient population—is vital to progress and constitutes the focus of this chapter. Included are considerations of the most effective ways to engage stakeholders through demonstration of the value of health information exchange in improving outcomes and efficiency, building confidence in security and privacy safeguards, and examining the learning health system–specific challenges posed in these areas. Examinations range from a focus on the sociotechnical components of privacy and the risk–benefit calculation in health information exchange to technical approaches to ensuring data privacy and security.

Edward Shortliffe of the American Medical Informatics Association addresses the need to build a strong fabric of trust among stakeholders by communicating and demonstrating value. Dr. Shortliffe states that in order for health information technology (HIT) to meet its full potential, patient and provider participation must be secure. This sense of security depends on an appreciation of the value presented by the HIT used as well as creating and maintaining proper security and safeguards. Sharing a personal anecdote about a provider who admitted that only patient demand would motivate him to adopt an electronic health record (EHR) system, Dr. Shortliffe observes that sufficient patient demand could even obviate the need for federal incentives. Using electronic banking as an example, he suggests that educational programs are necessary to inform stakeholders about the risks and benefits of EHRs, and predicts that with the establishment of an environment of trust, the value of increased convenience and quality offered by EHRs and data sharing will overcome concerns about privacy. Currently, however, the risks of adopting an EHR system are better understood and communicated, so the focus of stakeholder engagement activities going forward should be on communicating the benefits—most importantly, better care and lower costs.

The implementation of fair information practices to ensure privacy and security is the focus of the Center for Democracy and Technology's Deven McGraw. Citing surveys showing that while individuals desire electronic access to their health information, they have significant privacy concerns, she suggests that providing individuals with meaningful choices around privacy is an important approach to addressing these concerns. Ms. McGraw points to a comprehensive approach to patient privacy and data security based on the Markle Common Framework for Secure and Private Health Information Exchange. Key elements of the framework include an open and transparent process, specification of purpose, individual participation and control, and accountability and oversight. Closing with a warning that overreliance on consent leads to weak protection—shifting the burden of privacy protection to the individual—and that existing regulations are insufficient to cover the emerging issues of a learning health system, she notes the need for a trust fabric based on fair information practices.

Since its passage in 1996 and recent modifications, the Health Insurance Portability and Accountability Act (HIPAA), has served as the legal and policy framework for health information privacy. Bradley Malin of Vanderbilt University describes the current state of play around health data de-identification and highlights some of the relevant learning health system–related issues posed by HIPAA. Included among these are identity resolution while maintaining privacy and concern that de-identification could cause modifications to patient information that influence the meaning of clinical evidence. He asserts, however, that most of these challenges are not insurmountable, and that efforts to quantify risk are an important first step to mitigation. Dr. Malin suggests that use cases that better define health information uses, and progress in the area of distributed query-based research will be important in progressing toward a privacy-assured learning health system.

Ian Foster of Argonne National Laboratory addresses the technical components surrounding trust in the digital infrastructure for the learning health system. Dr. Foster lays out a number of challenges facing the a establishment of a secure digital platform. He points to the fact that a learning health system requires data sharing on an unprecedented scale, and that the purpose of this sharing be extended beyond individual patient care support to include research and population health. Identifying the challenge as one of a highly complex system with an unclear definition of security, Dr. Foster suggests some basic principles and technology solutions that can form a basis for progress: auditabililty (information can be mapped to an individual and data can be mapped to its origin); scalability; and transparency in terms of data usage, policies, and enforcement. Methods to achieve these principles include attribute-based authorization, distributed attribute management, and end-to end (scalable) security.

DEMONSTRATING VALUE TO SECURE TRUST

Edward H. Shortliffe, M.D., Ph.D.
American Medical Informatics Association

There is a widely acknowledged need for individuals to trust the use of EHRs in the management of their health and health care. People must believe that their personal data are being protected, and used consistently in their best interest. Formal studies in scientific journals that document the positive influences of electronic records on quality, safety, and efficiency—typically poorly communicated to the lay public—will not counter a deep concern that individual privacy can be compromised or that personal data will be used for nefarious purposes. Thus all the laudable goals we seek with the use of health information technology (HIT) that are under discussion at this workshop are dependent on a "fabric of trust"—the willingness of individuals and, by extension, society to contribute personal data and clinical experiences to the development of a learning healthcare system.

Individuals in the healthcare community bring a deep understanding of the health policy, financing, and quality issues that can be enhanced by the empowering use and effective implementation of HIT. We see strong advantages to society in the use of electronic health records (EHRs) and their adaptation to support a learning health system. Yet the individuals in our communities—and I fear this includes many members of the media—have a limited understanding of such issues and would find most of our work difficult to follow. What they can easily understand, however, are news stories that emphasize the way in which EHRs may threaten their privacy, the confidentiality of personal data, and general security issues (such as lost or stolen laptop computers containing private medical data regarding thousands of patients). We need to understand that the public's support for EHRs depends on their sense that their care is improved or their life is simplified when their provider uses the technology. The public needs to believe that all prudent measures are being taken to ensure that their personal data are protected from loss or inappropriate access.

Anecdotal Evidence of the Current Challenges

Like everyone else attending this workshop, I am a patient as well as a health professional. Long ago I made the personal decision, based on my understanding of the trade-offs, that I would greatly prefer to be cared for by a health system and by individual clinicians who had embraced the use of EHRs. When I recently moved to a new city and had to identify a primary care provider, I decided to rule out any physician or provider organization that lacked the infrastructure or philosophy that would allow me to communicate through e-mail with my physician and his office staff. Frustrated by my recent experience in another city, I swore that I would never again subject myself to a healthcare environment or physician who had not adopted modern electronic means of communication, data management, and information dissemination. I wanted to be sure it would be simple for me to book appointments online, to request prescription refills, to check lab results, and to review other aspects of my personal record. I also wanted to have reasonable faith in the authentication and authorization procedures that were in place before I or others could access my information online. I recognize that I am an early adopter of new information technologies by nature, but as I looked at the plethora of smart phones, Facebook pages, and laptops in airport security lines that surround me every day, I suspected that I was not alone in using such "digital literacy" criteria to guide my choice of physician and healthcare system. I have subsequently been pleased to find a suitably rigorous, electronically sophisticated physician and healthcare environment in my new city and realize that I personally associate such capabilities with quality of care, safety, and cost containment. Furthermore, I have minimal fear that my personal data are being indiscriminately accessed by others or being handled in ways that would make it easy for them to be lost or stolen.

It is natural to ask whether I am typical of patients with regard to my search for a physician who chooses to use EHRs. One indication that I am *atypical* was the conversation that I had with my previous physician when I asked him whether he had any plans to automate the practice in which he worked. He was surprised that any patient cared about such an esoteric topic. He told me that I was the first patient who had ever queried him on the matter, asserting that there was no demand from patients for him to use an EHR. Additionally, he was personally disinterested in the expense or the retraining that would be required. He noted that he would be retiring in 6–8 years and asked why he should go through this kind of transformation at the very end of his career. He had no interest in using an EHR and did not care what incentives were being offered by the government.

He did acknowledge that if all his patients were telling him that they really cared about automating the office, accepting e-mail, and providing EHR access for patients, then he might feel differently about the topic. One wonders whether federal incentives and the meaningful use criteria would have even been necessary if the average citizen was enamored of EHRs and warned their doctors that they would change providers if the practice did not implement electronic records. Under the current circumstances, however, he viewed the CMS incentives as a conspiracy in Washington, trying to force unproven technology upon him and his patients.

Public Use of HIT

Conversations with others have convinced me that my former physician is not atypical but that I, as a patient requesting that my providers use an EHR, am quite unusual. Seeking to better understand the public's attitudes toward EHRs, I was fascinated to come across a recent book that provides extensive survey data about the public and their access to and use of electronically available health information. Written by researchers at Brookings Institution and Brown University, *Digital Medicine* summarizes and interprets the results of many national e-health public opinion surveys. The emphasis is not on the technology per se but on current trends in adoption, acceptance, and pursuit of e-health solutions. Documenting relatively low use of information technology for health purposes by certain segments of society, the authors state a motivating argument that "in order to achieve the promise of health information technology, digital medicine must overcome the barriers created by political divisions, fragmented jurisdiction, the digital divide, the cost of technology, ethical conflicts, and privacy concerns" (West and Miller, 2009). I have described this volume in more detail elsewhere, noting that education—both of the public and of current and future health professionals—is viewed as a key element in any solution. There is evidence that this issue has been too often overlooked when others have assessed approaches to making better use of information technology in health care (Shortliffe, 2010). Given the economic determinants of e-health use and the digital divide, low-cost technologies and improved access through publicly available means continue to be key requirements.

Yet public familiarity with technology, and personal use of information resources in managing one's own health care, is not the same as having a society that understands and supports the use of EHRs by physicians and other health professionals. If we need educational programs to enhance the public's capabilities in the use of the electronic media for accessing health information, we also need to help them understand the risks and benefits of EHR use.

The Value Proposition: Convenience vs. Risk

I believe that convenience, quality, and perceived value of EHRs will trump concerns about privacy or other risks—but only if there is a climate of trust. The financial system has helped to demonstrate this social phenomenon to us. Consider, for example, the use of one ubiquitous financial technology, the automated teller machine (ATM). When ATMs were introduced, it rapidly became obvious to the public that there were huge advantages in using these machines rather than relying on the traditional interaction with a bank teller or the use of travelers' checks. We all know there are risks associated with electronic banking and ATMs—fraud, stolen PIN numbers, lost cards, and the like—but convenience and universal access to one's funds have clearly outweighed those concerns. In fact, individuals are even willing to *pay* for the convenience of an ATM, given the surcharges that are typically absorbed by the user. We perceive the value to be high, and the risks to be low—and most banks have explicit assurances about maximum losses in the case of documented fraud or theft. There is a *climate of trust* that, on balance, our funds are protected by the system with which we choose to interact.

But the acceptance of such trade-offs in the use of electronic banking clearly requires that the public appreciate the positive value of the innovation offered to them. The value proposition for EHR use is much less well understood by the public, and what they do know has tended to focus more on potential negatives (loss of privacy, government intrusion, etc.) rather than the benefits. Stories about threats to the safety and confidentiality of online health data have tended to dominate in the press; even when most organizations are taking measures to protect against the described threats, the public largely focuses on the negatives.

Engaging the Public

In educating the public about the ways in which the use of EHRs can be positive, the emphasis needs to be on aspects of their implementation that create a sense of value for individual patients or their families. The greater good—for public health, research, or a learning health system—must be viewed as secondary. Since we know that patients tend to trust their own doctors, one crucial source of trust in the health system is the individual's own physician. Thus, there is an important potential interaction between physicians and their patients that can help to inform the public about the clinical value of EHRs, and to assist in the creation of a climate of trust. That outcome, of course, requires that physicians themselves perceive the value of EHRs and believe that it outweighs the costs associated with adoption.

We know that the public appeal of EHRs will grow when they are viewed as convenient for patients, empowering them as partners in their own management, and providing a way to deal with the opacity of traditional healthcare interactions. Their consent for data use—and the subsequent steps toward a learning health system—will follow if there is a strong trust in the data stewardship that occurs when EHR data are shared, anonymized, pooled, and reused.

POLICIES AND PRACTICES TO BUILD PUBLIC TRUST

Deven McGraw, J.D.
Center for Democracy and Technology

Health information technology (HIT) and electronic health information exchange are engines of health reform and have tremendous potential to improve health, reduce costs, and empower patients. While some progress has been made on resolving the privacy and security issues raised by e-health, significant gaps remain and implementation challenges loom.

Many surveys show that people want to have electronic access to their health information, but these same surveys also demonstrate that people have significant privacy concerns about how their data will be used and protected. For example, a 2005 study by the California HealthCare Foundation revealed that a majority of the respondents (67%) have significant concerns about the privacy of their medical records (CHCF, 2005). More recent surveys by the Agency for Healthcare Research and Quality confirm these findings (AHRQ, 2009).

While most people acknowledge the importance of ensuring patient privacy in health information systems, many assume that providing a simple "opt-in" or "opt-out" option fully addresses the issue. Providing individuals with some meaningful choices is an integral part of any privacy system, but relying solely on a check box or blanket consent will not allay consumer fears or, more importantly, provide adequate safeguards against misuse of patient data.

The consequences of not ensuring privacy adequately can include failing to collect complete or adequate patient data. Without privacy protections, people may engage in "privacy-protective behaviors" to avoid having their information used inappropriately. A 2007 Harris Interactive survey revealed that one in six adults withhold information from providers due to privacy concerns (Harris Interactive, 2007). The frequency increases among people with poor health and among racial and ethnic minorities who report higher levels of concern and are more likely to engage in privacy-protective behaviors (CHCF, 2005).

A Comprehensive Strategy for Fair Information Practices

To counter these tendencies and to facilitate the collection of the most complete patient data possible, a comprehensive approach to patient privacy and data security is needed. It is important to note that privacy and security protections are not themselves obstacles to achieve these goals. Rather, enhanced privacy and security can enable higher levels of patient participation in health data collection and facilitate HIT and health information exchange.

The core elements of such a comprehensive strategy include commonly used fair information practices, such as those articulated in the Markle Common Framework for Secure and Private Health Information Exchange (Markle Foundation, 2006). The principles outlined seem so straightforward that, based on common sense, it would seem that everyone employs them. Unfortunately, this is often not the case. However, a serious application of these practices should serve as the lynchpin to building a trusted information-sharing infrastructure

Some of the key elements of fair information practices include: openness and transparency, purpose specification and minimization, collection and data use limitation, individual participation and control, data integrity and quality, security safeguards and controls, accountability and oversight, and remedies. Perhaps the most important element of a comprehensive approach is to develop an open and transparent process. Taking the time to educate patients about the purpose, uses, and goals of collecting their health information can go a long way toward building public trust. Such openness and transparency can reap higher rewards than simply presenting a consent form with little or no explanation and a vague guarantee of security and privacy.

Some elements of this framework are reflected in the Health Information Portability and Accountability Act (HIPAA) privacy and security rules, which provide important baseline protections for patient information. The recent rules added by the Health Information Technology for Economic and Clinical Health Act offer improvements, but existing regulations remain insufficient to cover all of the emerging issues in this new and rapidly evolving environment. For instance, there are now many entities involved in the health information infrastructure that are not covered by HIPAA and other federal regulations. There is also still some ambiguity on the roles, rights, and responsibilities of the various entities involved. For example, a prominent finding in the IOM study on HIPAA and medical research indicates that lack of clarity of the rules and their inconsistent interpretation often pose as much of an obstacle to research as the rules themselves (IOM, 2009).

Limitation of the Informed Consent Model

In this approach, consent is still important but, as noted, is only one element of a comprehensive approach. Indeed, it may not even be the most important component necessary to ensure data security and patient privacy since too much emphasis on consent can often lead to weak privacy protection in practice (CDT, 2009). In practice, an over reliance on consent provides weak privacy protection since it shifts the burden of privacy protection to the individual as opposed to requiring that data holders be good stewards of patient information that they use and maintain. The evidence is clear that individuals pay little attention to consent forms, and too often don't understand the full implications of what they have agreed to.

To ensure the highest level of privacy and security, we need fair information best practices to govern the digital infrastructure for a learning health system. Individual participation and control (consent) should play a role, but other principles (transparency; data minimization, collection, use and disclosure limitations, accountability, and oversight) are equally important in building trust.

HIPAA AND A LEARNING HEALTHCARE SYSTEM

Bradley Malin, Ph.D.
Vanderbilt University

In order to function efficiently and effectively, a learning health system requires reliable access to several critical pieces of information. First, it needs to be informed through knowledge that is derived from the healthcare system. This information must flow continually, so that the system can be updating through current patient experiences. The importance of this information is greater than simply ensuring the accuracy of a patient's EHR. Rather, the provision of this information enables the evolution toward a system that is flexible and able to continually evolve. Second, a learning health system needs to access, and analyze, health information on large populations to inform decision support models that allow for personalized approaches to care.

HIPAA and Data De-Identification

The Health Information Portability and Accountability Act (HIPAA) defines protected health information as information that is explicitly linked to a particular individual or could reasonably be expected to allow individual identification. The HIPAA Privacy Rule permits health information to be shared without patient consent for "secondary" purposes in two ways.

First, HIPAA permits data to be shared without oversight or contractual use agreements provided the data are "de-identified"—which is not the same as "anonymous." Rather, the regulation is designed to mitigate risk while facilitating the sharing of health information. De-identification can be achieved in two different ways: safe harbor and expert determination. Safe Harbor is satisfied when the data are stripped of 18 enumerated features. These include explicit identifiers (such as the individual's name and Social Security number), as well as potential quasi-identifiers (such as the date of birth, gender, and zip code). In contrast, expert determination (sometimes referred to as the statistical standard) states that health information is de-identified if an expert uses generally acceptable scientific principles and methods to certify that the risk of identifying an individual is sufficiently small. In doing so, the expert must document the methods and the results of any analysis used to justify this determination. Additionally, the covered entity is prohibited from revealing any mechanisms generated in the process that would allow an individual to be re-identified.

If a covered entity believes that de-identification would hamper the ability to support a learning system, then it could opt for an alternative: the HIPAA limited dataset. Under this model, the covered entity continues to be prohibited from sharing explicit patient identifiers, but can provide dates and geographic information. The caveat, however, is that the recipient of such information must enter into a data use agreement that states the recipient cannot use the information in a way that would harm, or attempt to identify, the corresponding individuals.

De-Identified Data in a Learning Health System

What is easy? One thing that is relatively easy to do is to build automated approaches to find and suppress patients' identifiers from structured health information. At the present time, there are currently no standards for representing identifiers, but there are various terminologies and message-based standards that we use to represent medical information. It would be fruitful to extend such languages to define types of identifiers.

What is not so easy? When repurposing an electronic medical record system, such as for clinical phenotyping of patients, we use natural language text. As a result, it is more challenging to guarantee the de-identification of this information. There exists software to automatically detect and suppress identifiers within natural language, but none are guaranteed to find all of the identifiers, all of the time. Even if the software is completely efficient, there is still no guarantee that the residual information would protect the corresponding individual from re-identification.

There are, however, alternatives to simply handing health information over to any interested recipient. For instance, we could construct an environment in which the clinical text is housed in a secure environment where an abstract programming interface allows users to submit programs to the system and retrieve aggregate statistics. This model has already been adopted by various statistical agencies around the world for providing access to sensitive governmental information.

What is hard? De-identification, and even aggregation, is not devoid of risks. The HIPAA safe harbor standard, for instance, leaves a certain portion of the population unique with respect to the residual demographics. Latanya Sweeney provided an example in her testimony before National Committee on Vital and Health Statistics several years ago, where she reported that 0.04% of the U.S. population is expected to be unique on residual demographics (NCVHS, 2007). The concern here is that such demographics have been linked to public resources that contain explicit identifiers to accomplish "re-identification." Moreover, when considering the expert determination approach for de-identification, there is no clear designation of what the statistical threshold should be or who can be designated as an expert. It would help greatly if there was a certification process, something similar to a Certified Information Systems Security Personnel program. Furthermore, and perhaps most challenging, is the fact that de-identification tools could suppress potentially useful clinical information. This is a great concern if it influences the meaning of clinical evidence. For example, if the evidence is changed from "no evidence of myocardial infarction" to "evidence of myocardial infarction," the statistics upon which the learning system is built could be subject to noise.

Common Challenges and Next Steps

Let us return to HIPAA from the perspective of challenges. At the present time, HIPAA does not make it easy to support longitudinal studies. If a patient was distributed across multiple covered entities, it would be difficult to resolve the patient's presence without access to identifiers. In the healthcare domain, we can execute some record linkage techniques without revealing patient identifiers through certain cryptographic mechanisms, but the interpretation of HIPAA is such that we are not allowed to apply those encryption technologies even though the keys never get revealed. This is somewhat strange, because it could be guaranteed with very strong evidence that a recipient of such information could not determine who the corresponding patient is.

One notion that I wish to make clear is that the challenges I have alluded to are not necessarily insurmountable. In particular, many of the risks that various studies have promoted (such as the risk of re-identification) may be less of a concern than initially anticipated. We can, and have, quantified risks prior to disclosing health information. Once such measurements are in hand, we can mitigate the risks. These are things we should do. Additionally, we must recognize that not every dataset of health information is susceptible to re-identification in the same way. In a study conducted by Latanya Sweeney, it was shown that one could use publicly available voter registration lists, for instance, to re-identify patients in a de-identified dataset because they shared common demographics (Sweeney, 2002). However, in 2008 we went back and surveyed all the state electoral commissions to see what you would actually get if you purchased or found their voter registration lists. In our investigation we found that the cost of conducting identification is completely different across the states. For instance, in Wisconsin it costs almost $13,000 to purchase such a list, whereas in the state of Minnesota it only costs $46. But it is equally, if not more, important to recognize that the information available in such resources varies. Date of birth is provided in voter lists in the states of Tennessee, Washington, and Illinois, but not in the list published by the state of Wisconsin. Additionally, in the state of Minnesota, only the year of birth is shown. There are always ways of intelligently surpassing, generalizing, or perturbing information such that you preserve the aggregate statistics or the statistics that a learning health system requires.

Conclusion

I will conclude with three parting statements on HIPAA, privacy, and the learning health system. First, as a society we must recognize that privacy risks are context dependent. There is no silver bullet ensuring that if a covered entity de-identifies data according to a particular recipe it is sufficiently protected. Second, the healthcare community must define use cases for the health information to be utilized. If there are no use cases, technologists will not know how the learning system should look, and will be unable to design protections for health information that support a learning system. We probably will not be able to develop methods that support all possible needs in healthcare within the next several years, but we may be able to orient technologies that address some of the bigger challenges first. Moreover, when providing such use cases, it needs to be made clear who needs access to the data. Is it the public? Is it the employees of covered entities? The amount of trust we have in the anticipated recipient influences the amount of health information that can be reported and the way in which it is reported. Finally, we need to determine if the system can learn from the health data remotely. Do we really need to share all of the data with all of the recipients? Or can we enable an environment that is built upon query-response systems? The more control we have over where health information goes and when, the better chance we have of ensuring that is appropriately secured.

BUILDING A SECURE LEARNING HEALTH SYSTEM

Ian Foster, Ph.D.
Argonne National Laboratory

A learning health system is "designed to: generate and apply the best evidence for the collaborative healthcare choices of each patient and provider; drive the process of discovery as a natural outgrowth of patient care; and ensure innovation, quality, safety, and value in health care" (IOM, 2007). The security challenge is to ensure that the wrong people do not learn the wrong things!

A learning health system requires data sharing on a far larger scale than today. This sharing must occur within a highly fragmented environment: most of the ~6,000 hospitals in the United States have restrictive and idiosyncratic data policies and practices, focused on avoiding risk rather than enabling learning. In this context, secure data sharing is as much a political as a technological challenge, and will require political as well as technological solutions. These comments are restricted to technology issues, and speak to the following questions: What can technology do and not do? What can we learn from other large-scale distributed systems in which sensitive data are shared on a large scale? What principles can guide us as we work to create systems that are sufficiently flexible to encompass not only today's applications but those of the future; scalable to a large number of participants; and robust to various threats, including not only malicious acts but also human error and the challenges of complexity?

Defining the Problem

Often the hardest step in building a secure system is characterizing what the system is and what we mean by security. In the case of the U.S. healthcare system, we are dealing with thousands of hospitals, millions of patients, and tens of millions of visits. Participants differ in their institutional structures, cost structures, incentives, capabilities, and regulatory environments. Information technology is often deployed and operated with a view to risk mitigation or avoidance rather than to enable a learning health system. Data sharing is needed not only for individual patients, but also for population health and research studies. Additionally, sharing needs evolve over time, as, for example, an individual patient moves from one caregiver to another or a research project is established linking different organizations. The overall situation is one of complexity, diversity, and constant change.

Further complicating the problem is the fact that the security needs of this system are not well defined. Policy statements tend to speak in generalities, stating, for example, that we should ensure security and privacy, offer patients options, maintain appropriate levels of privacy and security, and build in security and privacy from the outset (IOM, 2007). None of these prescriptions is precise. HIPAA regulations try to be specific, but are open to interpretation and can depend on statistical tests (Jajosky and Groseclose, 2004). We also have political and social considerations, such as objections to universal identifiers and different views on opt in vs. opt out.

Principles for Building Secure Systems

Overall, we have a system that is highly complex and a definition of security that is far from clear. Designing technical solutions to achieve security in this context is a challenging and, perhaps in some sense, impossible task. Nevertheless, there are basic principles that, if followed, can help improve the quality of security solutions.

Auditability means that all actions are mapped to individuals and the origin of all data is unambiguous. Any healthcare security and privacy solution must inevitably combine technical protections with appropriate regulatory frameworks (including penalties for release of data). Thus, we need to build in auditing at a foundational level so that any action performed on healthcare information can be mapped to the individual who performed that action. Equally important, both for research purposes and to protect from other sorts of attacks—for example, delivery of incorrect data—is to ensure that all data can be mapped unambiguously to their origin. This latter requirement becomes increasingly important as patients become more mobile.

Scalability means that the cost of adding participants—whether new institutions or new individuals—is small. Without this property, technological obstacles too easily impede the new connections required to support patient mobility and research studies.

Transparency is important from two perspectives. First, we require transparency with respect to what it done with data and where it is stored. Second, we need transparency with respect to the policies that are being enforced and the consequences of those policies. If multiple policies are being applied, it should be easy to work out what that actually means for an individual's data.

These principles may appear obvious, but it is striking how often systems deployed in healthcare settings ignore them. For example, we frequently see hospitals using virtual private networks (VPNs) to enable secure remote access. VPN technology is effective in protecting against snooping of messages transmitted between two points. However, it does not provide for scalability (every new participant requires an additional point-to-point VPN), auditability (there is no immediate control over who sees data when they are received from the remote location), or transparency (the policies that are enforced in this way are unclear, and the risks of information leakage hard to quantify). If, as is often the case, scaling is handled by adding more VPNs in an ad hoc manner, the result can easily become a complex system in which both usability and security are compromised.

Technology Success Stories

There are, fortunately, simple and well-understood methods that we can apply to help achieve auditability, scalability, and transparency. I describe three such methods here: attribute-based authorization, distributed attribute management, and end-to-end security. Each has been deployed and used on a large scale—for example, within grid systems such as the cancer Biomedical Informatics Grid (caBIG®), Biomedical Informatics Research Network, TeraGrid, and Open Science Grid—albeit for sharing either scientific data or clinical data for research purposes (Oster et al., 2008; Pordes et al., 2007). Many of these systems use technologies implemented within the Globus Toolkit (Foster, 2006).

Attribute-based authorization addresses the frequent (and fundamental) requirement in healthcare security to be able to control who can access a piece of data, software program, or other resource. This problem is often solved by associating an access control list—a list of authorized individuals—with each resource. However, the cost of change is then high. If Dr. X joins the team, Dr. X must be added to all relevant access control lists: a potentially complex and error-prone process.

Using attribute-based authorization, we express access control policies in terms of the properties that an individual must have in order to be allowed access. Properties can include the individual's identity, but more commonly will be properties such as "has Institutional Review Board (IRB) approval for participating in study 123" or "is a faculty member in the department of surgery." Attribute-based authorization provides scalability, because a single rule can govern any number of people that satisfy that rule. In addition, we end up with greater transparency. Instead of having to work out what Alice, Bob, and Chris have in common, we can read the access control rule to determine what condition applies. An important technology here is the eXtensible Access Control Markup Language, frequently used to express access control policies.

Distributed attribute management is an important adjunct to attribute-based authorization. The idea is that we rely on authoritative sources for all attributes. For example, an institution is likely the authoritative source for attributes concerning employment status and qualifications; the IRB for attributes concerning IRB approvals; and the National Institutes of Health for membership of study sections. Then, when an individual attempts to access a resource, the security system reaches out to each required authoritative source, each of which takes responsibility for ensuring that they are issued correctly. With the attributes in hand, the security system can then enforce appropriately the policies that apply at the individual resource. An important technology here is the Security Assertion Markup Language, which defines protocols and representations for requesting and communicating attribute assertions.

End-to-end security is a scalable, more capable alternative to VPNs. As we extract data from databases and move them to remote locations, there will typically be a set of things that we want to ensure happen: that the data are anonymized, that their provenance is documented, that they are not modified en route, and that privacy is preserved. We can achieve many of these things by wrapping the data in a cryptographic envelope that can then be processed appropriately as data move from one location to another. By thus packaging data in a manner that maintains key properties independent of context, we enhance our ability to achieve auditability, scalability, and transparency.

Summary

Security is a systems problem. Without clarity on the nature of the system we are securing, and what we mean by security, we will likely fail to create secure systems. We need to spend more time studying these issues within the context of a learning health system. Auditability, scalability, and transparency are all properties that we should seek to realize as we design a secure learning health system. In architecting security solutions, we can leverage attribute-based authorization, distributed attribute management, and end-to-end security—three methods that have been proven to scale and that tend to support these desirable properties.

REFERENCES

AHRQ (Agency for Healthcare Research and Quality). 2009. *Consumer engagement in developing electronic health information systems.* http://healthit.ahrq.gov/portal/server.pt/gateway/PTARGS_0_9442_909189_0_0_18/09-0081-EF.pdf (accessed January 31, 2011).

CDT (Center for Democracy and Technology). 2009. *Rethinking the role of consent in protecting health information privacy.* http://www.cdt.org/files/pdfs/20090126Consent.pdf (accessed January 31, 2011).

CHCF (California HealthCare Foundation). 2005. *National Consumer Health Privacy Survey 2005.* http://www.chcf.org/publications/2005/11/national-consumer-health-privacy-survey-2005 (accessed January 31, 2011).

Foster, I. 2006. Globus Toolkit version 4: Software for service-oriented systems. *Journal of Computational Science and Technology* 21(4):523-530.
Harris Interactive. 2007. *Many U.S. adults are satisfied with use of their personal health information.* http://www.harrisinteractive.com/vault/Harris-Interactive-Poll-Research-Health-Privacy-2007-03.pdf (accessed January 31, 2011).
IOM (Institute of Medicine). 2007. *The learning healthcare system: Workshop summary.* Washington, DC: The National Academies Press.
———. 2009. *Beyond the HIPAA privacy rule: Enhancing privacy, improving health through research.* Washington, DC: The National Academies Press.
Jajosky, R., and S. Groseclose. 2004. Evaluation of reporting timeliness of public health surveillance systems for infectious diseases. *BMC Public Health* 4(1):29.
Markle Foundation. 2006. *The common framework: Overview and principles.* http://www.markle.org/sites/default/files/Overview_Professionals.pdf (accessed February 25, 2011).
NCVHS (National Committee on Vital and Health Statistics). 2007. *Enhanced protections for uses of health data: A stewardship framework for "secondary uses" of electronically collected transmitted health data.* http://www.ncvhs.hhs.gov/071221lt.pdf (accessed February 25, 2011).
Oster, S., S. Langella, S. Hastings, D. Ervin, R. Madduri, J. Phillips, T. Kurc, F. Siebenlist, P. Covitz, K. Shanbhag, I. Foster, and J. Saltz. 2008. caGrid 1.0: An enterprise grid infrastructure for biomedical research. *Journal of the American Medical Informatics Association* 15(2):138-149.
Pordes, R., D. Petravick, B. Kramer, D. Olson, M. Livny, A. Roy, P. Avery, K. Blackburn, T. Wenaus, F. Würthwein, I. Foster, R. Gardner, M. Wilde, A. Blatecky, J. McGee, and R. Quick. 2007. *The Open Science Grid.* Paper presented at Scientific Discovery Through Advanced Computing (SciDAC) Conference.
Shortliffe, E. 2010. Tracking e-health. *Issues in Science and Technology* (Spring):92-95.
Sweeney, L. 2002. *k*-Anonymity: A model for protecting privacy. *International Journal of Uncertainty, Fuzziness, and Knowledge-Based Systems* 10(5):557-570.
West, D. M., and E. A. Miller. 2009. *Digital medicine: Health care in the Internet era.* Washington, DC: Brookings Institution Press.

6

Stewardship and Governance in the Learning Health System

INTRODUCTION

The growth and development of the digital infrastructure for health will depend on the effectiveness of its stewardship and governance mechanisms. This chapter focuses on a broad range of issues central to establishing a governance entity, such as the format and scope of authority of such an entity, and presents a case study from a similar effort in the United Kingdom. Remaining pieces focus on the types of governance issues raised when considering a learning health system, including leveraging ongoing efforts to accelerate development and approaches to mitigating potentially conflicting interests among stakeholders.

Drawing from her experiences—including leading the establishment of the Rhode Island Health Information Exchange—Laura Adams of the Rhode Island Quality Institute identifies and addresses fundamental questions posed in contemplating the governance of the digital health infrastructure. Focusing on the source and scope of authority, the mission, purpose, and primary goals, and the theoretical foundations for a governance structure, she lays out many options for consideration. Ms. Adams suggests that all potential models of governance structure and stakeholder participation should be considered, and that the scope of the governing bodies' authority should be succinctly communicated in a statement of purpose. She notes that this statement should draw on guiding principles such as transparency and commitment to the common good, and that consideration of guiding theories—such as complexity theory—could aid in providing an ethical and legal framework. Pointing to some of the unique governance challenges posed by a learning health system, including changing privacy considerations and accommodating new sources of data, Ms. Adams suggests drawing on past successes and experiences while incorporating the widest array of viewpoints possible.

Theresa Mullin from the Food and Drug Administration describes ongoing efforts to implement a systematic strategy for data standards development and adoption. This process will address heterogeneity in new drug applications, improve regulatory efficiency, and contribute toward the agency's public health mandate by facilitating exploration of safety and efficacy issues. Dr. Mullin suggests that, through the standardization of clinical data in electronic health records, this effort presents an opportunity to facilitate information exchange and analysis for learning, reducing costs, and reducing burdens on providers for adverse event reporting. Dr. Mullin also highlights some of the overarching governance principles driving this effort: an open, transparent, and inclusive process; and a requirement that the resulting requirements be practical, user-oriented, sensitive to costs, and sustainable.

Meeting patient expectations for privacy and security is central in developing a learning health system, explains Shawn Murphy from Partners HealthCare. He details how current limitations to privacy through de-identification could be overcome by a comprehensive security and privacy approach that does a better job of addressing patients' chief concerns around health information protection—avoiding embarrassment and economic risk. Citing an example of research program–based restrictions on physician access to data—whose risk to patient privacy is negligible given their otherwise broad access to patient information—Dr. Murphy suggests that the certified trustworthiness of the recipient should be a component of access control. He goes on to note that this, coupled with appropriate de-identification and secure data storage, provides a balanced approach to security that better matches the expectations of the patient while facilitating access for approved data users.

Guidance for approaches to governing the digital health infrastructure can be drawn from examples of similar efforts. Harry Cayton of the National Information Governance Board (NIGB) for Health and Social Care in the United Kingdom describes the approach they have taken in dealing with information governance issues facing the National Health Service. Mr. Cayton details the role played by the NIGB as an independent statutory committee to advise the government on the use of patient-identifiable data for clinical audit and research. He describes their philosophy that information governance (or stewardship) is the responsibility of every organization involved and provides a list of principles developed by the committee to guide their work. Stating that the purpose of the NIGB is to deal with the "wicked questions" that arise around use of health information,

Mr. Cayton affirms that there is no right or wrong answer, only the best answer at the time. In conclusion he suggests that all governance systems need the same things: mechanisms for agreeing on and applying consistent principles, checks for the practicality of guidance given, consistent procedures, and credibility with stakeholders.

GOVERNANCE COORDINATION, NEEDS, AND OPTIONS

Laura Adams, M.S., R.N.
Rhode Island Quality Institute

Establishing a governance structure for the learning health system calls for an open exploration that allows for emergence of structures perhaps not yet conceived, but advanced by consideration of several key factors to make it an effective and responsive function. Some important elements to be considered in establishing such a structure include the source and scope of authority; mission, purpose, and primary goals; operating procedures; the framework for evaluation and continual improvement; and the funding mechanism. For the purposes of this paper, only the following elements will be explored: source and scope of authority; mission, purpose, and primary goals; and special considerations such as a proposed theoretical foundation.

In terms of the broad organization of governance, several forms can be considered. It could be a centralized organization, a distributed system with no identified "center," a hybrid model, or one with few similarities to existing structures. Similarly, it could be established as a governmental agency, a private entity, a public–private partnership, or even a loose association. The scope of the governance structure could be national, international, or a combination of geopolitical considerations. It could be a formal organization, a virtual group, or reflect elements of both. Finally, the members of the governing body could be limited to the "usual suspects," or include patients and consumers as well.

The source (or sources) of authority for the governance structure, as well as the scope of this authority, will also be primary considerations. There are several models that can be drawn on as the source of authority. First, it could receive a direct official mandate by governmental statute or regulation. Alternatively, the governing structure could be created by a trusted neutral entity where authority is conferred by those being governed or by a private entity that receives official designation or mandate and is regulated by a government agency.

Ethical and Legal Foundations

Once these broad considerations are determined, the scope of the governing body's authority should be succinctly enunciated in a statement of purpose that encompasses the various purposes and goals. An example of such as statement is:

> To foster data utility for the common good, cultivating a bond of trust with the public and between data-sharing entities to accelerate collaborative progress toward the creation of a learning healthcare system.

The mission statement draws on the guiding principles for governance that consist of durable statements that represent a set of values and guide decision making. Such principles will include, for example, transparency of the governance functions and activities, a reflection of its commitment to the common good, and overarching respect for, and an intent to, protect privacy. As we have learned from similar efforts, these guiding principles can conflict. It is, indeed, one of the primary purposes of the organization to balance these competing concerns during the governing process.

In such cases, it can be useful to apply a particular guiding theory in developing governance processes and to help resolve such conflicts. One such theory is complexity theory, which posits that simple rules guide complex behavior and accommodate continuous evolution in complex adaptive systems. Surprisingly, these simple rules, once identified and applied consistently, can produce desired outcomes in very complex systems. Another aspect of complexity theory includes the acceptance of paradox and tension as natural and even desirable if managed properly. An example of such is the coexistence of a principle of widespread access to data alongside a commitment to privacy protection. The theories of complex adaptive systems offers guidance in understanding the need to become comfortable with tension and paradox and advance new approaches that acknowledge the existence and value of tension and paradox. Another example of managing paradox and tension is "giving direction without giving directives," and maintaining authority without having control (Zimmerman et al., 1998).

An emerging governance structure for the learning health system must also specify structures and relationships with other relevant entities. The legal and ethical framework guiding the activities of the governing body needs to be determined. In addition, the question arises as to whether there is to be a single governing body or several and, if the latter, how the different bodies will relate to each other and coordinate their activities. Other important questions include: What is the relationship of the governance structure with other existing governing bodies at the local, national, and international level? What are the inclusion criteria and selection processes for determining who will have a formal role in governance?

Ensuring Privacy and Promoting Trust

Once the legal and ethical framework is determined, the real work of governance begins. Some of the pressing governance challenges for the learning healthcare system include the changing locus of research and the changing nature of privacy considerations. Critical data sources are moving beyond the traditional clinical settings of large healthcare networks and academic medical centers. New sources of data—ranging from those collected in ambulatory clinical environments to the ever-growing sources of patient-supplied data—are becoming increasingly central to research. The changing landscape of trust as it relates to such issues as privacy also presents challenges. Consequently, governance activities will need to regard the nature, foundations, and manifestations of trust. Current privacy concerns could diminish over time (as a result of new methods of protection), but they could also grow and severely impact achievement of the goals of a learning health system.

Governance must understand that context plays an important role as it relates to a number of issues, including privacy. One iconic image from the aftermath of Hurricane Katrina is the photo of the driveway of a physician in Mississippi strewn with the medical records of his patients drying in the sun after his office had flooded. Records from many other physicians and hospitals were destroyed. In light of this reality, the local health information exchange (HIE) had relatively few problems with consent issues as they related to electronic health records, as people saw the value in moving away from paper records. The situation was different in Rhode Island, where from the beginning of the process of development of a statewide HIE, there was no contextual crisis, but a deep commitment to consumer engagement and addressing privacy concerns. The process included nearly 18 months of intense work and broad engagement of the community in order to produce the state's privacy framework, which included the passage of legislation mandating the voluntary nature of participation, consumers' rights to have the data in the HIE, State governmental oversight of the HIE, restrictions on the uses of the data, and stiff penalties for those convicted of misuse. The primary motivation in this endeavor was to respect and regard the differing viewpoints while using consumer control as the paramount guiding principle. The result was a community-supported consent model, as well as a significant degree of community trust and ongoing inclusion in the development of other aspects of the HIE.

Conclusion

These examples illustrate some of the elements that need to be incorporated into the governance structure of the learning health system. This is a complex system, and governance will confront many challenges in establishing sustainable procedures to oversee the implementation of a large-scale health information system. By drawing on the successes and experience of existing programs, a new governance structure can be established that has the requisite authority and framework to build partnerships among various data sources, ensure data integrity, address privacy issues, and establish policies for proper data use, auditing, and enforcement. By incorporating the widest possible array of viewpoints from competing stakeholders, the system can engender trust, foster adherence to common data models and standards, and garner financial support—all necessary for a sustainable governance function.

CONSISTENCY AND RELIABILITY IN REPORTING FOR REGULATORS

Theresa Mullin, Ph.D.
Food and Drug Administration

The information systems being developed to support health care have the potential to address critical questions related to public health, health policy, and healthcare delivery. These questions include

- How quickly and how well can we detect and interpret new safety signals?
- How do we maximize the value of what is learned in clinical trials?
- How do we ensure that key healthcare system participants have appropriate access to the information needed to make the best-informed decisions?

Policy makers and researchers can use data collected from the emerging digital health infrastructure to address these questions, as well as many more. Development and widespread adoption of information standards is essential for the use of health data for knowledge generation and expedited application of new knowledge in clinical care.

Building a learning health system requires governance and stewardship at many levels, particularly in the area of standards development for the format and content of patient data. Stewardship is necessary to ensure that the locus of these efforts is driven by the needs of healthcare decision makers rather than technical advances. Governance is necessary to ensure that relevant stakeholders, including potential end users of the data, are included in the standards development process. Together, stewardship and governance processes must ensure that electronic health data are reliable, available, and research-ready.

Within a narrower scope, the Food and Drug Administration (FDA) is engaging relevant stakeholders in the development of data standards for clinical trials data. These standards will facilitate a more transparent and reliable review process for new products as well as advance the agency's public health mission by providing a platform for consistent, science-based regulatory decisions. Although premarket clinical research yields only a fraction of the volume of clinical data generated by care delivery, stakeholders such as the FDA, sponsors, and standard-setting bodies have an active interest in developing data standards for clinical and preclinical data. Advances from these efforts may be useful leverage to jump-start the development of the digital infrastructure for the broader learning health system.

Background

FDA is responsible for the review of new drug applications (NDAs). Since 1938, every new drug has been the subject of an approved NDA before it could be sold in the United States. Since 1962, an NDA has included all animal and human data and analyses of those data intended to support claims of efficacy and safety. The data gathered during the animal studies and human clinical trials of an investigational NDA become part of the NDA. Under law, no pertinent data may be omitted.

The NDA submission should provide enough information to permit FDA reviewers to make the following judgments:

- The drug has been shown to be effective for its proposed use or uses.
- Safety has been assessed by all reasonably applicable methods.
- The drug is safe for its intended use; that is, the benefits of the drug outweigh the risks for the doses being proposed for approval.
- The drug's proposed labeling (package insert) provides adequate directions for use and whether other postmarket risk management is required.
- The methods used in manufacturing the drug and the controls used to maintain the drug's quality are adequate to preserve the drug's identity, strength, quality, and purity.

FDA currently receives and reviews approximately 140 original NDAs (Figure 6-1) and over 3,700 NDA supplements per year. There are no regulatory or statutory standards for the format of data submissions in NDAs. While an increasing proportion of submissions are being submitted in electronic format, some applications still contain paper documents. For wholly electronic submissions, the submissions and associated raw clini-

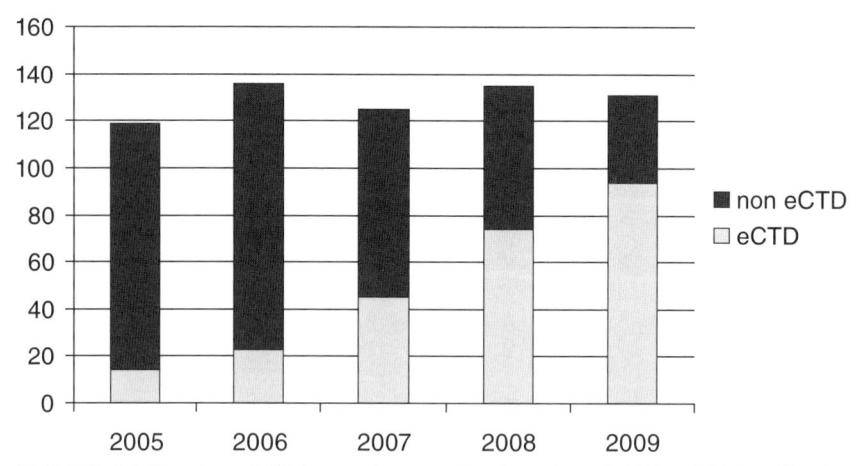

[Bar chart showing FDA new drug applications 2005-2009, with non eCTD and eCTD portions]

FIGURE 6-1 Number of FDA new drug applications from 2005 to 2009, indicating the proportion formatted according to the electronic Common Technical Document format.

cal data are large (the average size of an electronically submitted NDA is 10 gigabytes). Without a standardized structure, the application can be difficult to navigate. Fortunately, an increasing proportion of NDAs are being submitted electronically, and an increasing portion of the electronic submissions are being formatted according to the electronic Common Techical Document format.

The bigger struggle with electronic submissions is the format and content of the clinical and preclinical data included to support claims of efficacy and safety. Few submissions attempt to implement standards for the content of the subject-level data. The lack of standardized clinical data creates an impediment to rapid acquisition, analysis, and understanding of new drug performance. Furthermore, nonstandardized clinical data are difficult to integrate for analysis across datasets since each dataset requires formatting prior to integration. As a result, even a relatively straightforward review question can require extremely demanding data manipulations. This also increases the variability of reviews, and limits reviewers' ability to quickly address late-emerging issues.

Efforts to Address Data Challenges

To improve review efficiency and facilitate in-depth exploration of safety and efficacy questions, FDA is implementing a more systematic strategy for data standards development and adoption. FDA will need to address specific disease indications to identify the data elements and clinical terminology required for FDA reviewers to assess clinical benefits versus risks. A critical part of this effort involves FDA engagement with standards development organizations, other federal department and agencies, academic researchers, regulated industry, vendors, and others who will bring their data needs to the process.

Although this process is motivated by the FDA's own public health mission, addressing the agency's need for more standardized clinical data may provide leverage to support the development of other learning systems. Clinical data form a critical part of the content for records in the care setting, and the clinical data standards developed to meet FDA regulatory requirements can serve and support a transition to more standardized clinical data in electronic health records (EHRs). This would not only facilitate data analysis and enable learning from data generated in the healthcare system, but might also reduce the cost of clinical research and reduce the burden on healthcare providers for adverse event reporting. In the case of clinical research, an electronic case report form (the data collection tool for a clinical trial) might be automatically populated from an EHR that uses a specific data standard. With adverse event reporting, a standardized individual case safety report (the reporting form for adverse events) could also be automatically populated from the EHR. Pilots of these types of applications are already under way.

To fully benefit from the development of data standards for clinical data, FDA has identified the need to pursue data standards development collaboratively. FDA is including internal and external stakeholders in the development of standards for content, format, and exchange of electronic clinical data. Simultaneously, FDA will be developing regulatory policy changes that will outline new requirements for regulated industry, undertaking changes within FDA to gain significant business process improvements, and making technical infrastructure investments to ensure the capacity to do the advanced computing and data manipulations that standardized data would allow. Effective, continuing communication and stakeholder engagement will be critical in all of these endeavors, since all affected parties must be aware, involved, provide feedback, and be invested. As a practical consideration, sustained resources will also be necessary to ensure success.

Conclusions

Several general governance principles have emerged from FDA's experience to date, including

- The process must be open and inclusive of all stakeholders, respectful, transparent, and predictable.

- The standards, use policies, and formal requirements that result from the process must be practical, end-user oriented, cost-sensitive, and sustainable.

In summary, FDA's recent and ongoing work to develop health data standards is primarily driven by the agency's own public health mission and regulatory business needs. This work may also accelerate the readiness of clinical data standards for use in EHRs. Systems interoperability coupled with common data standards would facilitate data pooling to address questions across both premarket clinical research and postmarket clinical care. It would also enable more powerful and rapid application of data mining, semantic linking, meta-analysis, and other advanced methods intended to address continuing questions about the quality and effectiveness of therapeutic products. In a learning health system, a common language is the first requirement to facilitate widespread communication and knowledge sharing.

COMPLYING WITH PATIENT EXPECTATIONS FOR DATA DE-IDENTIFICATION

Shawn N. Murphy, M.D., Ph.D.
Partners HealthCare, Inc.

The use of patient data from electronic health record (EHR) systems can provide tremendous benefits to clinical research. However, the adequacies of measures to protect patient privacy while utilizing these records are constantly challenged. These challenges are rarely welcomed because they represent a seemingly endless set of technical constraints to be imposed upon our systems. But, could the answer to this situation not be a new technical solution but simply a more complete understanding of what the patients actually expect us to do to protect their privacy?

Patient Expectations

Overall, surveys have found that patients' opinions of how their data should be protected are on a continuum from the use of their health data where it may be distributed freely to a completely closed approach where it may hardly be used at all (Willison et al., 2007). Patients give several reasons for keeping their EHR data private. Some express a wish to control the purposes for which the data are used, although most patient surveys reflect a desire only to be informed of its uses. Others hope to avoid embarrassment with the revelation of medical information to people they know or will know in the future. Finally, there is a potential economic impact on the patient if insurance companies or employers obtain health data (Damschroder et al., 2007).

Meeting the patients' expectations for precautions to be taken to avoid embarrassment and economic loss is not the job of software tools, but the entire system. If one tries to describe the system for protecting medical records, we find it described as a method to restrict and determine the people allowed to view the data. A de-identification process that is appropriate for those allowed to view the data can be part of this system, but ultimately it is about restricting those who view the data. Patients will expect the entire system to work, and any valid approach needs to take this into consideration.

Limitations of Current De-Identification Protocols

Proper consideration of the needs of end users can determine the level of de-identification necessary. It is unrealistic to expect data to be properly de-identified for all audiences. Some of the algorithms developed will provide de-identification to line-item patient data to a degree known as k-level anonymity (Fischetti and Salazar, 1999; Sweeney, 2002). The number k represents the number of people's records that must be identical. If there are patient records that exceed this level of uniqueness, data values are removed from these patients' records until the records are no longer unique. Although superficially such methods seem like an adequate solution to the de-identification problem, such methods have proven to be subject to "reverse engineering," undoing the obfuscation (Dreiseitl et al., 2001). Furthermore (and somewhat obviously), they take out important attributes from the data (Ohno-Machado et al., 2001). De-identification methods are also quite actively used in "scrubbing" textual medical reports (Friedlin and McDonald, 2008; Uzuner et al., 2007). The patient names, dates, locations, and other potentially identifying information are removed by computer programs that search the text. These programs perform to various levels of accuracy, and involve trade-offs similar to those described above for structured data. The extent to which it can be assured that the data are de-identified and "unmatchable" to the original record is often dependent on removal of sentence structure, which is an important attribute of the data (Berman, 2003).

The failure of technology to offer a foolproof de-identification solution is not all that surprising. People are extremely resourceful and well accustomed to solving challenging problems. The bottom line is that the trust in who gets the data clearly needs to match the level of de-identification. If the receiver of the data is deemed to be unknown, then there is no amount of de-identification that can reliably protect the patient in all perpetuity unless the content is so simple and poor that it is rarely useful for clinical research.

A New Model for Protecting Health Data

It is possible to envision a better solution when one considers the two reasons patients are interested in preserving their privacy: embarrassment and economic risk. Patients expect the level of de-identification to comply with the risk, and the intentions of those who view the data to factor prominently into the risk. What we actually tend to see is that people who are extremely trustworthy with data and pose little risk of harm to the patient are restricted from data in illogical ways. For example, handling genomic data tends to be extremely restrictive. At Marshfield Clinic there is an enormous investment in a tissue bank of 20,000 consenting patients who get genotyped using the collected tissue. These genotypes are put together with de-identified data from their EHRs (McCarty and Wilke, 2010). The people who view the de-identified genomic data are not allowed to be the same people that have access to identified phenotypic data. This is due to the obvious potential that a person who can see both datasets could find a way to tie them both together. Since all the physicians at Marshfield Clinic must have access to the EHR, none of them are eligible to view these data. The result is that, although many are principal investigators of the studies, they cannot look at the data from their own study. In these cases, it seems highly unlikely that clinicians who are trusted with the lives of their patients, and see hundreds of patients' private information, really represent a risk to a patient's privacy.

The judgment used to manage a case such as the above should factor in the proper match of de-identification to the trustworthiness of its recipients. The trustworthiness of the recipients should not be taken for granted, but determined by a defined process. Criminal history checks, letters of reference, and credentialing systems have been used in many scenarios in society to perform an objective trust assessment. Ultimately, the ability to match trust to a data recipient should be a critical factor in all reviews of data distribution proposals. The greater the level of de-identification and the less the risk of economic harm and embarrassment, the less trustworthy the recipient needs to be.

Although an individual may be deemed trustworthy, technical competencies will vary. This factors into a third determinant of data privacy, the physical and policy platform upon which the data are to reside. The data must be protected so that they do not go beyond the recipients for whom they were intended. This leads to the concern of physically protecting the data, which will be implemented with a combination of policy and technology. At the University of California at San Francisco, there is a protected area inside a network firewall where data are kept and analyses are performed. People are encouraged to keep the data within the protected area by having legal coverage provided by the institution should the data be stolen from within the protected area. However, this approach requires a tremendous number of resources and limits the freedom of the individual to use "unsupported" software on privately funded platforms.

Other approaches, such as those used at Partners, put more responsibility upon the people who receive the data. A certain level of familiarity with security software and hardware platforms is assured by the necessity of taking a certified course. The data are then distributed behind a firewall in protected directories in an encrypted state, and the individuals manage their environments from this point. Protected network drives and computational resources are available for those who wish to use them—but it is not required—and private computational environments flourish behind the institutional firewall.

Conclusion

Data de-identification should not be considered a technical challenge, but rather a balance of three technical and human considerations: (1) techniques for de-identification, (2) the trustworthiness of the recipient, and (3) the physical security on which the data will reside. The first is indeed the way data can be changed to de-identify it, but the other two that should be balanced with this task are the trustworthiness of the data recipient and the physical security on which the data will reside. As an example, for a set of moderately sensitive de-identified text reports, it may only be possible to provide a 97% capability to truly scrub the identified data from the reports. In this case, the data will be authorized to be seen and shipped to the members of the community that are entrusted with this kind of identified data and have a reasonably secure location in which to place the data. Unlike the current scenario, the emphasis is not to keep the data within the entity, but to expose the data to trustworthy recipients in a physically secure environment. Intended use of the data is not factored in heavily to this algorithm, as it does not affect the risk to the patient.

The difference between this scenario and the current state is to consider every act of de-identification an achievement of balance between the level of data de-identification, the level of trustworthiness of the data recipients, and the level of security of the data location where it will reside. Although this will seem to make the process more complex, it is deemphasizing the institutional boundaries and uses of the data that can be equally complex and ambiguous. The principal merit of this recommendation is that it matches the expectations of the patient. They are entrusting us to "know their minds" and match the human expectations head on, rather than implement contrived polices that do not make them any more comfortable with the process. Answering patients' expectations with flawed technical de-identification approaches and legalistic restrictions will result in poor trust and a continuously changing set of technical and policy constraints from the community.

INFORMATION GOVERNANCE IN THE NATIONAL HEALTH SERVICE (UK)

Harry Cayton
National Information Governance Board for Health and Social Care (UK)

Information governance exists in the space between people and data. The legal and ethical framework for the public and private use of personal health information for care, clinical audit, management, and research in England has developed over time. The legal framework is both statutory—as set out in Data Protection Legislation and in the Human Rights Act—and based on legal precedent through the Common Law of England.

Ethical interpretations within the law are overseen at the local level by Caldicott Guardians, by clinical and research ethics committees, and nationally by the National Information Governance Board (NIGB). Of course information governance applies as importantly to paper records as it does to electronic systems. However, the introduction of a national electronic record system has presented new challenges to the application of both legal and ethical practice and required new applications of existing principles to ensure that information technology assists clinicians to provide better care. This short paper therefore deals primarily with the particular information governance issues facing the National Health Service (NHS) in England as electronic systems for gathering, storing, transmitting, and using patient data are developed.

NHS Connecting for Health

The NHS in England has been engaged in creating a health information and communication technology infrastructure since 2002. Initially known as the National Programme for IT and subsequently as NHS Connecting for Health, it has delivered growing interconnectedness of primary and secondary care records, a national personal demographics service using a unique identifier, nearly universal picture imaging and archiving system, a secure provider-to-provider network, a secure NHS e-mail system (NHSmail), e-prescribing and electronic transfer of prescriptions, electronic booking of appointments (Choose & Book), a summary care record, and a patient portal (HealthSpace). This ambitious program has been sometimes controversial and undoubtedly difficult—its benefits are not yet available across the NHS and its delivery is currently under review by the Coalition Government in the United Kingdom—but it has already achieved much.

The objectives of NHS Connecting for Health are

- Ready access to accurate, up-to-date patient information and a fast, reliable, and secure means of sending and receiving information.
- Streamlining clinical practice and smoother handovers of care, supporting multidisciplinary teamwork.
- Online decision support tools, easier access to best care pathways, and faster access to specialist opinions and diagnosis.
- Guidance on referral procedures and clear protocols for clinical investigations.
- More efficient referrals, alerts to conflicting medicines, and early detection of disease outbreaks.
- Reduced administration, paperwork, repetition, duplication, and bureaucracy.

Whatever is decided by the new government in relation to the implementation of the components of electronic health care, its commitment to "an information society" is explicit.

The National Information Governance Board for Health and Social Care

The NIGB is an independent statutory committee established by Act of Parliament in 2008. We advise the Secretary of State for Health on good practice in relation to information governance, specifically on the use of patient-identifiable data for clinical audit and research. The committee has 21 members, half nominated by national clinical and research bodies and half of them appointed from members of the public through advertisement and an independent public appointment system.

There are a number of ways you can define "information governance," but the NIGB used

> Information governance describes the structures, policies and practices which are used to ensure the confidentiality and security of records of patients and service users. Correctly developed and implemented it enables the appropriate and ethical use of information for the benefit of individuals and the public good. (Cayton, 2006)

The important word here is "enables." Privacy is a great enabler and we need to construct our thinking around this. It's also important to say that information governance in practice is the responsibility of each and every organization and data processor. The NIGB serves to advise, to support, and to develop standards and principles. Good information governance provides the framework of interoperability needed to be confident as professionals and as patients in sharing data with each other.

One of the most important things that the NIGB has done is establish a transparent set of principles. These are published, they are contestable, they are publicly viewable, and they set out the basis on which the NIGB approaches the problems (NIGB, 2008):

- People have personal interests and responsibilities.
- Informed consent and autonomy underpin health care.
- It is in people's interests to have safe accessible care, a sound research base, cost-effective well-managed services.
- Professionals must work within legal and professional frameworks.

We have also published two commitments to patients and the public: the NHS Care Record Guarantee and, more recently, a parallel document, the Social Care Record Guarantee. These set a framework for patients and service users, setting out what we will do with their data and how we will keep it safe. These two guarantees allow both professionals and service users to feel confident about sharing data. The NHS Care Record Guarantee states "this guarantee is our commitment that we will use records about you in ways that respect your rights and promote your health and well-being" (NIGB, 2010). Public trust is an absolutely essential building block of what the NIGB does. We have transparency in all of our business—all of our papers and minutes are published on our website, and we have regular meetings with patient and professional organizations.

Wicked Questions

If there were not wicked questions, there would be no need for the NIGB. Sometimes our principles are in conflict—sometimes the public good, and the individual good are in conflict—that's the point. These are the issues that the NIGB must resolve, whether it is a discussion about research or a discussion about how much a clinician respects a child's wishes that their parents do not know something intimate and personal. For these questions, there is no right or wrong answer, just the best answer at the time. That means that in applying our principles we can change our view if we keep consistent with the principles, but the circumstances or the information changes.

A few concrete examples illustrate the type of questions the NIGB has dealt with. We advised the Chief Medical Officer, giving him formal legal cover so that he could collect personal data from patients about swine flu in a way that did not breach either the law or best practice. We have done work on care records for children and young people dealing with difficult issues about confidentiality and security. We have produced a cartoon version of the Care Record Guarantee for children under 12 explaining to them what happens with their medical records. We have produced guidance on access to clinical information by social workers, and on how to correct or amend records (suppressing records that are wrong as a means of resolving disputes between clinicians and patients about what is in the record).

The Legal Use of Identifiable Data for Research

The NIGB advises the Secretary of State for Health to give researchers permission to use patient-identifiable data without consent. To gain permission, there are two tests applications must pass: (1) getting consent must be unduly onerous, and (2) the research has to be sufficiently important and in the public interest. Quite often we find that researchers can obtain consent and we are able to advise them how to do so. For example, one group wanted to do research looking at the quality of care of children who had recently died. They thought it would be too difficult to get consent from their parents. We were able to put them in touch with children's hospices who had experience of dealing sensitively with parents and in obtaining consent in these circumstances.

Conclusion

The model of a governance and oversight committee such as the NIGB is only one way of supporting legal, ethical, and confidential data sharing. However we have learned a lot from it. Information governance exists in the space between people and technology. Technology is not the solution; people are the solution. Getting people to use the technology wisely, ethically, and effectively is essential for professional confidence and public trust. All governance systems need the same things: a mechanism for agreeing on and applying consistent principles, checks to ensure that the guidance that you give people is practicable, procedures for promoting consistency, and creditability with both the public and professionals.

REFERENCES

Berman, J. J. 2003. Concept-match medical data scrubbing. How pathology text can be used in research. *Archives of Pathology and Laboratory Medicine* 127(6):680-686.

Cayton, H. 2006. *Information governance in the Department of Health and the NHS.* http://www.nigb.nhs.uk/about/publications/igreview.pdf (accessed September 10, 2010).

Damschroder, L. J., J. L. Pritts, M. A. Neblo, R. J. Kalarickal, J. W. Creswell, and R. A. Hayward. 2007. Patients, privacy and trust: Patients' willingness to allow researchers to access their medical records. *Social Science and Medicine* 64(1):223-235.

Dreiseitl, S., S. Vinterbo, and L. Ohno-Machado. 2001. Disambiguation data: Extracting information from anonymized sources. *Proceedings of the AMIA Symposium* 144-148.
Fischetti, M., and J. J. Salazar. 1999. Models and algorithms for the 2-dimensional cell suppression problem in statistical disclosure control. *Mathematical Programming* 84(2):283-312.
Friedlin, F. J., and C. J. McDonald. 2008. A software tool for removing patient identifying information from clinical documents. *Journal of the American Medical Informatics Association* 15(5):601-610.
McCarty, C. A., and R. A. Wilke. 2010. Biobanking and pharmacogenomics. *Pharmacogenomics* 11(5):637-641.
NIGB (National Information Governance Board) (UK). 2008. *The principles of the National Information Governance Board.* http://www.nigb.nhs.uk/about/meetings/principles.pdf (accessed September 10, 2010).
———. 2010. *The NHS care record guarantee.* http://www.nigb.nhs.uk/guarantee (accessed September 10, 2010).
Ohno-Machado, L., S. A. Vinterbo, and S. Dreiseitl. 2001. Effects of data anonymization by cell suppression on descriptive statistics and predictive modeling performance. *Proceedings of the AMIA Symposium* 503-507.
Sweeney, L. 2002. k-anonymity: A model for protecting privacy. *International Journal of Uncertainty, Fuzziness and Knowledge-Based Systems* 10(5):557-570.
Uzuner, O., Y. Luo, and P. Szolovits. 2007. Evaluating the state-of-the-art in automatic de-identification. *Journal of the American Medical Informatics Association* 14(5):550-563.
Willison, D. J., L. Schwartz, J. Abelson, C. Charles, M. Swinton, D. Northrup, and L. Thabane. 2007. Alternatives to project-specific consent for access to personal information for health research: What is the opinion of the Canadian public? *Journal of the American Medical Informatics Association* 14(6):706-712.
Zimmerman, B., C. Lindberg, and P. E. Plsek. 1998. *Edgeware: Insights from complexity science for health care leaders.* Irving, TX: VHA Inc.

7

Perspectives on Innovation

INTRODUCTION

Health information technology (HIT) is a rapidly developing field propelled by continual innovation. Participants in this session were invited to give informal remarks based on their observations of the workshop as well as personal experiences. These comments are summarized briefly in this chapter. The papers point to the need for novel approaches to the aggregation of health data to improve population health, offer observations on challenges and opportunities given the current state of HIT, and provide perspective on the opportunities afforded by the vast quantities of health and health-related information collected by individuals and available on the web.

Drawing from the assertion that population health is more than the aggregation of individual disease and, therefore, an understanding that population health cannot simply be gleaned by aggregating patient care data, Population and Public Health Information Services' Daniel Friedman advocates for the creation of a U.S. population health record. He emphasizes that while the United States has large amounts of publicly accessible population-level disease-related data, challenges for population health include a lack of that same level of granularity for functional status and well-being as well as problems of data integration and integrity. In order to address these issues he proposes the establishment of a single source of population health data backed by an overarching data model and theoretical framework. Data would be drawn from a number of different sources including those not typically integrated with clinical data, such as environmental sampling and census data.

In her remarks Molly Coye, formerly from the Public Health Institute (now the University of California, Los Angeles), identifies what she sees as three areas of opportunity for HIT innovation. Citing the need to improve the current state of clinical decision support she suggests areas where innovation could help meet this goal: how to recognize and deal with incorrect or missing data, integration of a single patient's data from multiple sources, and how to turn data into clinical guidance. Dr. Coye cites the need for research to be integrated into care processes and for evidence generated to be fed back in a continuous, seamless process that supports informed, shared decision making. Lastly, she points to the movement of healthcare delivery to integrated models—such as accountable care organizations—which increase the need for remote data collection, diagnosis, consultation, and treatment. Dr. Coye concludes by stressing that many of these challenges are social rather than technical in nature, and therefore successful approaches will need to take into account the complex character of these systems.

The growing prevalence of personal information ecologies provides the context for the remarks made by the Institute of the Future's Michael Liebhold. He notes that these ecologies are composed of digital artifacts not only related to health and fitness, but also to social activities, media use, and even civic life. Mr. Liebhold observes that citizens are ready and willing to collect and share their health information and, with the encouragement of industry and employers, to become more actively involved in their own health. However, effectively integrating information from all of these sources in a meaningful way presents a formidable challenge. Technologies such as those that underlie the semantic web hold much promise, but still face challenges, especially in the areas of privacy and security. Looking to the future, Mr. Leibhold notes the need for methods to curate web-based health information, for interoperable health app stores, and for the development of a web of linked, open healthcare information and knowledge interoperability.

CONCEPTUALIZING A U.S. POPULATION HEALTH RECORD

Daniel J. Friedman, Ph.D.
Population and Public Health Information Services

This paper presents a concept for a U.S. population health record (PopHR), an idea initially presented in a recent article coauthored with Gib Parrish (Friedman and Parrish, 2010). Before presenting the concept of a PopHR, it is necessary to define population health. Our definition is the level and distribution of disease, functional status, and well-being of a population. This definition focuses on (a) functional status and well-being as well as disease; and (b) the level and distribution of each, allowing for knowledge of disparities and equity.

Based on this definition, it becomes equally important to be explicit about what constitutes a population. We use the definition: all of the inhabitants of a given country or area taken together. In this definition, an area can be a province, state, neighborhood, city, or town and can include groups within the overall geography such as demographically bounded groups.

Health care is just one of many influences on population health. Influences such as the context of the population (natural environment, cultural context, political context) and community attributes (social and collective lifestyles, the environment, economic structures, education) all have a bearing on the health of a population. Simply put, population health is more than the aggregation of individual disease. As a result, the aggregation of patient care data provides only an incomplete understanding of population health.

Healthcare Data and Population Health

The United States has many blessings when it comes to population health data. We have rich disease-level data which allow researchers to look at causes of death, birth rates, and cancer prevalence down to the census track. However, we also have some burdens—what you cannot see at the local level is functional status and well-being. The level of granularity we have for causes of death does not exist for depression, disabling lower-back injuries, etc.

We are also blessed by a large amount of publicly accessible, web-based population-level disease data. Currently, roughly 28 states have web-based systems that provide public access to population health data. These systems vary in quality, but some are quite exceptional—employing sophisticated statistics and providing access to two dozen or more datasets. Additionally, the Department of Health and Human Services (HHS) has roughly two dozen web-based population health data systems that are publicly accessible. With so many different websites, datasets are often duplicative, resulting in different definitions for statistical measures or different definitions for the same variables.

The Population Health Record

These burdens could all be solved—not to mention the current benefits enhanced—if there was a single easily accessible source with an overarching data model and theoretical framework. This is the motivation behind a PopHR. The PopHR focuses on populations, not on individuals; it focuses on population health as defined above; and it focuses on the influences on population health enumerated above. Thus, we define PopHR as a repository of statistics, measures, and indicators regarding the state of and influences on the health of a defined population, in computer-processable form, stored and transmitted securely, and accessible by multiple authorized users.

Framework

Successfully developing a PopHR will require an explicit population health framework that includes a schematic representation of factors that will potentially influence population health. There are many different versions of this type of framework, with an example shown in Figure 7-1. Building the model around *population health* and not the *individual health* of members of the population will remedy gaps in our current knowledge such as functional status and well-being.

Information Model and Content

A logical and agreed upon information model will also be necessary for achieving a PopHR. As opposed to an individualized population health records system absent standards, adopting a standardized and agreed upon information model will reduce the burden of overlapping and inconsis-

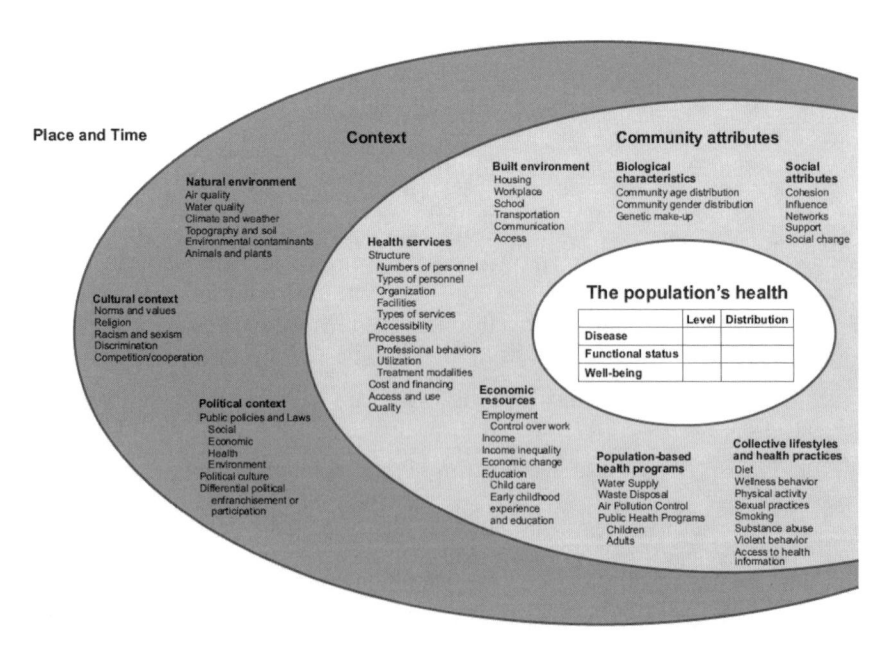

FIGURE 7-1 Influences on population health.
SOURCE: Friedman et al. (2005).

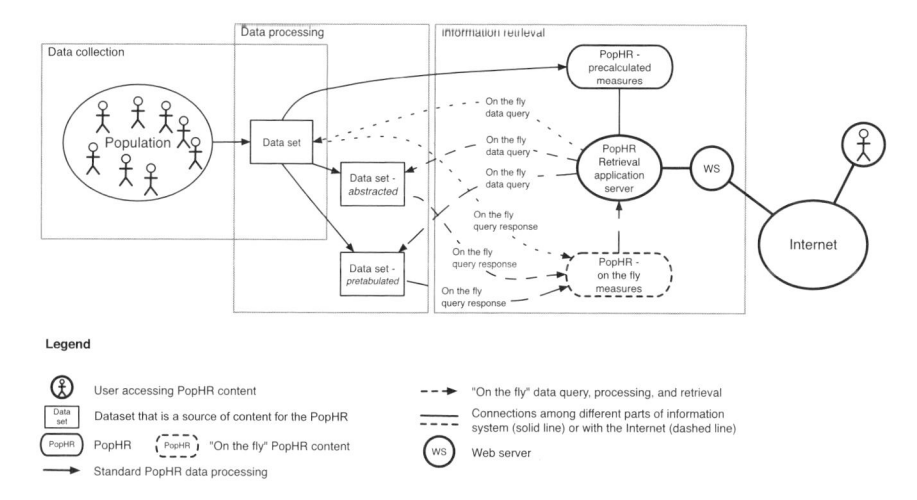

FIGURE 7-2 PopHR and PopHR system showing collection, processing, and retrieval of information content from a PopHR.
SOURCE: Friedman and Parrish (2010).

tently defined variables. A good example of such a model is the Australian Institute for Health and Welfare National Data Model and its more recent metadata directory called Meteor.[1] It is also important to consider information content. The PopHR would need to include information on health, and the determinants of health, from existing data sources such as ongoing population surveys; public health surveillance systems; environmental sampling; Medicare claims; and population census. These data sources could be either geographically or individually based, but would be aggregated to the population level in the PopHR—a process enabled by a standardized information model.

Conceptual Model

Figure 7-2 presents a conceptual model of a PopHR. Data for the population are collected using various methods—surveys, environmental monitoring, and abstraction of health records—and compiled and processed to form a population dataset. The dataset is then analyzed to produce a set of population health measures which are stored in the PopHR for later retrieval. To increase retrieval efficiency and speed, the PopHR system might use intermediate datasets in which one or more large datasets would be reduced in size by either selectively removing infrequently used data elements to form

---

[1] See www.aihw.gov.au/publications/hwi/nhimv2 (accessed March 2, 2011).

TABLE 7-1 Possible System Architectures for a Population Health Record (PopHR)

Model	Information Storage	Information Retrieval
1	Centralized	Centralized
2	Distributed	Centralized
3	Centralized	Distributed
4	Distributed	Distributed

SOURCE: Friedman and Parrish (2010).

an "abstracted dataset," or pre-tabulating and indexing the dataset on frequently retrieved data elements. In response to a user query of the PopHR, the PopHR system would retrieve information from either the PopHR with precalculated measures (a standard PopHR information retrieval), or one or more primary or intermediate datasets (an "on the fly" PopHR information retrieval). For some queries a combination of standard and "on the fly" retrievals might be necessary. The retrieved information would then be synthesized into a response and communicated to the user via the Internet.

Implementation

There are various types of system architectures that could be employed in a PopHR system (Table 7-1). In order to successfully implement a PopHR it will be useful to start with the most practical model, and then build to the nimblest and most versatile. In the near term (1 to 5 years) efforts should focus on developing a population health framework and logical information model as well as implementing Model 1 with core functionalities. Doing so will require leveraging the existing HHS web-based query systems. Efforts should be made to inventory the existing work and develop a logical information model and metadata directory for these datasets.

As time progresses, efforts can be made to shift to more advanced models—focusing first on developing and implementing Model 3 with core and enhanced functionalities, and then on doing the same for Model 4.

ACCELERATING INNOVATION OUTSIDE THE PRIVATE SECTOR

Molly J. Coye, M.D., M.P.H.
Public Health Institute (formerly)
University of California, Los Angeles

Currently there is tremendous innovation going on in the private sector, but we could be doing more to foster innovation in the public sector and at academic centers. This paper will address three challenges—which are not so much daunting as exciting—facing the healthcare system that can become loci for innovative projects. The first is decision support. Currently, we are very far away from the goal of not just producing an array of data but actually producing information that leads to change in the behavior of clinicians and patients. The second concerns consolidating a health information technology (HIT)-supported national knowledge base with parallel efforts in effectiveness research. This too is far off, but the Patient-Centered Outcomes Research Institute has the potential to help drive innovation. Finally, we will be undertaking these efforts to build the digital infrastructure amidst pivotal transformations in delivery of health care. While this certainly provides opportunities, we must also remain conscious of the context of the Patient Protection and Affordable Care Act (ACA) if these efforts are to be successful.

Decision Support

Decision support centers are turning healthcare data into healthcare information. The limitations of our current decision support systems have been very well described: they are klugy, physician-centric, and many physicians resist using them—often for good reason. Innovation in decision support will need to move through three stages: avoiding bad decisions caused by faulty or nonexistent data, integrating streams of data to provide optimally accurate and specific data, and supporting better decisions with clinical guidance. Many organizations are actively involved in work on all of these stages, with considerable progress being made on the first. However, the second—to have data about the same patient coming from multiple locations so that decisions are based on the most accurate and specific data—is proving more elusive and will likely remain a challenge for some time. While the meaningful use rules are encouraging progress, the third stage will require that every point-of-care decision is informed not by data, but by clinical guidance—again, turning data into information.

In order to activate innovation in decision support we need to do more to stimulate the development of small, close-to-the-ground decision support tools that will actually be used by physicians. To achieve this, it is necessary to develop explicit clinical performance benchmarks in consultation with physicians. Furthermore, it will be necessary to collaborate in design with employers and health plans to ensure that there is a business case for use. Unless providers who use these systems are rewarded for doing so, widespread adoption will be hard to achieve.

Comparative Effectiveness Research

Attempting to integrate HIT and comparative effectiveness research carries with it the unfortunate consequence of creating disillusionment. If we are able to build transparency about how little evidence base there is for much of our decisions into clinical decision support—and are transparent to patients on this risk, too—we risk considerable disillusionment. This could be ameliorated by integrating clinical research with the care encounter. Bill Press has outlined a possible approach to this situation (Press, 2009). In his model, when a patient comes to see a physician, the quality of evidence for different diagnostic and therapeutic options is arrayed as probabilities—the probability the diagnostic option will reveal, or the therapeutic option will resolve, the problem at hand. When the patient makes a decision—which, it should be noted, will be a shared and informed decision—the clinical encounter becomes part of a rolling clinical trial. As a result, the probabilities evolve as the results of individual encounters and treatments are recorded and reported. The result is a learning system, where evidence is continually generated and refined, and then fed back to clinicians and patients to promote informed, shared decision making.

The level of patient-fostered engagement in this approach is crucial to promote innovation. If patients can be convinced of the benefits in such a system they will not only be eager to participate, but will begin to demand such capabilities from the healthcare system. With consumer demand we might be able to accelerate work on the technical, political, social, and economic dimensions of facilitating the rich exchange of data necessary to enable such a system. This is an area of opportunity for academic medical centers (because of informatics resources) and large medical groups (because of capitated care and large databases) to design closed-loop learning systems that continually utilize data to evolve clinical understanding. Developing and refining this concept in small cases will begin to demonstrate the utility to the general public, stimulating larger efforts.

Remote Models of Care

The third challenge facing health care is the reconfiguration of the health delivery system toward integrated care models (such as accountable care organizations) as a result of ACA. One of the defining characteristics of these new delivery system models will be the remote nature of care. Functions, not just data, will be liberated and redistributed. Furthermore, we will likely see the rise of long-distance—or remote—diagnosis, consultation, and treatment. This will require advanced health information exchange between and among organizations. The evolution will be a fluid process, but it will also be rough. Considerable time and resources are being invested in the idea of distributed health information exchange, but this issue will continue to be a continual source of difficulty.

The challenge will not be so much technical, as it will be political and economic. Consequently, the Office of the National Coordinator for Health Information Technology (ONC) should partner with the most advanced systems using telemedicine, tele-ICU, tele-emergency and telehealth technologies to understand how the structures, regulations, and processes that we are setting up now facilitate, or complicate, delivering networked care.

Conclusion

Addressing these challenges will test the limits of data integration with electronic health records that live inside separate enterprises and support learning and the dissemination of principles gleaned from data exchange. Ultimately, successful approaches to these challenges will emerge from treating them as complex systems. Solutions will not involve rules and laws, but will be centered on processes for solving complex and evolving problems.

COMBINATORIAL INNOVATION IN HEALTH INFORMATION TECHNOLOGY

Michael Liebhold
Institute for the Future

The topic of this paper—combinatorial innovation—comes from a concept introduced by Google chief economist Hal Varian. He postulates that there is currently enough innovation available such that we do not have to invent anything new to create disruption. This paper will begin by addressing many elements that already exist today, but that in combination can be disruptive, and then move on to a discussion of work going on at the Institute for the Future as well as some priorities moving forward.

Capturing Personal Health Data

Discussions on the digital infrastructure for a learning health system tend to focus on clinical information ecologies and the notion of standardized and interoperable electronic health records (EHRs). Much attention, not to mention recent legislation, concerns the linkage between evidence-based science and an interoperable EHR, but this is really only half the picture. Something that is commonly ignored is personal information ecologies.

Citizens are constantly creating digital artifacts. These are not just health and fitness related, but come from their social life, shopping, media use, vocational activities, and civic life. There is enormous interest—not just in the healthcare community but across communities—in managing these digital artifacts. Doing so will necessitate a holistic program which, fortunately, has been acknowledged by the current administration. The recently released a multiagency recommendation for a national identity and security[2] that advocates for a federated model for identity management as an important step in harnessing the potential of these data.

When discussing patient engagement in health information technology, many argue that only a minority of people will collect their data and want to use it in their personal health record. Our indicators suggest that this is not going to be the case. In the Silicon Valley, leading companies like Intel, Cisco, Google, and others are providing real incentives for people to get involved with their own data—body mass index, blood pressure, cholesterol—and take control over their own health. This is viewed as a corporate health issue, making it reasonable to assume that it can spread to populations at large.

There are also growing stores of health-related information that many people do not normally consider. For example, since many people now carry GPS devices in their pocket, we can mine those data and forecast kinds of behaviors and activities in particular locations. Furthermore, some individuals are beginning to wear sensors—not just for their health but for fitness. In fact, there is a lot of new research in the area of using mobile devices as hubs for a wearable network of sensors.

Making Sense of Captured Data

All of these new technologies generate a surplus of information. We do not need all of the information, just the right information. Consequently, we need to combine or orchestrate information, devices, and infrastructure on a continual, real-time basis to deliver the right information to the patient/clinician at the right time. Fortunately, we are well on our way to doing so. In online social networks, we are seeing the rise of social graphs—a schematic that visualizes the kinds of linkages and relationships between people on a dynamic and real-time basis. This technique is based on a very common semantic web framework called Resource Description Framework (RDF), a simple grammar for describing relationships in terms of the subject, predicate, and object.

RDF is also the basis for almost all semantic web applications used for health information exchange. Soon, we will have a population of 500 million people who have a semantic web description of their relationships,

---

[2] See http://www.whitehouse.gov/blog/2010/06/25/national-strategy-trusted-identities-cyberspace (accessed March 3, 2010).

opening up unprecedented opportunities for data mining and sophisticated inference on a real-time and continuous basis. Of course there are problems with privacy and security if you put your data out there in a universal infrastructure—and there is a lot of work to be done on that front—but the opportunity is immense.

Institute for the Future

In this new climate there are several major contact points that need to be kept in mind: the relationship of our personal health information and the public health commons, the relationship of our personal information and contextual health information, the relationship of our clinical information and contextual health, and the relationship of the scientific evidence base with the clinical information. All of these pairs of relationships have to be explored as a coherent system, and at the Institute for the Future we are looking at what can be achieved with massive computing capability and an abundance of rich data.[3]

The examples discussed above are the types of technologies our teams have been working with—most recently in a project called Healthcare 2020—to develop tools for precise clinical health information and adaptive health coaching. The result would be that your mobile device would know, for example, that you are not supposed to drink and therefore advise you against going to a bar. Similarly, if you are a diabetic it could coax you to stay away from McDonald's and, instead, go for a run. With technologies like these we can optimize our health spans, not just prevent morbid conditions.

Priorities Moving Forward

As this field continues to grow, there will need to be a certification process for curating public health information on the web. With so many individuals getting health information on the web from dubious sources, there is a new stewardship role that has to be fulfilled. The government could take a leadership position and come up with standards to certify aggregators and curators of information on the web. Furthermore, the federal government can prime the pump by opening an interoperable health app store, providing tools for consumers to collect, report, generate, and analyze their health, behavioral, dietary, and fitness data. Finally, as these concepts are still in development, support for the development of a deep healthcare web of linked open data and open frameworks for knowledge interoperability, the roles and practices for real-time sensor data, and re-

---

[3] For more information, see http://www.iftf.org/health (accessed March 3, 2011).

search on therapeutic health information patterns are all needed if we are to harness the power of digital information for improvements in health and health care.

REFERENCES

Friedman, D. J., and R. G. Parrish. 2010. The population health record: Concepts, definition, design, and implementation. *Journal of the American Medical Informatics Association* 17(4):359-366.

Friedman, D. J., E. L. Hunter, and R. G. Parrish. 2005. *Health statistics: Shaping policy and practice to improve the population's health.* New York: Oxford University Press.

Press, W. H. 2009. Bandit solutions provide unified ethical models for randomized clinical trials and comparative effectiveness research. *Proceedings of the National Academy of Sciences* 106(52):22387-22392.

8

Fostering the Global Dimension of the Health Data Trust

INTRODUCTION

The ability to draw broadly from anywhere across the globe to provide relevant insights for health and healthcare improvement is a long-term goal for the learning health system. Meanwhile, the ability to learn from the experiences of other countries and to apply health information technology (HIT) for biosurveillance can actively facilitate progress toward this and other goals. This chapter reviews several activities relevant to exploring the global dimension of the digital infrastructure for a learning health system.

In his paper, Brendan Delaney from Kings College London describes the TRANSFoRm project. TRANSFoRm, a European Union (EU) effort to develop a learning health system driven with HIT, has been designed based on carefully chosen clinical use cases and is aimed at improving patient safety as well as supporting and accelerating clinical research. Dr. Delaney outlines several of the challenges that have arisen such as system interoperability, a need for advanced functionalities, and the support of knowledge translation. He also describes several techniques being employed to address these challenges, including clinical research information models, service-based approaches to semantic interoperability and data standards, detailed clinical data element representations built on archetypes, and an effort to prioritize electronic health record (EHR) and workflow integration in the development of clinical decision support systems that are designed to capture and present fine-grained clinical diagnostic cues.

Drawing from his involvement with SHARE, an EU-funded project to define the path toward greater implementation of grid computing approaches to health, Tony Solomonides, from the University of the West of England, discusses his current work to automate policy and regulatory compliance to allow health information sharing. He describes the implementation of attribute-based access controls to ensure enforcement of privacy obligations which—due to variations in their interpretation between EU countries—require a logic-based computed approach.

HIT holds great promise to increase quality and improve patient safety in developing and transitional countries. Harvard University's Ashish Jha describes how a dearth of reliable information has impeded efforts to better understand and design solutions to higher rates of adverse event–associated morbidity in developing countries, as well as obtain an accurate calculation of global disease burden. Dr. Jha describes an effort by the World Health Organization to maximize the impact of HIT in resource-poor settings through the development of a minimum dataset that would allow for systematic data collection to address safety issues.

David Buckeridge and John Brownstein from McGill University describe how HIT is enabling dramatic changes in domestic and international infectious disease surveillance. Detailing how the digital infrastructure can enhance existing systems through the use of automation and decision support, the authors also address novel approaches to surveillance enabled by recent informatics innovations. Using the DiSTRIBuTE project as an example of innovations in syndromic surveillance that drastically improve coverage and speed, they call for a renewed science of disease surveillance that embraces information technology as well as the potentially disruptive changes it brings to improve disease control.

TRANSFoRm: TRANSLATIONAL MEDICINE AND PATIENT SAFETY IN EUROPE

Brendan Delaney, M.D.
King's College London

The underlying concept of TRANSFoRm is to develop a "rapid learning healthcare system" driven by advanced computational infrastructure that can improve both patient safety and the conduct and volume of clinical research in Europe.

The European Union (EU) policy framework for information society and media, identifies e-health as one of the principal areas where advances in information and communications technology (ICT) can create better quality of life for Europe's citizens (Europe's Information Society, 2009). ICT has important roles in communication, decision making, monitoring, and learning in the healthcare setting. TRANSFoRm recognizes the need to advance the underpinning information and computer science to address these issues in a European and international context.

The Challenge of Interoperability

Providing interoperability between different clinical systems (which span national boundaries) and integrating those systems with the research enterprise lies at the heart of the eHealth Action Plan (Iakovidis and Purcarea, 2008). In both domains fragmentation of records and proprietary systems that do not adhere to uniform standards are as much of a challenge as the legal and ethical issues that complicate access to clinical data for researchers (Delaney, 2008). However, significant advances in international standards and in computational technology to support interoperability offer a way to overcome these challenges. Furthermore, advances in the understanding of clinical judgment and decision making—as well as the ways of supporting them via ICT—can inform the design of more "intelligent"electronic health record (EHR) systems.

Interoperability of data is underpinned by shared concepts and a common terminology (or at least an agreed and maintained mapping between terminologies). In research, interoperability of concepts between domains is promoted by the Biomedical Research Integrated Domain Group (BRIDG) Model (Fridsma et al., 2008). In primary care, the Primary Care Research Object Model defines the necessary domain-specific data classes, mapped to BRIDG (Speedie et al., 2008). In addition to terminologies, the system needs to enable multilanguage representations of the clinical terms, which is particularly important from an EU perspective.

However, simply providing a mechanism for the high-level interoperability of data will not provide sufficient functionality for a learning health system. System integration and shared detailed clinical data representations are also required. The system needs to have a common business model with a shared model of processes driven by a suite of open source middleware. Further, the integration of systems requires a much deeper level of interoperability than simple "diagnosis." Although SNOMED-CT has an underlying classification and allows for the concatenation of terms as well as representing diagnostic concepts such as clinical signs, it is probably not rich enough to represent all the symptoms and signs required for a diagnosis. Furthermore, these concepts need to be linked in an ontology rather than just a classification.

Building a Learning Health System

The single richest source of routine healthcare data lies within the records of Europe's general practitioners. Primary care providers are responsible for first contact, continuing, and generalist care of the entire population from birth to death (Schade et al., 2006). Any project that aims to comprehensively support the integration of clinical and research data should begin with primary care. In addition, even in countries where general practitioners do not fulfill a "gatekeeper" function—controlling access to specialist services—the quality of initial diagnosis at the primary care level determines much of the future course for an individual patient. In order to support patient safety in both clinical and research settings, significant ICT challenges need to be overcome in the areas of interoperability, common standards for data integration, data presentation, recording, scalability, and security (Ohmann and Kuchinke, 2009).

To explore these issues in more depth, it is useful to consider a list of requirements for a learning health system:

1. Supports complex queries of existing data, distributed and with support for various mapped terminologies.
2. Supports real-time recruitment of subjects with workflow-integrated prompts based on reason for encounter or any other data item within the clinical encounter.
3. Supports real-time prompts for data or sample collection based on data items within the clinical encounter.
4. Supports jointly controlled data entry into research and clinical records.
5. Supports real-time diagnostic and therapeutic decision support.
6. Supports all relevant requirements of data privacy, consent, and security.
7. Supports full audit and provenance of data.

To support this level of functionality a sharing of concepts at the very deepest level is required. The international standard CEN/ISO 13606 supports the use of archetypes (Kalra et al., 2005). Archetypes are computable expressions of a domain content model in the form of structured constraint statements based on a reference information model. They are often encapsulated together in templates, sit between lower level knowledge resources and production systems, and are independent of the interface and system. The latter is essential to the development of a sustainable business model whereby core shared work on archetypes can be deployed via a variety of commercial EHR systems.

Efficient support of knowledge translation is the final piece in the jigsaw. While decision support systems for management, quality improvement, and prescribing have all been shown to be effective, no system for diagnostic decision support has been positively evaluated or widely deployed (Garg et al., 2005). The principal reason for this is the failure of clinicians to use the systems routinely. Not only do they not integrate seamlessly with the EHR—for the technical reasons described above—but they have been developed without an understanding of the cognitive workflow involved in diagnosis. Much recent work in the field of medical decision making indicates that there may be specific points within the diagnostic process where decision support, in the form of alerts or prompts, may be effective. Accurate diagnosis has been shown to be related to the acquisition and interpretation of critical clinical cues. This process should be amenable to support by a well-specified ontology of diagnostic cues (Kostopoulou et al., 2008). In order for this to be achieved, it is necessary to provide an EHR interface that readily supports the capture and presentation of fine-grained clinical diagnostic cues. Given that "failure to diagnose promptly" is the single most common cause of litigation against primary care physicians, detailed justification of a diagnosis—richly recorded and linked to a knowledge base—will be one means by which clinicians may reduce the risk of litigation while improving patient care (Singh et al., 2007).

The TRANSFoRm Project

International cooperation in this area is essential. Working with and extending international standards for the representation of data and machine-readable clinical trial protocols, archetypes, and terminology services require international consensus and models of shared ownership. In addition, the market within which EHR systems are developed needs to be opened up to allow for widespread adoption of innovative user interfaces, decision support, terminology, and archetype services, and the export and linkage of data. The restriction of access to EHR data and systems is anticompetitive and restricts innovation in this field.

TRANSFoRm (Figure 8-1) brings together a highly multidisciplinary consortium where three carefully chosen clinical "use cases" will drive, evaluate, and validate the approach to the ICT challenges. The project will build on existing international work in clinical trial information models (BRIDG and the Primary Care Research Object Model), service-based approaches to semantic interoperability and data standards (ISO11179 and controlled vocabulary), data discovery, machine learning, and EHRs based on open standards (CEN/ISO 13606). We will extend this work to interact with individual EHR systems as well as operate within the consultation itself, providing diagnostic support as well as support for the identification and follow-up of subjects for research. The approach to system design will be modular and standards based—providing services via a distributed architecture—and will be tightly linked with the user community. Four years of development and testing will end with a fifth year dedicated to summative validation of the project deliverables in the primary care setting.

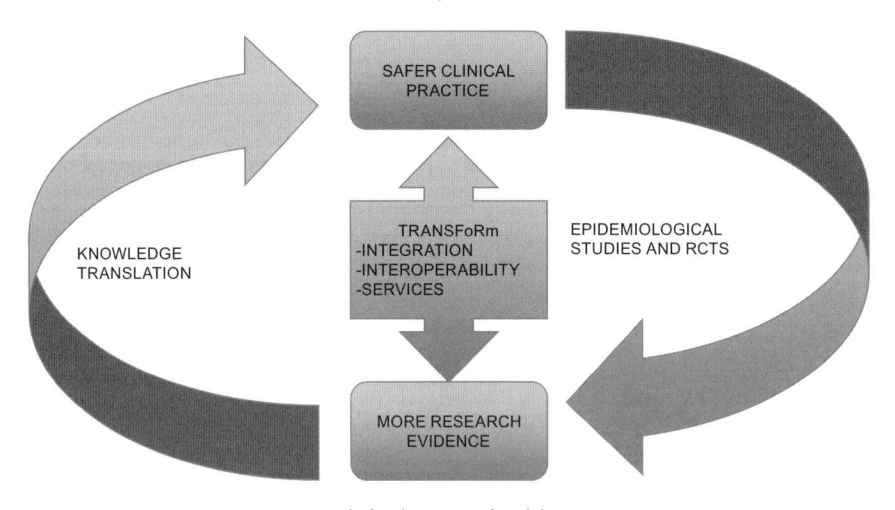

FIGURE 8-1 TRANSFoRm and the learning health system

HEALTHGRIDS, THE SHARE PROJECT, AND BEYOND

Tony Solomonides
University of the West of England

Grid computing was introduced in the late 1990s to serve as a medium of scientific collaboration and as a more immediate means of high-performance computing (Foster and Kesselman, 2004). If the Internet is an apparently inexhaustible information medium, the grid would also add rapid computation, large-scale data storage, and flexible collaboration by harnessing the power of large numbers of computers. As a computational paradigm, the grid was adopted for use in scientific fields—such as particle physics, astronomy, and bioinformatics—in which large volumes of data, very rapid processing, or both, are necessary.

The complementary idea of e-science arose from the observation that a scientist often has to juggle experiments, data collection, data processing, analysis of results, and their iteration and refinement. There is a need for intelligent conduit of information between these processes. Why not facilitate this through an informatic infrastructure that allows the scientist to pipeline activities in some way, leaving her free to concentrate on the science? If the work is being undertaken together with other scientists, this infrastructure should also support their collaboration but not expose their individual or joint efforts to anyone outside the specified group of collaborators.

Grids and Clouds in Health Care

There have also been several ambitious medical and healthcare applications of grids. While these initial exemplars have been mainly restricted to the research domain, there is a great deal of interest in real-world applications. However, there is some tension between the spirit of the grid paradigm and the requirements of healthcare applications. The grid maximizes its flexibility and minimizes overheads by requesting that computations be performed, and data stored/replicated, at the most appropriate node in the network. On the other hand, a hospital or other healthcare organization is required to maintain control of its confidential patient data and to remain accountable for its use at all times. The very basis of grid computing therefore appears to threaten certain inviolable principles: the confidentiality of medical data, the accountability of healthcare professionals, and the precise attribution of "duty of care."

Cloud computing is a more recent but related innovation. Like the grid, it arises from concepts and forces that were already present in the field, not least in the world of commercial computing. Precursors include the ideas of "application service provision" and "virtualization." Indeed, early adaptations of concepts from grid computing included the notion of utility computing—computing power distributed as if it were a "domestic" utility like gas of electricity. The advantage to a business that outsources its information systems to a cloud provider is that it need not own the infrastructure of servers and communications nor concern itself with maintaining the applications.

The current convergence of utility computing with social networking applications has led to several serious proposals to use clouds for patient-, or more accurately, carer-managed electronic health records (EHRs): commercial examples include Microsoft's *HealthVault* and *Google Health*, while in the United Kingdom there is debate on extending the use of *HealthSpace* along such lines. Indeed, the idea that personal EHRs could be "banked" originated with Dr. Bill Dodd in 1997 (Dodd, 1997). The opportunity to mine such records to the advantage of public health has also been noted (Bonander and Gates, 2010).

Healthgrids arose from the observation that healthcare and biomedical research share many of the characteristics of e-science. Consequently, many areas of biomedical research—medical imaging and image processing, modeling the human body, pharmaceutical research and development, epidemiological studies, genomic research, and personalized medicine—are expected to benefit from healthgrid technology. To use a familiar and successful example, consider a patient in a breast cancer screening program. If a mammogram gives cause for concern, it may be necessary to conduct further investigation or to seek a second opinion. There is already a powerful array of technological support for this, from image standardization software to computer-aided detection. The possibility of remote second opinion is also considered valuable if it does not take up too much time. If the patient is referred, the oncologist wants to know the history as succinctly as possible in order to review the diagnosis and begin with assessment and staging. If the patient needs to undergo surgery, the images from the diagnostic stage can be used in planning. In other cancers, radiotherapy planning may be assisted by review of imaging (Warren et al., 2007).

A powerful influence over the direction of these early projects was the *Bioinfomed* study which established a now familiar picture of the correspondences between biosocial organization (molecule–cell–organ–individual–community), pathologies and disciplines with different kinds of informatics (molecular modeling–imaging of cells and organs–electronic patient records–public health informatics) (Martin-Sanchez et al., 2004). It challenged the community to bring together information at these different levels into a coherent model. One of its most obvious successors is the Virtual Physiological Human, a program that seeks to provide a framework for the integration of different partial models of the human body, on different scales, toward an aggregate systemic study of human physiology.

HealthGrid and SHARE

HealthGrid was an EU-inspired initiative to support projects in the use of grid technology in health care and biomedical research. Incorporated as a not-for-profit organization in France, this collaboration edited a white paper setting out for senior decision makers the concept, benefits, and opportunities offered by healthgrids (Vincent et al., 2005). Starting from these conclusions, the EU funded the SHARE project aimed at identifying the important milestones toward wide deployment and adoption of healthgrids in Europe, perhaps as part of an action plan for a "European e-Health Area" (SHARE Collaboration, 2008). The project had to assess the status quo and set targets; identify key gaps, barriers, and opportunities; establish short- and long-term objectives; propose key developments; and suggest the actors needed to achieve the vision. The road map had to encompass issues regarding networks; infrastructure deployment; "middleware"; services to end users; standards; security; ethical, legal, and regulatory developments; social adjustments; and economic investments.

A draft road map was filtered through a number of "use cases" including drug discovery, large-scale public health emergency, imaging-based screening, and management of chronic conditions. The requirements arising from these different case studies led to differentiation between the development of (1) data, (2) computational, and (3) collaboration healthgrids. Indeed, the third category crystallized in the course of the project. The ultimate goal of a "knowledge grid" was then seen to emerge from the interaction of these three subparadigms, rather than to be an enhancement of the data grid, as had previously been thought.

Ethical, legal, social, and economic issues assumed increasing importance in the course of the project. The project mapped the legal and ethical landscape, identifying barriers to the wide adoption of healthgrids. Aspects of the law and emphasis on ethical requirements were initially considered to be inert constraints but were subsequently treated as parallel dynamic developments capable of being influenced by policy. These were therefore included in the road maps as areas in which fresh thinking and strategy were necessary. A project since undertaken at University of the West of England, Bristol, has demonstrated that it is possible for technology to incorporate goals such as regulatory compliance even in the face of potentially contradictory demands from different frameworks.

In relation to health care, SHARE identified evidence-based practice as the core requirement. As such, much of the work is underlain by assumptions about the dynamic nature of the evidence base, the need for biomedical advances to be translated into medicine, and for gold standard evidence to be interpreted in operational terms. Arguably, it paid less attention to the *business* of health care, including "internal markets" and commissioning (as in the United Kingdom) or actual markets (as in the United States). For example, the possibility of patients owning their data in real rather than in moral terms was considered but not fully explored. Developments in healthcare systems—including the halting progress of the English National Health Service National Programme for IT—have led governments to consider the role of cloud computing for the management of electronic patient records. This is regarded as a positive development that should help close the gap between healthgrids (for science and knowledge management) and clouds (for management, compliance, and business issues).

Technology and Regulatory Compliance

It has already been observed that the grid paradigm is in some ways at odds with the requirements of healthcare organizations. Although it featured significantly in subsequent research, security was not a top priority in its initial development. However, the complexity of medical data, the risk of disclosure through metadata, and the granularity of confidentiality are not readily accommodated in a raw grid environment. Healthgrids would have to take account of these constraints if they were ever to succeed in biomedical research or healthcare. Yet, all advantage would be lost if the very efficiency of grid computing was undermined by a constant need for human regulatory intervention.

The situation is somewhat reminiscent of the history of the motor car.

When the first motorized carriage was introduced in England in the mid-1890s, it was a legal requirement that a man walk ahead of any motorized vehicle with a red flag to warn pedestrians and to ensure that its speed did not exceed 4 mph.[1] It would be absurd to impose a restriction of that nature on healthgrids. The very idea behind the concept was to make sharing and exchange of data and workflows as smooth and uninterrupted as possible. Our goal in subsequent research was to show that technology could at least meet legal and ethical regulatory frameworks halfway. In doing so, technological innovation as well as ethical and legal policies would be framed in ways that acknowledged each other's legitimate concerns. Along with proposals for the mutual education of technologists and policy makers, this project was intended to be a demonstrator not only of technology *applied* to regulation, but of technology developed *in the light of* a sometimes uncertain and occasionally self-contradictory regulatory framework.

In the European Union, many areas of activity are controlled by what are known as "directives." For example, the European Working Time Directive restricts the number of working hours for different kinds of work. However, European directives are not legislation. Each directive has to be "transposed" as national legislation separately by each member state. Consequently, there is no guarantee of consistency. In our case, the relevant directive is 95/46/EC Data Protection Directive (European Parliament and Council of the European Union, 2010). The definitions of relevant terms (e.g., "personal data") and restrictions on data disclosure vary from country to country, even though all legislation is supposed to correspond to 95/46/EC. At the heart of the project reported here, therefore, is an assumption that text law is too complex to be interpreted by nonlegal expert users of healthgrids—whether they are biomedical researchers, clinicians, or technologists. Thus, we propose a twin-track approach: on one hand, the system may offer advice and decision support; on the other, it can ensure enforcement of privacy obligations at the process level (Figure 8-2).

At its most abstract, the initial question was this: given some legislation that has been translated into some sort of declarative framework, could we take that and map it to a deontic logic of permissions and obligations. In other words, can we develop an operational logic that could function at the infrastructure level? This begs the question: *What sort* of declarative framework would be suitable to encode legislation? The problem factors in a variety of ways. One of these is to distinguish between actionable advice and operational permissions/obligations. More importantly, the problem also factors into "preconditions for access to the data" and "postconditions for the treatment of the data." Finally, since much compliance checking is

---

[1] See http://www.datchethistory.org.uk/Link%20Articles/Ellis/evelyn_ellis.htm (accessed September 10, 2010).

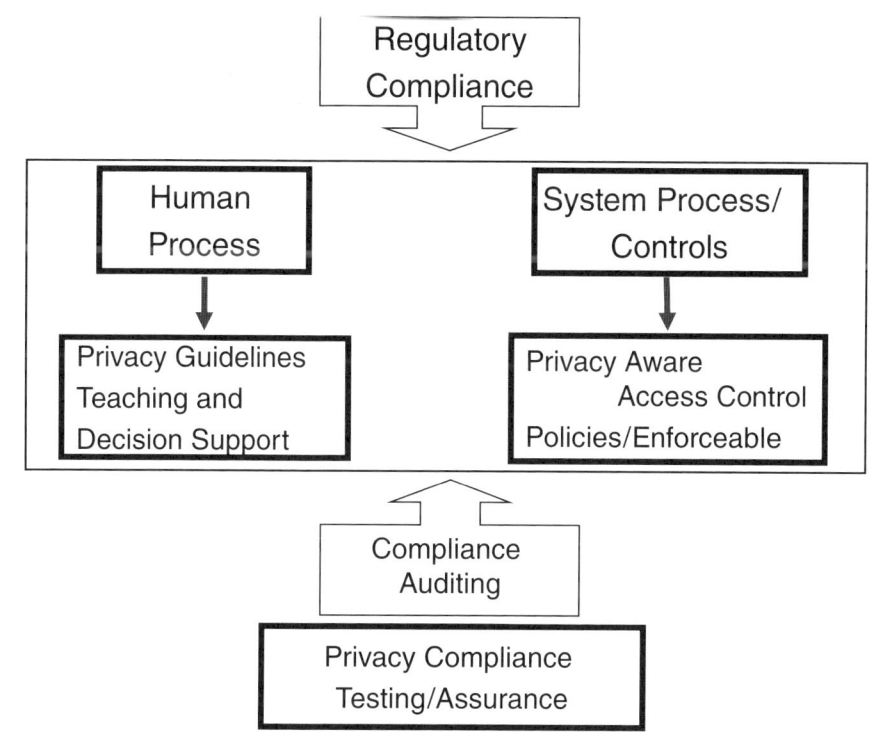

FOSTERING THE GLOBAL DIMENSION OF THE HEALTH DATA TRUST   207

FIGURE 8-2 Proposed regulatory framework for the HealthGrid.

done through audit, we need to determine what to document, and how, in order to provide evidence for audit.

A Proposed Ontology for Data Sharing

An approach through ontology allows us to (1) provide a semantic map of the directive and its "transposition" into UK, French, and Italian legislation; and (2) use the so-called Semantic Web Rule Language (SWRL) to reason with the ontology.

Figure 8-3 gives a diagrammatic representation of the Protégé ontology for rules on data sharing. At its center is an event of proposed DataSharing, which relates to certain data to be shared (SharedData) whose Privacy Status (*Anonymized*, *Encrypted*, or *Raw*) is also known. The DataSharing has a Sender and a Receiver, both of which, along with the SharedData, belong to a MemberState. The DataSharing has a SharingPurpose. Based on this information we can determine the ConsentNecessity (*Necessary* or *Unnecessary*), ConsentSpecificity (*Specific* or *Broad*), ConsentExplicitness

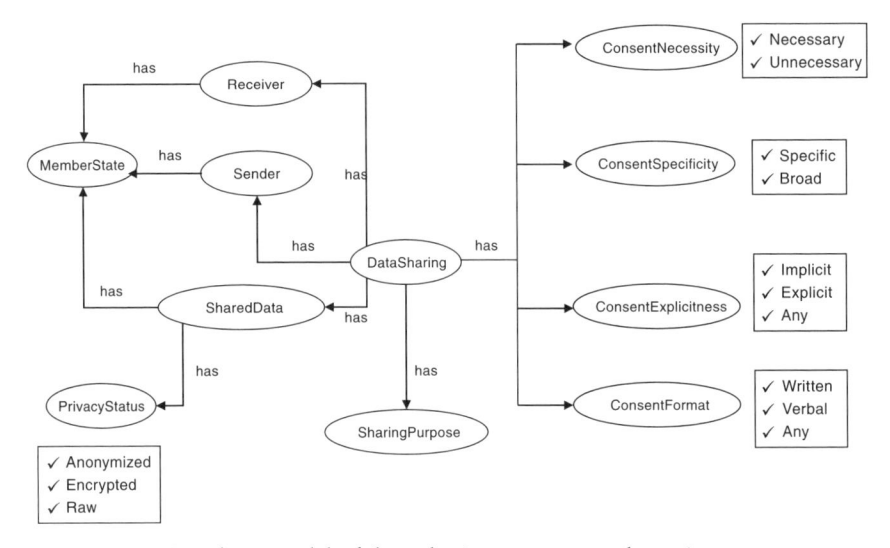

FIGURE 8-3 Ontology model of data-sharing contexts and requirements.

(*Implicit, Explicit,* or *Any*—that is, either or perhaps not even known), and the ConsentFormat (*Written, Verbal,* or *Any*).

Taking as our example a permissive clause, we consider the preconditions under which it is applicable and postconditions in the form of obligations or constraints on any subsequent processing of the data. The condition on the user(s), the data, and the purpose of any proposed sharing of the data are given in the Web Ontology Language (World Wide Web Consortium, 2009). SWRL is used to translate this knowledge into an if-then action rule, whose consequent involves an Action (e.g., *Allow*) and the imposition of certain further Obligation(s) on how the data should be processed once the permission has been enacted (World Wide Web Consortium, 2004).

A typical scenario may be the following: Patient Emma's mammogram series gives Dr. House some cause for concern; he believes that the mammogram includes certain features that Dr. Casa in Italy has reliably diagnosed with great accuracy in the past. Emma has provided consent for the mammograms to be taken and processed for the purpose of "breast cancer diagnosis and treatment." Dr. House's purpose in sharing the data with Dr. Casa is "to obtain second opinion on treatment options" which is compatible with the purpose for which Emma gave consent. The mammogram has been stripped of all obviously identifying information, but it could be traced back to Emma through secondary attributes and information about where and by whom she was treated. Nevertheless, for the strict clinical purpose for which the sharing is proposed, transmission of the mammogram to Dr. Casa is approved (provided he will destroy his electronic copy once he has completed his diagnosis). Thus, if Dr. Casa's insurance requires him to keep a record for his own protection, or if he wishes to use the mammogram in a text book, he must request further permission to do so. The SWRL representation of this example is shown in Figure 8-4.

Our intention was to translate our SWRL rules into an actionable logic. The choice for this is the eXtensible Access Control Markup Language (XACML) (OASIS, 2005). In XACML, a *Policy* is made up of *Rules* which may be combined through a *Rule Combining Algorithm* (it is also possible to have *Policy Sets* with *Policy Combining Algorithm*). A *Policy* may impose a certain *Obligation* as part of its response. A *Rule* has a *Target* and an *Effect* (e.g., *allow* or *deny*). A *Target* (i.e., the object of the *Rule*) includes a *Subject* (to whom the response is directed), an allowed or disallowed *Action*, a *Resource* to which the *Action* applies, and a *Purpose* for which the *Action* would be taken. Key structural elements in an XACML implementation are the *Policy Decision Point* and the *Policy Enforcement Point*. In our case, the *Policy Information Point* here has been implemented as our Semantic Web Knowledge Base and the Context Handler.

Figure 8-5 depicts this model and the numbered arrows indicate the sequential data flow that implements the rule we gave above. In the event that a whole set of data is to be shared, the same process takes place, except that the Context Handler classifies the data into sets with similar pre- and postconditions. The Context Handler now communicates directly with the *Policy Enforcement Point* to provide information, although the decision, as ever, is issued by the *Policy Decision Point*.

```
dataSharing(s1:sharing1)
    ∧    hasSender(s1, DrHouse) ∧ hasReceiver(s1, DrCasa)
    ∧    hasPurpose(s1, p1:SecondOpinionOnTreatment)
    ∧    locatedIn(, ) ∧ locatedIn( )
    ∧    concerning(s1, Data1) ∧ belongsTo(Data1, )
    ∧    isForPatient(Data1, PtId1)
    ∧    provided(PtId1, InformedConsent)
    ∧    hasCollectionPurpose(Data1, p2:BreastCancerDiagnosis)
    ∧    compatibleWith(p1, p2)
        →    hasSharingDecision(s1, Allow)
            ∧    hasObligation(s1, AttachSecondaryUsePolicy)
```

FIGURE 8-4 Semantic Web Rule Language representation of a data-sharing event.

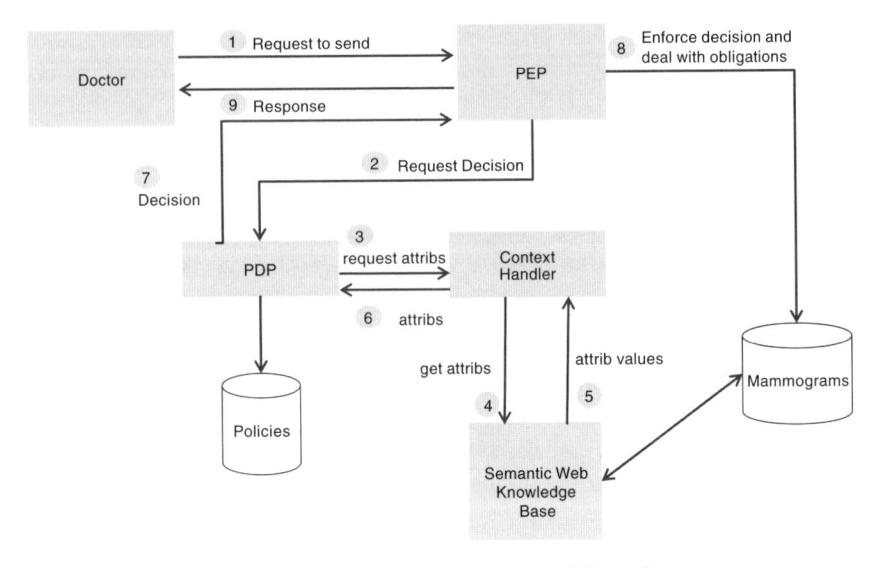

FIGURE 8-5 Extended XACML access control model/data flow.

Conclusion

These examples show how we may model contexts of medical data sharing by means of ontology, reason about which privacy requirements should be assigned to them, extend the ontology to allow the specification of adequate attribute-based access control policies, and map the semantic web policies to XACML to prove enforceability. The technological solution outlined above can handle the ambiguity of rules in the face of different interpretations of the same directive. The combining algorithm may be set to be conservative or liberal, maximal or minimal; in neither case does it violate any principles. In some circumstances it may not be able to reach an unambiguous decision, referring the user to authority.

Hopefully, this model points to a solution not only to the problem of automating compliance checks and speeding up the process of sharing medical data, but also to the issue of provenance management—that is, maintaining a metarecord with the data that provides details of where it came from, how it was constructed, what processes it has undergone since, and so on. This facilitates research through secondary use as well as the legal process of audit of compliance.

A GLOBAL PERSPECTIVE ON THE IMPORTANCE OF SYSTEMATIC DATA TO DRIVE IMPROVEMENTS IN CARE

Ashish K. Jha, M.D., M.P.H.
Harvard School of Public Health

There is broad consensus that improving patient safety is a critical component of advancing the health and well-being of citizens across the globe. Policy makers and clinicians increasingly view health information technologies (HITs)—and the data that underlie these systems—as a tool to drive quality improvement and improve patient safety. To date, the vast majority of global health efforts have focused on promoting access to care in developing and transitional countries. These efforts have further focused on specific conditions commonly viewed as the major global killers: HIV/AIDS, tuberculosis, and malaria.

Despite the successes realized by many of these initiatives, patient safety is an area of significant concern that warrants heightened attention among policy makers. Surprisingly, we know little about the safety of care delivered to patients and the magnitude to which care may cause harm. The available evidence indicates that unsafe care is a major cause of morbidity, mortality, and years of life lost, also carrying significant financial implications on health systems and society. Yet, due to the lack of systematic data sources, there is a dearth of data to inform actionable strategies aimed at improving the safety of care.

In this context, HIT may play a meaningful role. While the use of HIT systems to improve the safety and effectiveness of care delivered has received considerable attention in developed nations, the global debate on how HIT systems may be used to improve care in developing and transitional nations is in its infancy. The majority of key data needed to help policy makers and decision makers prioritize funding and allocate resources simply do not exist. Developing even the most basic form of information infrastructure is critical to thoughtfully push forward the policy debate. To better understand how HIT may be most effective, and to identify the best areas for intervention, more research is needed on the safety of care delivered in developing, transitional, and developed nations.

WHO World Alliance for Patient Safety

The World Health Organization (WHO) World Alliance for Patient Safety Working Group was charged with identifying global priorities for patient safety research. The group undertook two major initiatives: a report on the state of evidence on patient safety and calculating the global burden of unsafe care

Report on the State of Evidence on Patient Safety

The report, *Summary of the Evidence on Patient Safety: Implications for Research*, provides the most comprehensive picture of adverse events in health care (Jha, 2008). The report aims to not only describe the scope of challenges facing policy makers around patient safety, but also to provide recommendations and priorities for research. Members of the working group consisted of experts with multidisciplinary expertise in epidemiology, qualitative methods, and human factors and were from developing, transitional, and developed nations in all seven WHO regions.

Initially, the group identified the types of adverse events in health care and their causes. From these efforts, a list 23 major harms and their underlying causes was created (Table 8-1). Although these topics are not comprehensive of all epidemiological and clinical metrics, they are among the most important. The 23 patient safety topics were then categorized

TABLE 8-1 World Alliance for Patient Safety List of Common Adverse Events in Health Care

No.	Domain	Patient Safety Topic
1	Structure	Organizational determinants and latent failures
2	Structure	Use of accreditation and regulation to advance patient safety
3	Structure	Safety culture
4	Structure	Inadequate training and education, manpower issues
5	Structure	Stress and fatigue
6	Structure	Production pressures
7	Structure	Lack of appropriate knowledge, availability of knowledge, transfer of knowledge
8	Structure	Having measures of patient safety
9	Structure	Devices, procedures without human factors engineering
10	Process	Errors in care through misdiagnosis
11	Process	Errors in care through poor test follow-up
12	Process	Errors in care: counterfeit/substandard drugs
13	Process	Errors in care: unsafe injection practices
14	Process	Bringing patients' voices into patient safety
15	Outcomes	Adverse events and injuries due to medical devices
16	Outcomes	Adverse events due to medications
17	Outcomes	Adverse events due to surgical errors
18	Outcomes	Adverse events due to healthcare-associated infections
19	Outcomes	Adverse events due to unsafe blood products
20	Outcomes	Patient safety among pregnant women and newborns
21	Outcomes	Patient safety concerns among older adults
22	Outcomes	Adverse events due to falls in the hospital
23	Outcomes	Injury due to pressure sores and decubitus ulcers

SOURCE: Jha (2008).

into three groups: structural factors, processes of care, and outcomes. Lead experts in each topic area described the basic epidemiology of the topic, how the issue impacts patient care, and knowledge gaps to be addressed through future research.

Findings from the work are striking and identify large gaps in current data to inform priority setting. The overarching message of the evidence is that unsafe medical care continues to cause substantial morbidity, mortality, and years of life lost—particularly in the developing world. The majority of work has examined hospital care in developed nations and found adverse events rates of approximately 10% (Brennan et al., 2004; Davis et al., 2002, 2003; Thomas et al., 2000; Vincent et al., 2001). While few data exist on the care delivered in developing and transitional nations, these epidemiological studies suggest similar rates of adverse events but higher morbidity and mortality compared to developed nations (Jha, 2008). Thus, the consequences of unsafe care in the developing world appear to be much greater. Many of these events are not only preventable, but also expensive. Yet, safety remains low on the policy agenda.

While there is strong evidence on poor clinical outcomes as a result of unsafe care in developed nations and a small but growing number of smaller studies in developing and transitional nations, knowledge on structural factors and processes in care is not nearly as robust. The findings of the report underscore the need to fill the large gaps in data to inform the design of solutions and track strategies for improvement. Notably, understanding how to best address safety in different settings, determining which solutions are exportable among nations, and assessing the cost-effectiveness of specific solutions will be critical to guide policy makers as they make important, difficult decisions on how to allocate limited resources to improve health across the globe. Without more data, formulating effective solutions will pose a substantial challenge.

The Global Burden of Disease

Building on the work of the report, the World Alliance for Patient Safety focused on quantifying the global burden of unsafe care. The global burden of disease is the metric used by WHO, policy makers, and funders to allocate global health resources. The fundamental ability to accurately calculate the global burden of diseases is dependent on the types of data available. These results have vast implications for how big of a priority patient safety is deemed.

To calculate the global burden of disease, the 10 major types of preventable events that were identified in the report on global patient safety were used (Table 8-2). Using existing data, the group then developed two new analytical models: (1) health burden, measured by disability-adjusted

TABLE 8-2 Adverse Event Conditions Used by WHO to Calculate the Global Burden of Disease

Condition
Adverse drug events
Venous thromboembolism complications
Decubitus ulcers
Falls in the healthcare setting
Unsafe maternal/pregnancy care
Hospital-acquired infections
Surgical complications
Adverse medical device events
Unsafe blood products
Unsafe injection practices
Counterfeit medications

SOURCE: Jha (2008).

life years (DALYs) lost (due to injury and mortality) and (2) economic burden, measured by the financial impact (i.e., increased length of stay, repeated surgeries) on healthcare systems and society. The models included the number of people at risk, rate of hospitalization, average age at the time of acquiring the condition, four clinical outcomes (death, short-term disability followed by long-term disability, short-term disability then full recovery, no or minimal disability), average duration of the condition, average direct costs related to care of condition per episode, and disability weights.

The findings were again powerful and indicate that unsafe care is one of the major causes of disability and death in the world. Initial estimates suggest that over 34 million adverse events in hospitals occur among the conditions examined (over 60 percent from developing and transitional countries), and that the global burden of unsafe care from these conditions may account for as many as 20 million DALYs lost per year (approximately 60 percent of which are from developing and transitional countries). The number of estimated DALYs lost due do unsafe care falls directly behind top major global causes of disability and death, such as lower respiratory infection (94.5 million DALYs), unipolar depression disorders (65.5 million DALYs), ischemic heart disease (62.6 million DALYS), and cerebrovascular disease (46.6 millions DALYs) (WHO, 2008a). However, unlike these conditions, much unsafe care is preventable. Furthermore, these results are likely to be conservative since not all types of adverse events were included in the calculations. Thus, designing and implementing successful interventions to curb unsafe care may be an important area to prioritize global health efforts.

While the models were based on the most current and comprehensive data available, the research methodology further highlighted the reality that there is a paucity of systematic data sources globally. Particularly in developing and transitional nations, there is extensive variability in the data. For example, rates of hospitalization among these nations ranged from 8 percent to 98 percent. While hospitalization estimates in developed nations were between 113 and 147 million, the estimates were between 111 and 469 million in developing and transitional countries. The data, still qualified in developing nations, only exists on the prevalence of injury (how often patients are injured in the hospital). The global burden of disease models requires more key data on patient demographics, the severity of disability, and injury duration. Until we have these data elements and more robust information infrastructure that facilitates the collection and analysis of these data, precise estimations to inform policy makers will be a major challenge.

WHO Resource-Poor Setting Initiative

Given the acute need for better data to help policy makers make decisions in poor, resource-lacking countries, WHO has begun thinking about identifying the minimum dataset needed in the developing world. Implementing comprehensive electronic health records and health information exchange infrastructure in the developing world is not a realistic strategy at the present date. Thus, WHO has convened an expert consensus group to identify the major causative structural factors (i.e., lack of protocols or systematic monitoring) that drive a few key patient safety issues and then determine a systematic method to collect the data elements hospitals need to overcome structural failings. This is an important initial step to obtaining the basic information that will help paint a broader picture on the scope of patient safety issues and understand how these issues may be resolved.

Conclusion

In summary, we find that the much of the developing and transitional world faces challenges similar to those of the United States and other high-income countries: ensuring the delivery of high-quality, safe care in an efficient way. While the issues of access to health care feel paramount to developing nations, ensuring access to safe, effective care is critically important. Our preliminary work suggests that millions of the world's citizens—a majority in developing countries—are injured or killed due to unsafe health care. Information systems, whether they be rudimentary or advanced, are central to helping resource-poor nations develop an approach to improving patient safety, and building the trust of patients in the healthcare system in order to ensure that all of the world's citizens have access to safe, effective care.

INFORMATICS AND THE FUTURE OF INFECTIOUS DISEASE SURVEILLANCE

David L. Buckeridge, M.D., Ph.D., and John S. Brownstein, Ph.D.
McGill University

Advances in information technology are enabling dramatic changes in domestic and global infectious disease surveillance. Understanding the nature of these changes is critical to ensuring that existing and novel surveillance systems contribute effectively to disease control. In this paper, we describe how information technology is altering the surveillance landscape and identify how public health should harness these changes for effective disease control.

Traditional Domestic and International Surveillance Systems

Infectious disease surveillance has evolved over the last century to exploit many sources of information, but even where capacity is sufficient, systems based upon laboratory-confirmed diagnoses remain the preferred approach (Van Beneden and Lyndfield, 2010). Recent epidemics and pandemics, however, have highlighted the limited sensitivity and timeliness of laboratory-based systems. Since a case can be detected only if an infected person seeks medial care, sensitivity is limited by patterns of healthcare utilization. During the clinical encounter, sensitivity can be further reduced if a clinician does not order a laboratory test that can identify the organism under surveillance, or if a test is not routinely available.

The reporting of a laboratory-confirmed case of infection to a public health department is usually a manual process, which can take a week or longer to occur. Moreover, subsequent reporting between public health jurisdictions tends to follow a hierarchical pattern: a local health department informing a regional public health authority which then informs the national public health authority, a process that often takes 2 to 3 weeks (Birkhead et al., 1991; Jajosky and Groseclose, 2004; Jansson et al., 2004; Yoo et al., 2009). Finally, the national public health authority may inform the World Health Organization in accordance with the International Health Regulations (WHO, 2008b).

In the context where lab resources are constrained, systems for public health surveillance face similar limitations. Existing networks of traditional surveillance efforts—managed by health ministries, public health institutes, multinational agencies, and laboratory and institutional networks—have wide gaps in geographic coverage, capacity, and training, often resulting in poor and sometimes suppressed information flow.

Using Information Technology to Enhance Existing Systems

Advances in information technology are beginning to alter the landscape of infectious disease surveillance by addressing the limitations of traditional surveillance approaches. For example, large-scale telephone consultation lines that rely upon computerized decision algorithms (such as National Health Service Direct in the UK) attempt to direct patients to the appropriate level of clinical care (Snooks et al., 2009). Such streamlining of care may benefit laboratory-based surveillance by increasing the likelihood that those with diseases under surveillance seek care. Another application of information technology that may enhance existing surveillance systems is the use of decision support to prompt clinicians to order tests for conditions under surveillance (Lurio et al., 2010).

One of the more concerted attempts to apply information technology to modernize existing surveillance systems has aimed to automate the reporting of positive results from laboratories to public health departments. Evidence suggests that such automation can enhance sensitivity and improve the timeliness of reporting, reducing delays in initial reports from laboratories by 4 to 7 days (Effler et al., 1999; Overhage et al., 2008; Panackal et al., 2002; Ward et al., 2005). In the United States, considerable resources are being directed toward the acquisition of clinical information systems that support such electronic laboratory reporting (Blumenthal and Tavenner, 2010).

These applications of information technology have the potential to improve existing surveillance systems but they cannot resolve some of the most important limitations of surveillance. In resource-poor settings, they cannot address the issue of laboratory testing capacity. Even where laboratory resources are sufficient, improving test ordering and reporting does little to address the delays inherent in hierarchical reporting among public health jurisdictions after initial reports are received from laboratories.

Using Information Technology to Disrupt the Traditional Approach

In addition to enhancing existing surveillance systems, advances in information technology are also disrupting the traditional public health surveillance model by enabling new approaches to data sharing. Data are increasingly available from sources other than laboratories and these novel types of surveillance data are often shared outside of traditional public health channels. In contrast to the hierarchy that typifies reporting of laboratory-confirmed cases, data are increasingly shared more broadly, with decreased control over data sharing by governmental agencies.

The DiSTRIBuTE project[2] is one example of an innovative approach to sharing surveillance data extracted from sources other than laboratories (Buckeridge et al., 2011). This project builds on the growing adoption of syndromic surveillance systems (Buehler et al., 2009), which allow public health departments to follow the reasons for visits to emergency departments (EDs) in their jurisdictions (Mandl et al., 2004). Although these ED data lack the specificity of laboratory-confirmed reports, they are sensitive, available immediately, and have been shown to correlate well with laboratory-confirmed reports for diseases such as influenza (Marsden-Haug et al., 2007). The DiSTRIBuTE project allows health departments with syndromic surveillance systems to rapidly share information from their systems. Over one-third of ED visits in the United States are now captured by the DiSTRIBuTE system, and information extracted from these data to support influenza surveillance are made publicly available with a delay of less that 72 hours for the majority of participating health departments (Buckeridge et al., 2011).

HealthMap is another example of using information technology to expand the scope of surveillance sources and free the flow of surveillance information. HealthMap harnesses and organizes the enormous amount of valuable epidemic intelligence found in web-accessible sources such as discussion sites, disease reporting networks, and news outlets (Freifeld et al., 2008). These resources provide current, highly local information about outbreaks—even from areas relatively invisible to traditional global public health efforts. These web-based data sources not only facilitate early outbreak detection, but also support increasing public awareness of disease outbreaks prior to their formal recognition (Brownstein et al., 2010).

A Renewed Science of Surveillance on the Road to Effective Disease Control

Applications of information technology are enhancing existing systems and disrupting current surveillance models to make more information about infectious diseases available with less delay. Although some applications of information technology that influence infectious disease surveillance are under the control of the public health system, many are not. This reality is both exciting and challenging for the future of public health surveillance. It points to a future where disease information is available broadly and quickly, but raises the questions of how, and by whom, this information will be used to further effective disease control.

Public health workers use surveillance data to assess population health status and project the likely evolution of that status in the face of available

---

[2] See http://www.ISDSDistribute.org (accessed January 14, 2011).

interventions (Buehler et al., 2009). To accomplish these tasks, data from different surveillance sources must be combined (Khan et al., 2010). Such combination could make the most of highly specific laboratory data, when available, and more sensitive and timely data from other sources. Combining data to support decision making, however, requires an understanding of the nature and quality of the data, something that is not always available for novel data sources.

While concern about the nature and quality of data is appropriate, public health authorities cannot and should not avoid novel sources of data and rest complacent with traditional models of surveillance. Instead, public health surveillance as a discipline must extend its theoretical and practical foundations to embrace the opportunities presented by information technology. In other words, a renewed science of disease surveillance is needed; one that starts from public health principles and embraces information technology enhancements as well as disruptive changes on the road to improved disease control (Thacker et al., 1989).

REFERENCES

Birkhead, G., T. Chorba, S. Root, D. Klaucke, and N. Gibbs. 1991. Timeliness of national reporting of communicable diseases: The experience of the National Electronic Telecommunications System for Surveillance. *American Journal of Public Health* 81:1313-1315.

Blumenthal, D., and M. Tavenner. 2010. The "meaningful use" regulation for electronic health records. *New England Journal of Medicine* 363(6):501-504.

Bonander, J., and S. Gates. 2010. Public health in an era of personal health records: Opportunities for innovation and new partnerships. *Journal of Medical Internet Research* 12(3):e33.

Brennan, T. A., L. L. Leape, N. M. Laird, L. Hebert, A. R. Localio, A. G. Lawthers, J. P. Newhouse, P. C. Weiler, and H. H. Hiatt. 2004. Incidence of adverse events and negligence in hospitalized patients: Results of the Harvard Medical Practice Study. *Quality and Safety in Health Care* 13(2):145-151; discussion 151-152.

Brownstein, J. S., C. C. Freifeld, E. H. Chan, M. Keller, A. L. Sonricker, S. R. Mekaru, and D. L. Buckeridge. 2010. Information technology and global surveillance of cases of 2009 H1N1 influenza. *New England Journal of Medicine* 362(18):1731-1735.

Buckeridge, D. L., J. S. Brownstein, W. B. Lober, D. R. Olson, M. Paladini, D. Ross, L. Finelli, T. Kass-Hout, and J. W. Buehler. 2011. The DiSTRIBuTE Project: Rapid sharing of emergency-department surveillance data during the 2009 influenza A/H1N1 pandemic. *(Submitted)*.

Buehler, J. W., E. A. Whitney, D. Smith, M. J. Prietula, S. H. Stanton, and A. P. Isakov. 2009. Situational uses of syndromic surveillance. *Biosecurity and Bioterrorism* 7(2):165-177.

Davis, P., R. Lay-Yee, R. Briant, W. Ali, A. Scott, and S. Schug. 2002. Adverse events in New Zealand public hospitals: Occurrence and impact. *New Zealand Medical Journal* 115(1167):U271.

———. 2003. Adverse events in New Zealand public hospitals: Preventability and clinical context. *New Zealand Medical Journal* 116(1183):U624.

Delaney, B. C. 2008. Potential for improving patient safety by computerized decision support systems. *Family Practice* 25(3):137-138.

Dodd, B. 1997. An independent "health information bank" could solve data security issues. *British Journal of Healthcare Computing and Information Management* 14(8):33-35.

Effler, P., M. Ching-Lee, A. Bogard, M. Ieong, T. Nekomoto, and D. Jernigan. 1999. Statewide system of electronic notifiable disease reporting from clinical laboratories: Comparing automated reporting with conventional. *Journal of the American Medical Association* 282:1845-1850.

European Parliament and Council of the European Union. 2010. *Directive 95/46/ec.* http://eur-lex.europa.eu/LexUriServ/LexUriServ.do?uri=CELEX:31995L0046:en:NOT (accessed September 10, 2010).

Europe's Information Society. 2009. *I2010—A European information society for growth and employment.* http://ec.europa.eu/information_society/eeurope/i2010/index_en.htm (accessed November 16, 2010).

Foster, I., and C. Kesselman. 2004. *The Grid 2: Blueprint for a new computing infrastructure.* Oxford, UK: Elsevier Science.

Freifeld, C. C., K. D. Mandl, B. Y. Reis, and J. S. Brownstein. 2008. HealthMap: Global infectious disease monitoring through automated classification and visualization of Internet media reports. *Journal of the American Medical Informatics Association* 15(2):150-157.

Fridsma, D. B., J. Evans, S. Hastak, and C. N. Mead. 2008. The BRIDG project: A technical report. *Journal of the American Medical Informatics Association* 15(2):130-137.

Garg, A. X., N. K. Adhikari, H. McDonald, M. P. Rosas-Arellano, P. J. Devereaux, J. Beyene, J. Sam, and R. B. Haynes. 2005. Effects of computerized clinical decision support systems on practitioner performance and patient outcomes: A systematic review. *Journal of the American Medical Association* 293(10):1223-1238.

Iakovidis, I., and O. Purcarea. 2008. eHealth in Europe: From vision to reality. *Studies in Health Technology and Informatics* 134:163-168.

Jajosky, R., and S. Groseclose. 2004. Evaluation of reporting timeliness of public health surveillance systems for infectious diseases. *BMC Public Health* 4(1):29.

Jansson, A., M. Arneborn, K. Skorlund, and K. Ekdahl. 2004. Timeliness of case reporting in the Swedish statutory surveillance of communicable diseases 1998-2002. In *Scandinavian Journal of Infectious Diseases* 36(11-12):865-872.

Jha, A. K. editor. 2008. *Summary of the evidence on patient safety: Implications for research.* Geneva, Switzerland: World Health Organization.

Kalra, D., T. Beale, and S. Heard. 2005. The openEHR Foundation. *Studies in Health Technology and Informatics* 115:153-173.

Khan, A. S., A. Fleischauer, J. Casani, and S. L. Groseclose. 2010. The next public health revolution: Public health information fusion and social networks. *American Journal of Public Health* 100(7):1237-1242.

Kostopoulou, O., J. Oudhoff, R. Nath, B. C. Delaney, C. W. Munro, C. Harries, and R. Holder. 2008. Predictors of diagnostic accuracy and safe management in difficult diagnostic problems in family medicine. *Medical Decision Making* 28(5):668-680.

Lurio, J., F. P. Morrison, M. Pichardo, R. Berg, M. D. Buck, W. Wu, K. Kitson, F. Mostashari, and N. Calman. 2010. Using electronic health record alerts to provide public health situational awareness to clinicians. *Journal of the American Medical Informatics Association* 17(2):217-219.

Mandl, K. D., J. M. Overhage, M. M. Wagner, W. B. Lober, P. Sebastiani, F. Mostashari, J. A. Pavlin, P. H. Gesteland, T. Treadwell, E. Koski, L. Hutwagner, D. L. Buckeridge, R. D. Aller, and S. Grannis. 2004. Implementing syndromic surveillance: A practical guide informed by the early experience. *Journal of the American Medical Informatics Association* 11(2):141-150.

Marsden-Haug, N., V. B. Foster, P. L. Gould, E. Elbert, H. Wang, and J. A. Pavlin. 2007. Code based syndromic surveillance for influenzalike illness by International Classification of Diseases, ninth revision. *Emerging Infectious Diseases* 13(2):207-216.

Martin-Sanchez, F., I. Iakovidis, S. Nørager, V. Maojo, P. de Groen, J. Van der Lei, T. Jones, K. Abraham-Fuchs, R. Apweiler, A. Babic, R. Baud, V. Breton, P. Cinquin, P. Doupi, M. Dugas, R. Eils, R. Engelbrecht, P. Ghazal, P. Jehenson, C. Kulikowski, K. Lampe, G. De Moor, S. Orphanoudakis, N. Rossing, B. Sarachan, A. Sousa, G. Spekowius, G. Thireos, G. Zahlmann, J. Zvárová, I. Hermosilla, and F. J. Vicente. 2004. Synergy between medical informatics and bioinformatics: Facilitating genomic medicine for future health care. *Journal of Biomedical Informatics* 37(1):30-42.

OASIS (Organization for the Advancement of Structured Information Standards). 2005. *eXtensible Access Control Markup Language (XACML) version 2.0.* http://docs.oasis-open.org/xacml/2.0/access_control-xacml-2.0-core-spec-os.pdf (accessed September 10, 2010).

Ohmann, C., and W. Kuchinke. 2009. Future developments of medical informatics from the viewpoint of networked clinical research. Interoperability and integration. *Methods of Information in Medicine* 48(1):45-54.

Overhage, J. M., S. Grannis, and C. J. McDonald. 2008. A comparison of the completeness and timeliness of automated electronic laboratory reporting and spontaneous reporting of notifiable conditions. *American Journal of Public Health* 98(2):344-350.

Panackal, A. A., M. M'ikanatha N, F. C. Tsui, J. McMahon, M. M. Wagner, B. W. Dixon, J. Zubieta, M. Phelan, S. Mirza, J. Morgan, D. Jernigan, A. W. Pascule, J. T. Rankin, Jr., R. A. Hajjeh, and L. H. Harrison. 2002. Automatic electronic laboratory-based reporting of notifiable infectious diseases at a large health system. *Emerging Infectious Diseases* 8(7):685-691.

Schade, C. P., F. M. Sullivan, S. de Lusignan, and J. Madeley. 2006. E-prescribing, efficiency, quality: Lessons from the computerization of UK family practice. *Journal of the American Medical Informatics Association* 13(5):470-475.

SHARE Collaboration. 2008. *Share roadmap II.* http://www.healthgrid.org/documents/pdf/SHARE_roadmap_long.pdf (accessed September 10, 2010).

Singh, H., E. J. Thomas, M. M. Khan, and L. A. Petersen. 2007. Identifying diagnostic errors in primary care using an electronic screening algorithm. *Archives of Internal Medicine* 167(3):302-308.

Snooks, H., J. Peconi, J. Munro, W. Y. Cheung, J. Rance, and A. Williams. 2009. An evaluation of the appropriateness of advice and healthcare contacts made following calls to NHS Direct Wales. *BMC Health Services Research* 9:178.

Speedie, S. M., A. Taweel, I. Sim, T. N. Arvanitis, B. Delaney, and K. A. Peterson. 2008. The Primary Care Research Object Model (PCROM): A computable information model for practice-based primary care research. *Journal of the American Medical Informatics Association* 15(5):661-670.

Thacker, S. B., R. L. Berkelman, and D. F. Stroup. 1989. The science of public health surveillance. *Journal of Public Health Policy* 10(2):187-203.

Thomas, E. J., D. M. Studdert, H. R. Burstin, E. J. Orav, T. Zeena, E. J. Williams, K. M. Howard, P. C. Weiler, and T. A. Brennan. 2000. Incidence and types of adverse events and negligent care in Utah and Colorado. *Medical Care* 38(3):261-271.

Van Beneden, C., and R. Lynfield. 2010. Public health surveillance for infectious diseases. In *Principles and practice of public health surveillance*, edited by L. M. Lee, S. M. Teutsch, S. B. Thacker, and M. E. St. Louis. Oxford: Oxford University Press. Pp. 236-254.

Vincent, B., D. Kevin, and S. Tony. 2005. The healthgrid white paper. In *From grid to Health-Grid: Proceedings of HealthGrid 2005.* Oxford, UK: ISO Press. Pp. 249-321.

Vincent, C., G. Neale, and M. Woloshynowych. 2001. Adverse events in British hospitals: Preliminary retrospective record review. *British Medical Journal* 322(7285):517-519.

Ward, M., P. Brandsema, E. van Straten, and A. Bosman. 2005. Electronic reporting improves timeliness and completeness of infectious disease notification, the Netherlands, 2003. *European Surveillance* 10(1):27-30.

Warren, R., A. E. Solomonides, C. del Frate, I. Warsi, J. Ding, M. Odeh, R. McClatchey, C. Tromans, M. Brady, R. Highnam, M. Cordell, F. Estrella, M. Bazzocchi, and S. R. Amendolia. 2007. Mammogrid—a prototype distributed mammographic database for Europe. *Clinical Radiology* 62(11):1044-1051.

WHO (World Health Organization). 2008a. *Global burden of disease: 2004 update.* Geneva, Switzerland.

———. 2008b. *International health regulations.* http://www.searo.who.int/LinkFiles/International_Health_Regulations_IHR_2005_en.pdf (accessed January 14, 2011).

World Wide Web Consortium. 2004. *SWRL: A Semantic Web Rule Language combining OWL and RULEML.* http://www.w3.org/Submission/SWRL/ (accessed September 10, 2010).

———. 2009. *OWL: Web Ontology Language—overview.* http://www.w3.org/TR/owl-features/ (accessed September 10, 2010).

Yoo, H. S., O. Park, H. K. Park, E. G. Lee, E. K. Jeong, J. K. Lee, and S. I. Cho. 2009. Timeliness of national notifiable diseases surveillance system in Korea: A cross-sectional study. *BMC Public Health* 9:93.

9

Growing the Digital Health Infrastructure

INTRODUCTION

Drawing on the collective expertise represented in the presentations and discussions of the first workshop, in the two subsequent workshops participants focused on four crosscutting priority domains: promoting technical advances and innovation, knowledge generation and use, engaging patients and the population, and fostering stewardship and governance. Encouraged to give due consideration to "out of the box" approaches and to use examples from health and nonhealth fields to illustrate and test key needs and opportunities through small group sessions, participants identified and presented for discussion a number of strategic elements important to progress in each domain. They are included in Box 9-1 and described in more detail in the sections below.

Participants called out a number of elements for consideration surrounding the strategic opportunities for technical progress. They included the need to address health as a complex sociotechnical system and therefore apply an approach that addresses both characteristics. Discussions noted the need to focus strategic thinking around the functionalities desired by such a system, including the ability to produce a complete longitudinal patient record at the point of care and the ability to use records for research purposes. Participants cautioned of the importance of taking a parsimonious approach to systems specifications and suggested one that tolerated the use of "dirty data" with context maintenance as a starting point. Usability was discussed as an important strategic consideration, and the need to address workflow integration as a crucial component of this consideration.

> **BOX 9-1**
> **Strategic Elements**
>
> **TECHNICAL PROGRESS . . . activities that advance:**
> - Ultra-large-scale system perspective
> - Functionality focus
> - System specifications/interoperability
> - Workflow and usability
> - Security and privacy safeguards
> - System innovation
>
> **KNOWLEDGE GENERATION AND USE . . . activities that advance:**
> - Shared learning environment
> - Point of decision support and guidance
> - Research-ready records for data reuse
> - Patient-generated data
> - Integration and use of data across sources
> - Distributed data repositories
> - Sentinel indicators
> - Query capacity
> - Analytic tools and methods innovation
>
> **PATIENT AND POPULATION ENGAGEMENT . . . activities that advance:**
> - Value proposition and patient confidence
> - Shared learning culture
> - Patient-clinician outcomes partnerships
> - Person-centric, lay-oriented health information access
> - Closing the disparity gap
> - Continuous evaluation
>
> **GOVERNANCE . . . activities that advance:**
> - The vision
> - Guiding principles
> - Participant roles and responsibilities
> - Process and protocol stewardship
> - Implementation phasing
> - Continuous evaluation

Attention to the technical aspects of security and privacy concerns were highlighted as major contributors to the building of trust among system stakeholders. Finally, the need to drive continuous innovation of technical approaches through constant testing and refinement and the creation of a supporting multidisciplinary research ecosystem were suggested.

Discussion of the strategic elements needing attention for the creation of a robust knowledge generation and use engine for the learning health system encompassed issues ranging from cultural changes to the need for innovative methods development. Workshop participants suggested that a learning health system would not be possible without patients and clinicians buying into a shared learning culture. Consideration of approaches to facilitate the use of clinical records for research, such as the identification of core research-related components, was also discussed. Leveraging the full potential of health information by including sources other than just clinical records—such as patient-generated data and nonmedical health-related data—was discussed as an important strategic element. Finally, participants stressed the need to better develop innovative analytical methods to use distributed data repositories in order to address security and privacy concerns.

Maximally leveraging the digital infrastructure to better engage patients and the population in health was another principal focus of the discussions. Conveying the value proposition for stakeholder participation and creation of a shared learning culture among patients and the population were prominent themes. Participants discussed using the digital infrastructure to strengthen patient–clinician outcome partnerships through better patient portals and increased availability of lay-oriented, user-friendly clinical and nonmedical health data. Participants highlighted the need to call out the opportunity presented by a learning health system to aid in the elimination of health disparities and the role that a digital infrastructure could play to that end. Finally, the need for constant improvement through evaluation and innovation was discussed as an important component of an approach to patient and population engagement.

Explorations of the possible approaches to governance of the digital infrastructure for the learning health system were approached through the ultra-large-scale (ULS) lens, and drew from examples outside health care. Beginning with a discussion of the need to set a vision as a reference point for progress, participants explored the need to work toward identifying a minimal set of guiding principles to meet this vision while allowing for autonomy and innovation. Participant roles and responsibilities as well as delineation of the processes and protocols to be managed in support of the core learning functionalities were also identified as important components of a strategic plan. Finally, the incorporation of continuous evaluation and improvement in the approach to governance was also highlighted.

TECHNICAL PROGRESS

A *ULS system* is complex, constantly growing, and evolving, much like an organic, biological ecosystem. The digital infrastructure needed to support the U.S. healthcare system can be classified as a ULS system given its enormous scale including the numbers of agents, lines of code, and ever-expanding diverse sources of data; the preponderance of legacy systems that must be incorporated; the local nature of health care and the corresponding requirement that each institution have autonomy; the specific regulatory, legal, and social requirements that must be met; and the understanding that it is too complex to be subject to effective central control. Introduced to the digital health information conversation by colleagues from the computer science field, hallmarks of a ULS system include preservation of local autonomy through decentralization of data, development, and operational authority. This allows for local innovation, personalization, and emergent behaviors without requiring consensus from all nodes. In discussions focused on developing a set of strategic scenarios for technical progress, the ULS system approach emerged as an appropriate framework since it would allow for empowerment through knowledge and control of health and health information; support a broad diversity of data sources and processes; support evolution and change; contain minimal, extensible standards; and leverage past work toward long-term goals.

In discussing the implications and issues surrounding this approach, participants identified the relevance and appeal of the engineering approach to health care—systems analyses, design, implementation, and evaluation plans—inherent to the ULS system perspective. Specifically, they noted the potential of a collaborative effort between the computer science and health information technology (HIT) communities to develop a deliberate and systematic engineering analysis—characterized by iterative testing and development of prototypes—to set technical and sociotechnical system goals, requirements, specifications, and architecture. This could be supported by a multidisciplinary research community, armed with clarified terminology for ease of collaboration, and with participation from a wide array of both private and public stakeholders (computer science, health informatics, law, policy, ethics, etc.). Similarly, workshop participants stressed the need for technical policies that support experimentation and innovation and allow for the progressive adoption and evolution of system requirements, specifications, and architecture choices.

Participants pointed to a *focus on functionalities* consistent with ULS systems, and their application to the digital health system, as a potential starting point in advancing the ULS approach. Definition of the ULS principles and characteristics that support learning system functionalities, including the feedback and feedforward nature of the learning engine, such as identification strategies, privacy controls, the availability of a complete longitudinal record at the point of care, inferential capacity, and research-readiness, were highlighted as critical foundational steps in the development of this technical enterprise. Noted as similarly important to system functionality was the mechanism for developing and maintaining an approach to information structure, classification, and storage.

Promoting these targeted functionalities requires advancing parsimonious *system specifications and interoperability*. Discussions centered on the need to specify the minimum set of standards to allow for partial interoperability. A focus on semantic comparability, maintenance of context and provenance, architectural consistency, and transportability were discussed as potential starting points. In congruence with the priorities laid out subsequently in the PCAST report (see Appendix E), particular attention was paid to the use of metadata to facilitate interoperability and information exchange—including to maintain data context and provenance, authentication, and privacy. This, in concert with a fast-prototyping component, can allow for incremental specification and system growth with the opportunity for functional enhancement, such as refinement of semantic interoperability, to meet specific requirements depending on use.

Part and parcel with the need to address the technical specifications of the digital utility for the learning health system is consideration for how these interface with users. Considerations for *workflow integration* were discussed by workshop participants as important to ensure that the technology is not only innovative and useful but also useable. To date, this disjuncture between established workflow patterns and an unfamiliar, often awkward, overlay of HIT tools has proved a substantial barrier to adoption.

Security and privacy safeguards were an important consideration in all areas of discussion. Participants often pointed to a lack of trust as being one of the major impediments to health information exchange. Therefore, attendance to the technical aspects of these issues was emphasized as a crucial part of building trust among stakeholders. Discussions and presentations (see Foster, Chapter 5, and Solomonides, Chapter 8) described technical approaches such as attribute-based authorization and distributed identity management, and provided examples of how they could be deployed to address these concerns and achieve a state of secure data liquidity. Additionally, innovations around data security and privacy in alternative environments such as hosted, web-based systems were suggested in order to build capacity.

Finally, the need for *continuous innovation* was a recurring theme in technical discussions. Participants suggested strategies such as creating a test-bed network for assessment of innovative system functionalities, the use of challenge problems to test ULS system issues and opportunities, and the cultivation of interdisciplinary research initiatives among academic, industry, and government stakeholders.

KNOWLEDGE GENERATION AND USE

Discussions of the generation and use of knowledge fell into three areas: the availability and capture of reliable data, the tools to analyze the data, and seamless feedback of knowledge to the system. Research, quality improvement initiatives, and public health surveillance efforts are all examples of uses and drivers for these learning-associated processes.

A necessary precondition for successful progress on any of these dimensions is a *shared learning environment*. Technical advances and innovative research methods make it possible to bring clinical research and clinical practice much closer together. However, it was noted that the ability to take advantage of that opportunity depends on a healthcare culture in which both patients and clinicians are compelled by the prospects of clinical data to improve understanding, care delivery, and outcomes as well as provide reliable, just-in-time information to assist decision making. For these reasons, participants highlighted the need for a learning environment that is supported, shared, and nurtured by both patients and clinicians.

Several tools and approaches currently exist to provide *point-of-decision support and guidance*. In the face of the number of interacting factors, competing priorities, and an ever-growing set of diagnostic and therapeutic options, "best practice" can only be a theoretical notion without the ability to bring the best available information to the decision process. On the other hand, it was noted that reminders and decision prompts not successfully engineered into natural workflow patterns will be little more than ignored distractions. Consequently, approaches are needed to better marshal reliable clinical information and guidelines in time, form, and content that is seamlessly accessed and used by clinicians and patients.

Participants identified a number of needs to be addressed in order for the digital health infrastructure to reach its full potential as a source of real-time clinical research insights. For example, clinical research activities require enlisting clinician support and involvement in *research-ready clinical records* on both quality and content dimensions for reuse in knowledge generation. The identification of a limited set of standardized core research-related components as basic elements across vendors and systems was one suggestion to facilitate individual and cooperative clinical research activities as well as sentinel event surveillance. Concerns over the reliability and heterogeneity of data in clinical records were underscored as an important rate-limiting factor for both quality of care and clinical research activities, again highlighting the importance of the mechanisms for information structure, classification, and storage. This is particularly important for repurposing data collected for other uses, such as Food and Drug Administration (FDA) clinical trial–associated data, in order to maximally leverage efforts and investments already in place.

Discussions on the increased utility of clinical records for research went hand in hand with those on the need to take advantage of information from patients and other sources. *Patient-generated data* can provide a level of context that is impossible to capture through more traditional data collection methods. Initiatives to better develop, test, and improve the capture and use of these data so that they can be used to support research, quality improvement, public reporting, and patient care were suggested as priorities.

Similarly, efforts to promote the *integration and use of data across various sources*—clinical, public health, commercial—were emphasized as central to effectively leveraging the full range of information for progress in improving efforts aimed at populations as well as individuals. Included in this, and considered with a longer term vision, were growing information sources outside of "mainstream" health care, such as online forums and communities. In order for such proposals to be successful, it was noted that protocols must be developed to build interoperability as a natural and seamless element of data sources.

Storage and aggregation of data for the purpose of analysis and knowledge generation have been problematic given the security and privacy issues they entail. Discussions of current and ongoing efforts in the creation of *distributed data repositories*, such as those being used in FDA's Sentinel Initiative and the HMO Research Network, suggest a promising approach. Coordination between these ongoing efforts, additional support and incentives for their use for clinical research activities, and the support of coordinated intervention-specific patient registries were discussed as potential approaches moving forward. Prospects for the use of scalable, distributed, hosted, storage solutions—such as those used by Amazon—were also noted as promising future directions. These discussions, however, were often punctuated with caution around privacy and security, components that participants felt needed further exploration and development.

Finally, considerable attention was paid to the development of methods, tools, and *query capacity* for the generation of knowledge needed to sustain a digital learning health system. In line with the ULS system architecture approach, and the creation and support of distributed data repositories, the development of capacity for national, distributed query-based research—including the ability to identify and track *sentinel* events and indicators—was identified as a strategic priority. To support this, and the continuing development and *innovation around other analytical approaches*, the importance of collaborative interdisciplinary networks of researchers was underscored. This was discussed not only for cooperative studies, but for cooperative engagement of issues such as strategies on consistent identifiers for patients, the use of modeling and simulation for knowledge generation, evaluation of approaches for the use of diverse data types and varying data quality, and development of methods for the use of information from mobile consumer devices and patient-generated data.

PATIENT AND POPULATION ENGAGEMENT

Discussions on the roles of patients and the public in growing the digital infrastructure for the learning health system were anchored strongly in the concept of reengineering the care culture to ensure the centrality of the individual patient in the care process—a concept underscored in the *Quality Chasm* report (IOM, 2001) that remains elusive. Signs of change are only beginning to appear as appreciation increases for the use of web-based information and the clinical and outcome advantages of a patient who is better informed and more involved. Often referenced in the discussions was the need for the establishment of a "new norm" around engaging patients and the population in health—both theirs and that of the population—through the use of the digital infrastructure. Basic to this "re-norming" is a deepened appreciation by patients and the general population for the personal and public benefits that are likely to occur, as well as a strong measure of confidence in the security of the system.

The *value proposition* must be apparent to the stakeholders. Communication of the value of a digital health infrastructure in the improvement of care coordination, quality, and, ultimately, the health of the population at large, was identified in workshop discussions as a fundamental priority. Furthermore, participants pointed out that, in order to be successful, the value proposition should be approached in the context of transparent conversations about privacy, security, and other impeding concerns. The use of case studies and quantitative assessments of the contribution of HIT to improved patient experiences and outcomes was discussed as a potential starting point.

A common theme across several workshop discussions was the value in fostering a *shared learning culture* among system stakeholders—in particular, a culture that recognizes the unique contributions that patients and the general population can make to the learning system as collaborators, not subjects. Activities that foster patient involvement in and support of knowledge generation, including illustrating the importance of patient preference information to improving care, were discussed as potential approaches to this issue.

Following the theme of "renorming" participation of patients and the population in health improvement, and building on the framework established by previous Institute of Medicine work in this area, discussions of the opportunity for strengthening *patient–clinician outcome partnerships* through the digital infrastructure were discussed. The development of templates and protocols that support the use of HIT to engage patients in decision making as well as tools for more effective provider–patient communication were proposed. An important element in this respect is providing patients with secure access to and control of their health information. This includes further development of *patient portals*, building on technologies already widely accepted by consumers, and supporting efforts for increased information liquidity and control such as the Veterans Health Administration/Centers for Medicare & Medicaid Services Blue Button initiative.

In concert with these efforts, participants discussed the need to increase the availability and access to *lay-oriented, user-friendly clinical and nonmedical health information*. Investing in templates for form and content of information for the lay consumer, as well as gathering patient-derived data for care and delivery improvement were suggested as areas of focus. Indeed, the "new norm" was discussed as involving a focus on improving patients' health, not just health care, by emphasizing health maintenance as a lifelong process that includes a patient's actions and decisions outside of the clinical care setting. To this end, participants proposed providing individuals with useful information concerning their clinical encounters and the relevant state of evidence, as well as giving them more responsibility for utilizing this information in their own decision making.

HIT provides an opportunity for engaging populations not historically well served by the traditional healthcare community. For this reason, the potential of the digital health utility in the elimination of *health disparities* was discussed as a strategic priority for further attention and action. The impact of facilitating patient and population contribution to, and control of, their health information has the potential to address disparities in underserved populations.

The importance of a component of *continuous evaluation* and improvement in efforts for patient and population engagement in the digital health learning system was again emphasized. Areas of focus that were highlighted include ongoing assessment of patient preferences for use in tailoring of health plans, innovative approaches to confidentiality and privacy issues, and assessments of opportunities to use contemporary sociotechnical approaches (e.g., social networking and smart phones) for patient and population engagement.

GOVERNANCE

Discussions of governance strategies for the digital infrastructure for the learning health system focused on facilitating activities to advance some very basic components and principles of the ULS digital health information system. Participants often struggled with the question "what are we proposing to govern?" and certainly the health information system as it exists now does not easily fit into most established governance models. On the other hand, upon applying the ULS lens to this issue, and considering innovative governance approaches in cases outside of health (such as

VISA and the Smart GRID, see Appendix B for more information), certain governance-related strategic elements emerged. Participants often pointed to the example of the Internet Engineering Task Force as one example of a governance approach that, while created under different circumstances, reflects many of the same governing principles.

Of principal concern is the issue of the *vision*. As a means of establishing a reference point for progress, workshop participants articulated the need for work to establish a shared vision of the digital health utility for the learning health system. Prospective components noted for this vision include expectations, guiding principles, modus operandi, and an appreciation for the global perspective. Considerations of the differences between a structure that governs versus one that provides guidance were included in these discussions.

Participants noted that a governance model in line with the ULS approach would be one that identified and depended on a minimal set of *guiding principles* with which all stakeholders must comport, maximizing local autonomy over all other decisions. Tolerance of change and adaptability were additional characteristics that participants felt were important to incorporate. Exploring the most decentralized level at which these standards might be delegated and focusing standards on major functional requirements were proposed as starting points. Additionally, the importance of tailoring the governance approach to the local situation and needs was emphasized. A focus on the ability to use an inclusive (both/and) rather than a deterministic (either/or) approach was discussed as a foundational principle that encapsulated this thinking. A related issue discussed was the broader context of the governance enterprise. Participants discussed the need to include societal values such as trust, privacy, and fairness; fair information practices such as transparency and data collection and use limitations; goals of the health sector to improve quality of care and enhance clinical knowledge; technical concepts such as innovation; and economic aspects such as promoting efficiency and reducing costs.

Possible *participant roles and responsibilities* in the governance structure were identified as an important early step, and different approaches were considered. These included broad participation by all stakeholders, which was pointed out to be logistically very difficult; very narrow participation, which participants felt was unlikely to be successful; or a hybrid model, that incorporated both broad and narrow participation depending on the needs at that particular level. Some participants noted that multiple layers of governance were likely to be required to address concerns at the appropriate level whether local, regional, national, or international.

Several approaches to the establishment of a governance model were considered and discussed by workshop participants. Leveraging lessons through collaborative discussions among ongoing efforts—at both the national and local levels—and establishing a working group to begin collecting initial input were suggested as starting points. To enhance the efficiency of deliberative efforts, participants suggested coordinating these activities, potentially through the Office of the National Coordinator for Health Information Technology's Health IT Policy Committee's Governance Working Group; building upon and aligning existing policies, such as Health Insurance Portability and Accountability Act, agency regulations, and informed consent processes to encourage learning health system activities; and nurturing the interfaces with the international community.

A potential responsibility discussed for the governance structure was the *stewardship of processes and protocols* associated with learning health system functionalities. Participants noted that developing processes for proposing, reviewing, and validating protocols on key elements including data gathering, security, and use is an integral part of this approach. Ongoing stewardship responsibilities for the governing entity will involve monitoring and maintaining protocols, managing variability across participants, and devising an approach to provide incentives to stakeholders to conform to stated goals and principles. A related element discussed as a governance challenge was that of *implementation phasing*, or sequencing protocol development activities so that barriers to progress in an entrepreneurial environment are not presented by premature initiation of activity bounding exercises.

In the spirit of a continuously improving learning health system, a process for *continuous evaluation and improvement* of the governance entity and approach was emphasized as important. Areas highlighted included establishing an approach to ongoing assessment of progress and problems, systematic assessment of value realization for recognition and promotion of successful practices, and the support of research on governance and orchestration of the ULS digital health utility in the United States and globally.

COMMON THEMES AND PRINCIPLES

Several common themes recurred throughout the rich and varied discussion. These themes, included in Box 9-2 and summarized below, were reflected in discussions of each of the four focus areas (technical progress, knowledge generation and use, patient and population engagement, and governance), as well as the discussions around various strategic elements. They ranged from issues related to the culture and environment for learning to the centrality of the patient and the importance of flexibility and trust.

- *Build a shared learning environment.* HIT provides an opportunity to change the current environment in which health decisions are made to one of shared input and active participation from patients,

> **BOX 9-2**
> **Common Themes and Principles**
>
> - Build a shared learning environment
> - Engage health and health care, population, and patient
> - Leverage existing programs and policies
> - Embed services and research in a continuous learning loop
> - Anchor in an ultra-large-scale systems approach
> - Emphasize decentralization and specifications parsimony
> - Keep use barriers low and complexity incremental
> - Foster a socio-technical perspective, focused on the population
> - Weave a strong and secure trust fabric among stakeholders
> - Provide continuous evaluation and improvement

caregivers, and the population at large. Approaches discussed to developing this shared learning environment include the direct involvement and support of patient and population roles in the generation of knowledge through the incorporation of user-generated data, understanding the benefits of information use in patient care and population health improvement, and improving patient access to health information to allow for a more active role in care decisions.

- *Engage health and health care, population, and patient.* Many participants reiterated that in order to improve health outcomes for the nation, thinking must extend beyond clinical encounters, and even beyond the individual patient, to the population as a whole. This shift of scope brought into clearer focus several issues discussed, including the opportunity to use HIT and its associated information to build a concept of health that is about more than medical care and draws on seamless interface with information from nonmedical health-related sources to generate knowledge that allows for a more inclusive view of population health improvement.
- *Leverage existing programs and policies.* A foundational assumption during the discussions was the advantage provided by building on, and accelerating, the substantial recent progress, both nationally and internationally, with an emphasis on the importance of fostering coordination among these efforts to capture efficiencies and prevent unnecessary duplication and waste going forward. Participants often noted that recent policies and legislation have laid a foundation for this work, and that the resulting investments and progress can be leveraged to move toward long-term system goals.

- *Embed services and research in a continuous learning loop.* Meeting participants often underscored that a digital infrastructure that supports both the generation and use of knowledge cannot be effective unless it is integrated seamlessly within the processes from which it draws and is meant to support care delivery, research, quality improvement, and population health monitoring. Ease of use for health system stakeholders, attention to the effects on workflow, and the delivery of useful decision support at point of care were often mentioned in discussions.
- *Anchor in an ultra-large-scale systems approach.* One of the most prominent features of the discussions was the notion that the health system is a complex, sociotechnical ecosystem, and therefore necessitates a unique conceptual approach. Grounding this approach to coordination and integration of the digital infrastructure for the learning health system in the principles of a ULS systems approach was suggested by several workshop participants from the computer science community (see Box 9-3). The term "ultra-large-scale system" refers to the existence of a virtual system that has bearing on a social purpose—for example, improving health and health care—and in which a few key elements, such as interchange representation, may be standardized, but whose many participants have diverse and even conflicting goals, so adaptability is key. Institutions retain flexibility for innovation in their choices, and evolutionary functional change can be shaped by architectural precepts, incentives, and compliance assessment, but not by centralized control. ULS functionality is therefore facilitated by protocols that allow maximum practical flexibility for participants. Incorporating decentralization of data, development, and operational authority and control, this approach fosters local innovation, personalization, and emergent behaviors. Participants felt that this approach was well suited to the complex adaptive characteristics of the health system, and that it could serve as an anchoring framework for approaching both the social and technical components of the overall infrastructure.
- *Emphasize decentralization and specifications parsimony.* In line with the complex adaptive qualities of the health system outlined in the *Quality Chasm* (IOM, 2001) report and reiterated during the workshops, both the social and technical components of the digital health infrastructure require a framework that allows for tailoring to specific needs, local innovation, and evolvability. In this respect, the commonly repeated refrain was a call for the principle of parsimony and minimizing centralization that might constitute a barrier to entry: specify only the minimal set of standards or requirements

> **BOX 9-3**
> **Ultra-Large-Scale (ULS) System Characteristics**
>
> The ULS approach can be best described by a set of characteristics that tend to arise as a result of the scale of the system (in this case health and health care) rather than a prescriptive set of required components. Previous work on the ULS concept has identified the following key characteristics of ULS systems:
>
> **Decentralization:** The scale of ULS systems means that they will necessarily be decentralized in a variety of ways—decentralized data, development, evolution, and operational control.
>
> **Inherently conflicting, unknowable, and diverse requirements:** ULS systems will be developed and used by a wide variety of stakeholders with unavoidably different, conflicting, complex, and changing needs.
>
> **Continuous evolution and deployment:** There will be an increasing need to integrate new capabilities into a ULS system while it is operating. New and different capabilities will be deployed, and unused capabilities will be dropped; the system will be evolving not in phases, but continuously.
>
> **Heterogeneous, inconsistent, and changing elements:** A ULS system will not be constructed from uniform parts: there will be some misfits, especially as the system is extended and repaired.
>
> **Erosion of the people/system boundary:** People will not just be users of a ULS system; they will be elements of the system, affecting its overall emergent behavior.
>
> **Normal failures:** Software and hardware failures will be the norm rather than the exception.
>
> **New paradigms for acquisition and policy:** The acquisition of a ULS system will be simultaneous with the operation of the system and require new methods for control.
>
> SOURCE: Northrop et al. (2006).

necessary for key functional utility, and push the maximum amount of control to the periphery. This approach is in line with strategies such as those suggested in the PCAST report for use of metadata for wrapping individual information packets to facilitate interoperability and health information exchange, in which a primary focus would be on development of the metadata standards.

- *Keep use barriers low and complexity incremental.* Similarly, incentives for broad participation in the digital infrastructure by all stakeholders was discussed as a crucial factor to its success. The proposal to keep the barriers for use of the infrastructure, such as deployment and operational complexity, low was articulated by workshop participants in order to allow for maximum participation at a baseline level, and allow for incremental complexity and sophistication where possible or necessary.
- *Foster a sociotechnical perspective, focused on the population.* From the outset of the discussions, participants pointed out that the major barriers to technical progress often lie in social and cultural domains. Acknowledging and engaging this fact was described as being crucial to success, with discussions centering on an approach that reorients future efforts to engage the patient more directly in the collection and use of information in a way that is most useful to them.
- *Weave a strong trust fabric among stakeholders.* Security and privacy concerns represent a strong threat to participation in, and therefore the success of, the sociotechnical ecosystem. Accordingly, they must be dealt with from both the social and technical perspectives. Participants emphasized the need for systems security to comply with all current requirements and regulations and retain an ability to evolve to meet future needs. In addition, continued honest communication to the public and other involved stakeholders about risks and benefits will be crucial to building a foundation of trust.
- *Provide continuous evaluation and improvement.* A learning system is one that assesses its own performance against a set of goals and uses the results of that evaluation to change future behaviors. Workshop participants articulated the importance that all components of a digital infrastructure must themselves function as learning systems.

REFERENCES

IOM (Institute of Medicine). 2001. *Crossing the quality chasm: A new health system for the 21st century.* Washington, DC: National Academy Press.

Northrop, L., P. H. Feiler, B. Pollak, and D. Pipitone. 2006. *Ultra-large-scale systems: The software challenge of the future.* Pittsburgh, PA: Software Engineering Institute, Carnegie Mellon University.

10

Accelerating Progress

INTRODUCTION

Throughout the workshop discussions—and most prominently at the third meeting in the series—participants identified several specific, cross-cutting action targets as priority elements for future work. These activities were presented as actionable next steps necessary to accelerate progress on the issues and domains outlined in Chapter 9. This chapter begins by presenting 10 priority action targets (summarized in Box 10-1) that were most often cited throughout discussions. These activities represent participants' views on the necessary next steps to accelerate progress in four domains: stakeholder engagement, technical progress, infrastructure use, and governance. When discussing necessary follow-up activities, participants continually referenced the potential held by the next stages of the meaningful use guidelines for growing the digital health infrastructure. Participants' views on key possibilities to be considered when developing and releasing stage 2 and 3 guidelines are summarized in Box 10-2 and elaborated on in this chapter. Finally, due to the cross-cutting nature of the priority action targets identified, discussions often focused on delineating specific stakeholder responsibilities and opportunities for action. This chapter concludes with a summary of participant views on the near-term steps that private and public stakeholders can take to accelerate progress on the follow-up areas identified.

BOX 10-1
Priority Action Targets Discussed

Stakeholder Engagement

The case: Analyses to assess the potential returns on health and economic dimensions

Involvement: Initiative on citizens, patients, and clinicians as active learning stakeholders

Technical Progress

Functionality standards: Consensus on standards for core functionalities—care, quality, public health, and research

Interoperability: Stakeholder vehicle to accelerate exchange and interoperability specifications

ULS system test bed: Identify opportunities, implications, and test beds for ULS system approach

Technical acceleration: Collaborative vehicle for computational scientists and HIT community

Infrastructure Use

Quality measures: Consensus on embedded outcome-focused quality measures

Clinical research: Cooperative network to advance distributed research capacity and core measures

Identity resolution: Consortium to address patient identification across the system

Governance

Governance and coordination: Determination and implementation of governing principles, priorities, system specifications, and cooperative strategies

STAKEHOLDER ENGAGEMENT

The case: Analyses to assess the potential returns on health and economic dimensions. Because of the centrality of broad-based support to progress, and the "public good" nature of many of the activities, the need to demonstrate a value proposition or business case for participation by stakeholders in a digital learning health system was a topic of much discussion during the workshop series. This emphasis was reinforced by the approach taken by the President's Council on Science and Technology report to encourage the development of a market around digital health information exchange. Support of methods that apply serious analytical rigor to these issues and generate both technical and policy suggestions were identified as being crucial to this effort. Researchers and organizations such as think tanks were discussed as likely being the best positioned to undertake the necessary analyses with support of a commissioning resource.

Involvement: Initiative on citizens, patients, and clinicians as active learning stakeholders. Many workshop discussions considered that stakeholder investment to be a necessary component of any successful strategy. Participants identified the need to redefine the roles of citizens, patients, and clinicians in a way that activates their participation in their own health, and the health of the population at large, through the facilitative properties of the digital infrastructure. It was noted that patient and clinician groups can play a crucial role in this effort by helping convey the value proposition and ensuring that the interests of their constituents are represented in the development and evolution of the system. Efforts that facilitate stakeholder participation—such as increased control of health information by patients and the use of patient-generated data in care plans and knowledge generating processes—were discussed as priority next steps in stakeholder engagement. Additionally, to attend to concerns around privacy, security, trust, and additional work burden, participants stressed the importance of honesty and transparency in facilitating support and understanding. Ultimately, discussions noted that demonstrating the value of a digital health infrastructure through the use of case studies that point to improved outcomes and efficiency was likely the most compelling strategy to appeal to stakeholders.

TECHNICAL PROGRESS

Functionality standards: Consensus on standards for core functionalities—care, quality, public health, and research. Progress on the technical standards necessary to support the core functionalities of the learning health system was continually referenced in workshop discussions. Participants focused on the standards necessary not only to improve, monitor, and guide care decisions but also to accelerate research, quality efforts, patient monitoring, and health surveillance. Related requirements include the ability to exchange information through the use of minimal standards (such as those to enable use of metadata-tagged information packets), query and analyze distributed repositories of data for research purposes, ensure care decision support, and enable quality improvement initiatives and public health surveillance and reporting. Discussions also touched on the need for the digital infrastructure to interface with next-generation systems including mobile health applications and the way in which these and other capacities could help engage patients and the public through improved information access. Participants also underscored the strategic importance of adhering to a minimal set of standards that support core functions but do not introduce unnecessary barriers to progress.

Interoperability: Stakeholder vehicle to accelerate exchange and interoperability specifications. System interoperability remains a major obstacle to realizing a digital learning health system. When applying the ultra-large-scale (ULS) system lens to this challenge, participants stressed the need to develop a parsimonious set of standards—such as those for metadata—to allow for practical interoperability and information exchange across systems. Noting that this issue lies in the realm of both technical capacity and governance structure, participants often compared this effort to the evolution and governance of the Internet. While the differences between the digital health infrastructure and the Internet were acknowledged, it was suggested that the establishment and work of the Internet Engineering Task Force might provide guidance for an industrial institution for the governance of interoperability-related standards. Additionally, leveraging and coordinating existing progress and ongoing efforts in the areas of standards development and facilitation were underscored as strategies to ensure activities progress as efficiently as possible.

ULS system test bed: Identify opportunities, implications, and test beds for ULS system approach. As discussions focused on the characterization of the health system as a complex sociotechnical ecosystem, analysis was suggested on how the ULS approach might be applied to the health system in both the short and long term. Mapping of a key ULS system report (Northrop et al., 2006) to the learning health system through a collaborative effort between software engineers, computer scientists, medical informaticians, and clinicians was offered as a starting point for this effort. Furthermore, performing a rigorous engineering systems analysis leading to a concept paper was suggested to clarify further the opportunities and implications for the ULS system approach. Integral to the ULS approach is the need to support rapid prototyping for continuous innovation. It was suggested that test beds for the development, assessment, and dissemination of these prototypes would be central to continual innovation. In this vein, several participants pointed to the opportunity presented by the creation of the Center for Medicare & Medicaid Innovation (CMMI). Certain communities of excellence already provide some capacity in this area, and participants often referenced ongoing activities at these institutions (see Appendix B).

Technical acceleration: Collaborative vehicle for computational scientists and HIT community. Much of the work in the development of a digital learning health system will necessitate interdisciplinary collaboration between academic, public, and private partners across the computer science, HIT, science, and engineering communities. Participants suggested establishing a collaborative forum where these efforts can be initiated and developed. This forum could catalyze the interdisciplinary research program necessary to develop the digital health infrastructure, and some participants suggested that funding for such a forum and its associated activities might best be served by collaborative efforts across relevant federal agencies (such asthe National Institutes of Health (NIH) and the National Science Foundation (NSF)), relevant private sector partners, or both.

INFRASTRUCTURE USE

Quality measures: Consensus on embedded outcome-focused quality measures. Participants noted that the first step in determining the usefulness of data collected by the digital health infrastructure is to identify the necessary elements to collect. It was stated several times that in order to support the quality improvement and research activities required for a learning system, consensus around useful outcome-based measures is needed. Participants suggested that this would motivate vendors and users to incorporate these measures into their systems, driving seamless integration of quality measurement and reporting into the digital infrastructure. Work at the National Quality Forum, through the Office of the National Coordinator for Health Information Technology (ONC) HIT Policy Committee, and at the Centers for Medicare & Medicaid Services (CMS) has already begun addressing these needs.

Clinical research: Cooperative network to advance distributed research capacity and core measures. Discussions often highlighted the centrality of ongoing and continuous generation of knowledge from clinical data as a central feature of the learning health system. Efforts to do research on data held in distributed repositories, such as the HMO Research Network and the Food and Drug Administration's (FDA's) Mini-Sentinel program, were pointed to as important early-stage efforts in building systematic, larger scale capacity.

Participants suggested that a multidisciplinary, cooperative network of the relevant stakeholders—principally computer scientists, clinical researchers, and data holders—could be a starting point in accelerating progress in this dimension. It was noted that this network would need to consider development of core datasets to facilitate research and quality efforts, fostering consensus on levels of consent and de-identification strategies necessary for effective re-use of data, development of methodologies for query-based and automated research and signal detection across distributed systems, development of standards for distributed queries across the system, implications for a ULS approach to existing and future distributed networks, and implications for distributed research from possible advances in data structure and packaging strategies for data interoperability and exchange across systems.

Identity resolution: Consortium to address patient identification across the system. One of the major barriers discussed for several key system functions—care appropriateness, continuity, quality assessment, and research—relates to the current inability to track and link individual patients with their associated information reliably across the health system. This poses a problem for issues around care coordination, including the goal of being able to make care decisions based on comprehensive health information, as well as the development of a useful knowledge generation engine that can incorporate all relevant information and deliver useful, accurate support. Privacy and system security are paramount, but participants noted that approaches are available to address these issues responsibly and the barrier appears to be one of cultural hesitancy rather than a lack of technical capability. Targeting this issue through a consortium approach was proposed as a way to provide the opportunity for stakeholder representation and engagement in an honest, transparent conversation about the component value issues involved.

GOVERNANCE

Governance and coordination: Determination and implementation of governing principles, priorities, system specifications, and cooperative strategies. Workshop participants articulated the idea that governance principles and priorities for a learning health system will require breaking new ground both organizationally and functionally. Discussions identified the need to improve coordination among key stakeholders to accelerate progress in identifying and sharing lessons, examining commonalities, and exploiting opportunities for efficiencies. It was noted that broad agreement will need to be cooperatively marshaled to attend to principles and priorities that support learning system functionalities such as data integrity, policies for data use, human subjects research issues, and proprietary interests. In addition, discussions highlighted the role of governance in planning for and mitigating system failures, an inevitable occurrence in all systems, but one particularly well tolerated within the ULS system. Such failures would, of course, be opportunities for learning, but are potentially alarming in the context of health- and healthcare-associated information. An interdisciplinary consortium of computer scientists and health infomaticians, such as the one mentioned above, was suggested as a suitable place to engage this issue on a technical level. However, addressing system failures in the health system also has a deeply sociocultural component for which approaches that emphasize honesty and transparency with patients and the public were suggested. Education and outreach about this issue were identified as being crucial in preventing irreparable tears in the trust fabric necessary to support a digital learning health system. In this respect, participants noted the important contributions and potential of the HIT Policy Committee's Governance Working Group. Discussions also underscored the potential advantages of establishing a novel nongovernmental or public–private venture to foster the necessary governance capacity in this country and to work with similar efforts internationally.

OPPORTUNITIES IN THE NEXT STAGES OF MEANINGFUL USE

In line with these priorities, discussions often focused on the ongoing meaningful use requirement development process. Workshop participants discussed the "beyond meaningful use" issue as key to increasing the utility of digitally embedded clinical records in a learning health system. Specifically, since meaningful use is now such a well-established benchmark process, elements of particular importance to the development of a learning health system might not otherwise be addressed in the meaningful use process if they are not called out for explicit attention in the upcoming stages. Depicted in Box 10-2 is a brief description of the meaningful use stages, the current expected focus of the requirements for stages 2 and 3, and bullet points highlighting some key possibilities proposed by workshop participants.

Stage 2. Items that workshop participants felt were of particular importance in enhancing the impact that stage 2 of meaningful use could have on the progress of the digital learning health system cut across several dimensions. Flagged as especially key were actions to accelerate standards for semantic interoperability and exchange, as well as approaches for consistent identification of patients. In order to further the utility of EHRs in clinical research and population health, participants suggested core data elements for EHRs and seamless access to information from immunization registries. Reflecting the extensive discussion on the opportunity for using the digital infrastructure to better engage patients in their health care, participants suggested the addition of lay-interpretable language for patient-accessible

BOX 10-2
Meaningful Use and the Digital Learning Health System Infrastructure

Stage 1: 2011-2012

Stage 1 of meaningful use established 14-15 (eligible hospitals or eligible professionals) required core functional components, focused on data capture and sharing, along with a menu set of 10 additional components, from which 5 are to be selected by the eligible hospitals or eligible professionals.

Stage 2: 2013-2014

Stage 2 of meaningful use is under development by the Health Information Technology (HIT) Policy Committee, including consideration of further focus on advanced clinical processes such as: clinical decision support, disease management, patient access to health information, quality measurement, research, public health, and interoperability across information technology (IT) systems. The following are items underscored in Institute of Medicine (IOM) discussions as being of particular and immediate importance to the impact of Stage 2 enhancements on progress toward the digital infrastructure for the learning health system:

- Integration of semantic interoperability and exchange standards, including data provenance and context
- Elements fostering seamless integration of clinical decision support
- Use of lay-interpretable language for patient-accessible electronic health record (EHR) information
- Incorporation of patient generated data, including patient preferences
- Inclusion of core data elements that facilitate use of EHR data for clinical research.
- Strategy for seamless access to immunization history from immunization registries
- Strategy for consistent identification of patients

Stage 3: 2015+

Stage 3 of meaningful use is expected to expand on requirements from stages 1 and 2, with more direct emphasis on improved patient outcomes through sharpened focus on quality, safety, efficiency, population health, and interoperability. Following are items, in addition to those noted above for stage 2, underscored in IOM discussions as being of particular and immediate importance to the impact of Stage 3 enhancements on progress toward the digital infrastructure for the learning health system:

- Ability to access comprehensive, longitudinal patient record at point of care
- Incorporation of patient editing ability
- Demonstration of baseline semantic interoperability and exchange capacity among IT systems
- Integration of nonmedical, health-related information
- Seamless clinician–public health agency exchange on case-level information and alerts

information and incorporation of patient-generated data. Finally, discussions emphasized the need for clinical decision support to be seamlessly integrated into HIT systems to speed adoption.

Stage 3. Looking ahead to stage 3 of meaningful use, workshop participants suggested deepening the focus on requirements related to demonstrating semantic interoperability and exchange capacity among systems, the ability to access comprehensive patient records at the point of care, and seamless exchange of cases and alerts between clinicians and public health agencies. Additionally, participants suggested strategies for including additional types of data—including nonmedical, health-related data—as well as providing patients with an annotated editing ability over their own records.

STAKEHOLDER RESPONSIBILITIES AND OPPORTUNITIES

Throughout each workshop, frequent reference was made to leadership responsibilities that fell naturally to individual stakeholders, or groups of stakeholders, to advance progress in developing the digital infrastructure for the learning health system. In many cases, this involved leveraging ongoing efforts or building upon them with an orientation toward a continuous learning system. Summarized below are some of those most often noted. These responsibilities are summarized in Appendix C.

Federal Government

Even though participants noted the decentralized manner in which localized innovation is likely to contribute to system progress, many of the central strategy elements and priority action targets discussed require strong leadership from federal agencies. Since a clear lead responsibility was given to ONC and the Secretary of the Department of Health and Human Services by the Health Information Technology for Economic and Clinical Health (HITECH) Act, ONC was noted as the natural leadership locus for activities needing coordination at the national level. Opportunities to build on the foundation laid by the HITECH requirements for work on standards, requirements, and certification criterion in meaningful use of EHRs include cooperation with other federal agencies in the development of a strategic plan for national HIT efforts; establishment of a governance mechanism for the Nationwide Health Information Network; accelerating, in cooperation with the National Institute for Standards and Technology, work on standards for exchange and interoperability; and work with the Federal Communications Commission, FDA, and CMS to identify standards and reconcile regulations to facilitate wireless transmission of medical information. Participants noted that, as the HITECH funds are used, the coordinating capacity of ONC will take on even greater importance, as coalitions will be needed to harmonize various key activities geared at developing the standards, policies, governance, and research projects necessary for effective progress toward a learning health system.

With respect to technical innovation, as the leading federal agency for funding computer science and engineering research, the NSF was noted as a logical locus to work with ONC and NIH in the development of test beds for the rapid deployment and evaluation of innovative technological approaches. This work would have the potential to transform the functionality and capacity of the digital health infrastructure, as well as to shepherd the establishment of collaborative vehicles for the ongoing partnerships between the HIT and computational science communities.

Similarly, it was noted that progress in the quality and knowledge generation dimensions of the digital platform will require leadership from federal health agencies. The Agency for Healthcare Research and Quality (AHRQ), working with ONC, professional societies, and groups such as the National Quality Forum and the National Committee for Quality Assurance, is a natural steward for initiatives that enhance the utility of the digital infrastructure for quality improvement and health services research.

The Centers for Disease Control and Prevention's (CDC's) focus on population health places it at the center of extending the scope of the digital infrastructure beyond health care. This carries implications for almost all elements of the system, but will be especially important for the support of public health processes and research as well as public engagement. To these ends, participants suggested developing templates and protocols for the integration of nonmedical population health and demographic information into the system.

As the nation's largest healthcare financing organization, CMS currently serves as the principal vehicle for applying economic incentives and standards to accelerate application of the meaningful use requirements. Furthermore, much promise for future innovation in HIT to support a learning system resides in the CMMI, which provides an opportunity for testing innovative approaches suggested by workshop participants. These approaches include test beds for ULS-associated programs and new approaches to integrating clinical decision support with care coordination and delivery models.

On the research front, both NIH and NSF have mandates and networks to develop and demonstrate methods of improving the functionality of the digital infrastructure for health research applications. NIH, the Veterans Health Administration, the Department of Defense, FDA, and AHRQ all have active programs under way that can evolve into cooperative leadership efforts to expand the use of EHRs for research into the clinical effectiveness of health interventions.

To build support and engagement among patients and the general population, AHRQ, FDA, NIH, and ONC each has established links to patient communities that can serve as the building blocks for a collaborative initiative to better characterize and communicate the health and economic advantages of public involvement in a digital platform for health improvement.

Given this level of activity, and the number of central stakeholders, the importance of ONC's coordination mandate was often underscored. Similarly emphasized was the need to cultivate strong counterpart capacity outside of government to partner in coordination and governance responsibilities.

State and Local Government Leadership

Given the regional emphasis of many of the ongoing efforts related to the digital learning health system—such as the establishment of regional health information exchanges—state and local governments and health departments have experience establishing governance structures and developing programs for engaging local stakeholders. As a result, participants noted, state and local bodies can function as resources and foundation stones for broader efforts. By collaborating with ONC, CMS, the Health Resources and Services Administration, and other federal initiatives, best practices and lessons learned can be leveraged from state and local efforts. Additionally, it was suggested that some of the more advanced local initiatives could serve as test beds for some of the innovative ULS-associated approaches suggested by participants.

Initiatives Outside Government

Outside of government, the entrepreneurial capacity of the commercial sector will certainly be a major driver of progress. Similarly, the full potential of the learning health system can only be achieved through the full engagement of patients and the public. Workshop discussants frequently underscored the roles of patient and clinician groups to facilitate dialogue between stakeholders and mediate public engagement. In particular, by using case studies to demonstrate the value of the digital infrastructure, participants felt these organizations could help develop the shared learning culture and trust necessary for the learning system to function. Many patient and clinician groups—such as the American College of Physicians, the American College of Cardiology, the Society of Thoracic Surgeons, and the National Partnership for Women and Families—are already involved in this type of work. Participants noted that these existing activities could be built upon to include issues of particular importance to the learning system approach.

Delivery systems, particularly those integrated across healthcare components, have been at the cutting edge of innovative EHR use, quality improvement, clinical data stewardship, patient engagement, quality initiatives, and distributed research efforts. Workshop conversations often pointed to these efforts, such as those at Kaiser Permanente and Geisinger Health System, suggesting that continued coordination between these delivery systems and relevant federal government agencies would be important in growing the digital health infrastructure.

As the stewards of the largest stores of clinical and transactional information outside of the federal government, insurers, payers, and product developers have an essential role to play in development of the digital infrastructure. Their use of transactional health data to assess utilization patterns, effectiveness, and efficiency is a foundational block on which strategies for broader knowledge generation can build. Furthermore, companies such as UnitedHealthcare have begun engaging the public in the use of data in health. These efforts often were cited during discussions as crucial first steps in establishing a learning culture.

Research is a fundamental aspect of the learning health system. Consequently, participants noted the fundamental role researchers have in developing the infrastructure necessary for continuous knowledge generation and application. Formation of multidisciplinary research communities was often cited as a critical step in accelerating many of the strategies discussed. Funding for these communities was noted as a clear opportunity for collaboration between NSF and NIH. Additionally, discussions highlighted that much work remains to be done in order to maximize the knowledge generation capabilities of the digital infrastructure, and that clinical research and product development communities have an essential role in building this capacity.

As much of the progress to date is a result of initiatives from many independent organizations, their continued efforts as facilitators and innovators were noted as crucial to accelerating progress. Reference was often made to the importance of these organizations as the foundational elements for coordination and governance leadership from outside government.

Finally, and ultimately of paramount importance, is the global perspective. As highlighted during workshop discussions and presentations (see Chapter 8), meeting the goals of a learning health system will inevitably require drawing upon resources and leadership of similar efforts throughout the world. Some of this activity has begun in the limited arena of infectious disease surveillance and monitoring, and offers a hint of the potential opportunities—and challenges—in developing a truly global clinical data utility for health progress.

REFERENCE

Northrop, L., P. H. Feiler, B. Pollak, and D. Pipitone. 2006. *Ultra-large-scale systems: The software challenge of the future*. Pittsburgh, PA: Software Engineering Institute, Carnegie Mellon University.

A

The Learning Health System and the Digital Health Utility

Foundational Elements	Learning Health System Characteristics		
Data utility: data stewarded and used for the common good	*Digital technology:* the engine for continuous improvement	*Trust fabric:* strong, protected, and actively nurtured	*Leadership:* multi-focal, networked, and dynamic
Care: starting with the best practice, every time	*Health information:* a reliable, secure, and reusable resource	*Outcomes and costs:* transparent and constantly assessed	*Knowledge:* ongoing, seamless product of services and research
Culture: participatory, team-based, transparent, improving	*Design and processes:* patient-anchored and tested	*Patients and public:* fully and actively engaged	*Decisions:* informed, facilitated, shared, and coordinated
	Meaningful Use Requirements[a]		
Core structured personal data (age, sex, ethnicity)	Core list of active problems	Core structured clinical data (VS, meds, [labs])	Clinical decision support	Care coordination support/ interoperability
Outpatient medicines electronically prescribed	Automated medication safeguard/ econciliation	Visit-specific information to patients	Automated patient reminders	e-Record patient access (copy or patient portal)
Embedded clinical quality measures	Security safeguards	[Condition-specific data retrieval capacity]	[Public health reporting (reportable conditions)]	[Advance directives for ages >65]

Next-Generation Digital Infrastructure

	LHS Digital Health Utility Next generation requirements	Strategy Elements Activities that advance:	Stakeholder Responsibilities[b]
Technical Progress	Ultra-large-scale system perspective Distributed, local data maintenance Virtual interoperability Reliable use and system security protocols Standards vehicles for setting/revising, metadata, vocabulary, data transport, common core datasets, sentinel indicators, access authorization/authentication, data quality review protocols	Ultra-large-scale system perspective Functionality focus System specifications/interoperability Workflow and usability Security and privacy safeguards System innovation	ONC works with NIST, other agencies and IT community to advance interoperability and security protocols NSF works with ONC/NIH on test beds for digital infrastructure component technologies including ULS system approach Interoperability agreements among delivery systems utilizing EHRs CMS develops test beds for digital infrastructure application in care coordination/delivery model innovation
Knowledge Generation/Use	Core clinical data elements available for quality improvement and research Channels and protocols for integrating clinical and public health data Capacity and protocols for query-driven data use in quality and research and monitoring of sentinel indicators Novel statistical and database tools for reliable new insights	Shared learning environment Point of decision support and guidance Research-ready records for data reuse Patient-generated data Integration/use of data across sources Distributed data repositories Sentinel indicators Query capacity Analytical tools and methods innovation	NIH, NSF, AHRQ, and FDA work on innovative approaches to research insights from clinical data CDC develops templates/protocols for integrating population and clinical data Healthcare organizations form research collaboratives

continued

Patient/Population Engagement	"New norm" for patient involvement Facilitated personal record interface Clinician–patient electronic partnership Patient information access/control Updated best practices delivered at point of decision Active patient support for data use in care improvement Clinician–public health e-partnership	Value proposition and patient confidence Shared learning culture Patient–clinician outcome partnerships Person-centric, lay-oriented health information Closing the disparity gap Continuous evaluation	AHRQ, FDA, NIH, and ONC use established links with patient community to foster active embracing of the digital health utility Patient and clinician groups mediate public engagement and facilitate dialogue among stakeholders to develop shared learning culture/trust
Governance	Progressively evolving requirements, specifications, process protocols for exchange, interoperability, and research Cross-national harmonization to foster the global e-health utility Broad ongoing evaluation capacity	The vision Guiding principles Participant roles and responsibilities Process and protocol stewardship Implementation phasing Continuous evaluation	ONC works with other agencies, the HIT community, and patient/clinician groups to foster development of a governance mechanism that encourages dynamic entrepreneurial growth while safeguarding personal security and the common good

[a] Optional elements denoted with [ ]. See Appendix B for details.
[b] Sample list, neither definitive nor complete. See page xxiii for list of acronyms.

Appendix B

Case Studies for the Digital Health Infrastructure

THE caBIG® INITIATIVE

Prepared by Ken Buetow (National Cancer Institute)

Overview

The National Cancer Institute (NCI) has developed an informatics program designed to improve patient care and accelerate scientific discoveries by enabling the collection and analysis of large amounts of biological and clinical information and facilitating connectivity and collaboration among biomedical researchers and organizations. Called caBIG® (cancer Biomedical Informatics Grid), this program is developing the foundational informatics infrastructure to improve health and combat disease emerging at the intersection of life sciences, information technology, and medicine. The caBIG® program has three core components: community, connectivity, and content.

The caBIG® Community

The caBIG® program has been from the start a collaborative endeavor. Its community has grown dramatically in size and scope since the program began in 2004. More than 2,200 individuals representing more than 700 different organizations are actively engaged in caBIG®, and participation is steadily increasing. These individuals include basic and clinical researchers, consumers, physicians, advocates, software architects and developers, bioinformatics specialists, and executives from academe, medical centers, government, and commercial software, pharmaceutical, and biotechnology companies from the United States and in 15+ countries around the globe. In support of the development of a Rapid Learning Health System, the caBIG® participation includes both academic and community cancer centers.

The caBIG® program is organized into workspaces focused on specific domains such as medical imaging, IT architecture, and clinical trials. Subject matter experts and developers within each workspace use virtual conferences and regular face-to-face meetings to work collaboratively on domain-specific issues and projects. The entire caBIG® community meets once per year for the Annual Meeting, whose growth in size and scope year-over-year has mirrored that of the caBIG® program. More than 1,100 individuals representing more than 300 organizations and 13 countries attended the 2009 meeting, held in Washington, DC, where participants celebrated the first 5 years of the caBIG® program by planning new applications and research uses.

While the caBIG® community is highly diverse, its members have similar needs for data management and analysis.

Through participation in the caBIG® program, they are able to access the informatics infrastructure required to work productively, advancing the knowledge of the underlying causes of disease and providing improved patient outcomes.

Connectivity

From a technology perspective, caBIG® is centered on four key principles:

- *Open development*—Planning, testing, validation, and deployment of caBIG® tools and infrastructure are open to the entire research community, and contributions from many organizations ensure applicability to a wide range of common research problems.
- *Open access*—caBIG® is open to all individuals and organizations interested in solving their data management and connectivity challenges, thus ensuring widespread access to tools, data, and infrastructure.
- *Open source*—The underlying software code of caBIG® tools is freely available for use and modification by any organization, public or private, thus encouraging commercial partnerships.
- *Federation*—Data and analytical resources can be controlled locally or integrated across multiple sites. Control of secure access to those resources is retained by the originating organization. This federated approach obviates the need for a central authority and reduces data management overhead.

Together, these four organizing principles ensure the availability of robustly designed tools that address a wide range of basic and clinical research requirements. Central to these needs is the requirement for interoperability—the ability to access and make meaningful use of data and information by multiple systems. By building and deploying IT based on industry-recognized standards, and providing application programming interfaces and software development kits for third-party developers, the process of creating new caBIG®-compatible software or adapting existing software to become caBIG®-compatible is simplified, encouraging partnerships across the IT community.

At the heart of the caBIG® program—invisible to the end user and customized for the specific needs of biomedical researchers—is caGrid, a model-driven, service-oriented architecture that provides standards-based core "services," tools, and interfaces so the community can connect to share data and analyses efficiently and securely. More than 120 organizations are connected to caGrid. The number continues to expand as more NCI-designated Comprehensive Cancer Centers, as well as academic and commercial organizations set up nodes on the grid, making caGrid the largest biomedical research network in the world today.

Such caBIG®-enabled connectivity is not limited to organizations conducting cancer research. In partnership with the American Society of Clincal Oncology, caBIG® is developing specifications and services to support oncology-extended electronic health records (EHRs) that are being deployed in community practice and hospital settings. caBIG® tools and technology are also being used by researchers working on cardiovascular health, arthritis, and AIDS. In addition, pilot projects have successfully connected caGrid to other networks, including the Nationwide Health Information Network, the CardioVascular Research Grid, and the computational network TeraGrid.

Ultimately, the vision of the caBIG® program is to provide the technical infrastructure for a resource called the Biomedical Knowledge Cloud. The Biomedical Knowledge Cloud is a means of using the Internet to connect massive amounts of individual and organizational biomedical data, software applications with which to handle and analyze all those data, and the computational horsepower to do the work. The Cloud is bounded with patient privacy and other data-sharing protections.

Although the components of the Cloud are not new, the concept of joining them together to provide seamless, secure access to biomedical information is just being realized today.

Simply connecting organizations and individuals would be of little value if they were not able to access and understand the data and information created by different laboratories. Currently, many software systems, either commercial or created in-house to serve the needs of a particular institution, are based on proprietary data formats and, as a result, cannot readily exchange data. They lack the ability to be interoperable.

Since its inception, the caBIG® program has worked with key healthcare industry organizations to create or expand standards and common vocabularies that describe data types, analytical processes, and even clinical procedures. By developing tools that adhere to these standards and leverage these vocabularies, institutions can exchange data seamlessly, much the same way that agreed-upon interoperable standards enabled the global banking system to develop the interconnected network of ATMs for consumer use.

caBIG® is based on the belief that strong confidentiality, privacy, and security measures are both necessary and feasible in any electronic health information exchange environment, and that the measures can be scaled to accommodate a broad range of participants without unnecessarily impeding scientific discovery and medical progress. The program has developed robust computer security measures to ensure that only researchers with the appropriate credentials have access to data, as well as guidelines to assist those researchers in determining the sensitivity of their data for sharing.

Content

As scientific understanding of the complexities underlying most diseases increases, the interconnectedness of biological systems becomes more and more obvious, and researchers must apply multidisciplinary analysis techniques to large, diverse datasets to make new discoveries. For example, by correlating the activity of a specific set of genes with observed outcomes from large groups of patients on the same treatment protocol, cause-and-effect relationships can be found that would be missed when examining the expression patterns alone, or when looking at a small group of patients.

By enabling researchers to work collaboratively—leveraging large, diverse datasets—all constituents of the health care community reap the benefits. Biomedical researchers can ask and answer more complex questions that help uncover the underlying causes of disease, speeding the development of novel diagnostics and therapeutics. Healthcare providers can stay current on new treatments and outcome information gathered from large populations of patients who have similar diseases. This capability allows them to provide the best treatment options for their patients, ultimately improving patient outcomes. The patients themselves are assured of receiving optimal treatment regardless of their physical location, since their complete medical history is secure yet available as needed to guide their treatment.

FDA'S SENTINEL INITIATIVE

Prepared by Judy Racoosin (Food and Drug Administration)

Background

In May 2008, the Department of Health and Human Services (HHS) and the Food and Drug Administration (FDA) announced the launch of FDA's Sentinel Initiative, a long-term program designed to build and implement a national electronic system (Sentinel System) for monitoring the safety of FDA-approved drugs and other medical products. The Sentinel System will function as an active postmarket safety monitoring system, augmenting FDA's existing safety monitoring systems. The launch of the Sentinel Initiative followed passage of the Food and Drug Administration Amendments Act (FDAAA), which became law in September 2007. Section 905 of FDAAA mandates FDA to develop an enhanced ability to monitor the safety of marketed drugs using automated healthcare data sources. The Sentinel Initiative is designed to manage the development and implementation of the Sentinel System while ensuring that it fulfills the mandates included in FDAAA.

Once developed and implemented, the Sentinel System will enable FDA to monitor the safety of drugs and other medical products with the assistance of a wide array of collaborating institutions throughout the United States. Data partners in the Sentinel System will include organizations such as academic medical centers, healthcare systems, and health insurance companies. As currently envisioned, participating data partners will access, maintain, and protect their respective data, functioning as part of a "distributed system." Collaborating organizations will also include patient and healthcare professional advocacy groups, academic institutions, and regulated industry, among others.

In the active surveillance environment of the Sentinel System, FDA will prioritize safety questions that have emerged from premarket or postmarket safety data sources (e.g., clinical trial data, postmarket adverse event reports) and submit them to a Coordinating Center for evaluation by data partners that are participating in the Sentinel System. Data partners will securely access their databases to evaluate the submitted question and return Health Insurance Portability and Accountability Act (HIPAA)–compliant result summaries to the Coordinating Center. The Coordinating Center will then aggregate and/or summarize these results and forward them to FDA for their use in assessing the safety question.

Mini-Sentinel

In September 2009, FDA awarded a contract to Harvard Pilgrim Health Care, Inc. (Harvard Pilgrim) to develop a smaller working version of the future Sentinel System. The pilot has been dubbed "Mini-Sentinel." Harvard Pilgrim's Mini-Sentinel Coordinating Center (MSCC) is creating a kind of laboratory, giving FDA the opportunity to access disparate automated healthcare data sources and test epidemiological and statistical methodologies in the evaluation of postmarket safety issues. Through this pilot, FDA will learn more about some of the barriers and challenges, both internal and external, to establishing a Sentinel System for medical product safety monitoring. The MSCC is leading a consortium of more than 20 collaborating institutions.[1]

The MSCC and participating data partners are using a common data model as the basis for their analytical approach. The approach requires the data partners to transform their data into a standardized format. Based on this standardized format, the MSCC will write a single analytical software program for a given safety question and provide it to each of the data partners. This will allow each data partner to run the program on its standardized data. Data partners will conduct analyses behind their existing, secure firewalls and send only summary results to the MSCC for aggregation and further evaluation. The MSCC will provide FDA with both the aggregated results and the summary results from each data partner. The use of a common analytical program will minimize the potential for differences in results across data holders resulting from differences in the implementation of an active surveillance protocol. As this pilot is being implemented, a governance structure is being developed to ensure that the activity encourages broad collaboration within appropriate guidelines for the conduct of public health surveillance activities. In order to accomplish that, the MSCC is developing a Statement of Principles and Policies that will include descriptions of the organizational structure and policies related to communication, privacy, confidentiality, data usage, conflicts of interest, and intellectual property.

Also, with the launch of Mini-Sentinel, a Privacy Panel was formed to provide expertise regarding patient privacy-related regulations that pertain

---

[1] The collaborating institutions in the consortium include the following organizations: CIGNA Healthcare; Cincinnati Children's Hospital Medical Center; Brigham and Women's Hospital; Duke University School of Medicine; HMO Research Network sites (includes Group Health Cooperative, Harvard Pilgrim Health Care Institute, HealthPartners, Henry Ford, Lovelace Clinic Foundation, Marshfield Clinic Research Foundation, Meyers Primary Care Institute [Fallon]); HealthCore; Humana-Miami Health Services Research Center; Kaiser Permanente (includes KPNC, KPSC, KPCO, KPNW, KPG, KPHI, KPOhio, KPmidatlantic); Outcome Sciences, Inc.; University of Illinois at Chicago; University of Iowa, College of Public Health; University of Pennsylvania School of Medicine; Vanderbilt University School of Medicine; Weill Cornell Medical College.

to the conduct of Mini-Sentinel. The panel members are independent privacy experts with extensive knowledge of legal and ethical issues related to the use of protected health information (PHI), including applicable laws and regulations, data privacy and confidentiality, and the use of PHI for public health surveillance activities. The panel is

- Providing expertise on application of relevant laws and regulations governing the privacy and security of health information for Mini-Sentinel's purposes. The panel advises specifically on the applicability of laws, including HIPAA and other relevant laws and regulations.
- Making recommendations on creation of appropriate policies and procedures to guide specific uses of PHI in Mini-Sentinel.
- Assisting the MSCC in reviewing documents, agreements, and contracts to ensure that they adequately incorporate the panel's discussions regarding the issues delineated above.

Federal Partners' Collaboration

FDA is furthering the science of medical product surveillance by broadening existing pilot programs that use federally held data sources. The effort, known as the Federal Partners' Collaboration (FPC), involves the Centers for Medicare & Medicaid Services (CMS), the Veterans Administration (VA), and the Department of Defense. FPC is an expansion of the SafeRx project, a collaboration between FDA and CMS that uses Medicare and Medicaid data for medical product safety surveillance. The FPC is similar to the Mini-Sentinel pilot in that it will use an active surveillance approach and involves a distributed system. However, unlike Mini-Sentinel, the FPC will not use a common data model. Rather, the FPC will develop a common active surveillance protocol, and then each data partner will write analytical code to run the protocol in their database. Lessons learned from this pilot will be compared to lessons learned as part of Mini-Sentinel (i.e., using a common data model where centralized analytics are employed). In this way, FDA can compare the potential benefits and drawbacks of every data partner running a single analytical program based on a common data model versus each data partner developing its own analytical program based on a common protocol.

Outreach Related to Active Medical Product Surveillance

Continuing a high level of stakeholder involvement is key to maintaining broad-based support and momentum for effective, responsive, active medical product surveillance through FDA's Sentinel Initiative. FDA has awarded a cooperative agreement to the Brookings Institution (Brookings) to convene a broad range of stakeholders to explore and address methodological, data development, technical, and communication issues related to active medical product surveillance.

These meetings encompass a range of formats including webinars on active surveillance–related topics, expert panels on targeted topics central to the development of the Sentinel System, public meetings on the progress of the Sentinel Initiative, and meetings intended to interweave lessons learned by various active surveillance initiatives.

In addition to convening and moderating each meeting, Brookings is synthesizing findings and making them publicly available in order for other organizations and individuals to use the information to further develop active medical product surveillance methods and systems.

In addition, FDA has sought to foster transparency through the creation and maintenance of a Sentinel Initiative Website, which provides information on the background of the initiative, relevant news and events, presentations, completed deliverables from contracted work, and updates on ongoing projects and funding opportunities. A docket is open to allow for public comment on any of this information. The agency also piloted a web-based discussion room to encourage public comment and promote transparency. Sentinel Initiative staff also foster transparency by speaking about the Sentinel Initiative to external stakeholder groups including academia, regulated industry, patient and consumer groups, and medical professional societies, as well as doing internal outreach to FDA staff.

Contracts and Cooperative Agreements Informing FDA on the Development of the Sentinel System

The following documents are now available in the FDA docket and on the Sentinel website http://www.fda.gov/Safety/ FDAsSentinelInitiative/default.htm.

- *Developing a Governance and Operations Structure for the Sentinel Initiative*, an eHealth Initiative Foundation report.
- *Engagement of Patients, Consumers, and Healthcare Professionals in the Sentinel Initiative*, an eHealth Initiative Foundation report.
- *Defining and Evaluating Possible Database Models*, a Harvard Pilgrim Health Care, Inc. report.
- *Evaluation of Existing Methods for Safety Signal Identification*, a Group Health Cooperative Center for Healthcare Studies report.
- *Evaluation of Potential Data Sources for a National Network of Orthopedic Device Implant Registries*, an Outcome Sciences, Inc. report.

- *Evaluation of Timeliness of Medical Update for Surveillance in Health Care Databases*, an IMS Government Solutions report.
- *Evaluating Potential Network Data Sources for Blood and Tissue Product Safety Surveillance and Studies*, a Pragmatic Data report.
- *Evaluation of State Privacy Regulations and Relation to the Sentinel Initiative*, a Qual-Rx report.

Work on the following projects is ongoing.

- *Evaluation of Potential Data Sources*, a Booz Allen Hamilton report.
- *Evaluation of Potential Data Sources for Animal Drugs Used in Veterinary Medicine*, an Insight Policy Research, Inc. report.
- *Detection and Analysis of Adverse Events to Regulated Products in Automated Healthcare Data: Efforts to Develop the Sentinel.*

Additional Background

FDA's Sentinel Initiative, launched in 2008, is a long-term program designed to build and implement a national electronic system (the "Sentinel System") for monitoring the safety of FDA-approved drugs and other medical products. The Sentinel System will fulfill, and go beyond, the congressional mandate put forth in the FDAAA of 2007 that requires FDA to create a system for postmarket risk identification and analysis using public and private automated data sources.

Engaging Patients and the Public

Broad engagement of all stakeholders is essential to developing a governance framework that addresses the many issues that need to be considered for the successful implementation of a system that leverages secondary use of automated healthcare information to improve the public health.

- Early activities of the Sentinel Initiative included meetings with a broad range of stakeholders including other government agencies, potential data partners, patient advocacy groups, professional societies, academia, and regulated industry.
- To ensure continued input of all stakeholder groups, in 2009 FDA awarded a cooperative agreement to the Brookings Institution to function as a convener on topics related to active medical product safety surveillance. They have sponsored large public meetings on the Sentinel Initiative, smaller expert panel discussions on focused topics, and webinar-style roundtables to discuss new methodologies and findings.

Paramount to this effort is safeguarding the privacy and security of the data leveraged for these activities, and ensuring that patients and consumers understand that their privacy is being protected. This includes compliance with federal and state laws and regulations and consideration of additional forms of protection.

- As part of the Mini-Sentinel pilot, a privacy panel consisting of established experts in the field, including patient advocates, has been convened to address privacy and security concerns.

Promoting Technical Advances and Innovation

After careful consideration of all options, FDA concluded that a distributed system is essential to the success of efforts such as the Sentinel Initiative. The key benefits of this distributed approach include the following:

- Patient privacy is maintained by keeping directly identifiable patient information behind local firewalls in its existing protected environment.
- Data partners' involvement in running analyses ensures an informed approach to interpreting results because they are aware of the changes that have occurred in their healthcare systems that result in the unique character of their database.
- Patient and consumer concerns about potential misuse are greatly reduced. A distributed system can operate efficiently, compared to a centralized system, by having the data partners adopt a common data model and then creating the capability for efficient distribution of queries (executable computer programs) and return of their output.
- Through the Mini-Sentinel pilot, FDA has developed the first stage of such a system, which will ultimately include administrative claims, EHRs, and registry data.

We must develop methods to link information about patients between data sources (e.g., inpatient hospital records, outpatient records, and patient registries) in order to produce a complete longitudinal profile of patient care. We must train the next generation of statisticians and epidemiologists to ensure that we will have a workforce with the skills to support active medical product safety surveillance.

Fostering Stewardship and Governance

Governance and stewardship should allow multiple activities, including both public health practice and research, to share a common national resource that allows the use of automated healthcare data for secondary uses, such as safety surveillance, comparative effectiveness research, and quality assessment.

HEALTHWISE

Prepared by Cartherine Serio and Don Kemper (Healthwise)

About Healthwise

Nonprofit mission: Help people make better health decisions (since 1975) 110 million user sessions with Healthwise content in 2009

Current Clients:

- The top 10 U.S. health plans (Kaiser, Aetna, Cigna, Wellpoint, etc.)
- 300-plus U.S. hospitals (Mass General, Sutter, Sisters of Mercy, Health Partners, etc.)
- Leading disease management companies (Health Dialog, Alere, etc.)
- Government agencies (Department of Veterans Affairs, Department of Defense, State Medicaid, British Columbia, etc.)
- Most large health portals (WebMD, AOL, Yahoo, MSN, Health.com, etc.)

Innovation History

- 1970s: Medical self-care handbooks and workshops (28 million books sold)
- 1980s: Wellness books and workshops
- 1990s: Healthwise Knowledgebase for Websites and nurse call centers
  o Patient decision aids (now 158)
  o Symptom guides, action plans, tests, treatments, and self-care
- 2000s: Information therapy, interactive conversations, guided self-management

Promoting the consumer as the greatest untapped resource in health care.

Healthwise Engagement Tips

1. Think like a consumer (patient-centric engagement)
   - Understand consumers' motivation for engagement
   - Anticipate consumers' needs
   - Design toward those needs
2. Engagement ingredients
   - Establish trust
   - Use plain language
   - Allow choice
3. Engagement strategies
   - Pull: How to engage people who are ready to "pull" information from the Web.
   - Push: How to engage people by "pushing" information relevant to their needs.
   - Pay: How to engage even more people through incentives for active patienthood.
4. Engage the consumer's community
   - Social networking allows consumers to get, and give, emotional support

KAISER PERMANENTE[2]

Health Information Technology (HIT) at Kaiser Permanente

Kaiser Permanente has been using information technology for more than 40 years to improve clinical and administrative functions. Its use of electronic health records (EHRs) dates from the 1990s in some regions. Building on this experience, and with the active participation of its physicians, Kaiser Permanente in 2003 launched a $4 billion health information system called KP HealthConnect that links its facilities nationwide and represents the largest civilian installation of EHRs in the United States. As of April 2008, the system was successfully implemented in outpatient clinics in all eight Kaiser regions. Every Kaiser hospital has the essential components of the system and 25 had implemented all modules as of December 2008.

---

[2] Prepared by Roundtable Staff using the following sources:

Healthcare Information and Management Systems Society (HIMSS) Analytics. *Kaiser Permanente—EHR Adoption Model.* http://www.himssanalytics.org/hc_providers/stage7casestudies_KP.asp.

McCarthy, D., and K. Mueller. 2009. *Kaiser Permanente: Bridging the Quality Divide with Integrated Practice, Group Accountability, and Health Information Technology.* The Commonwealth Fund. http://www.commonwealthfund.org/~/media/Files/Publications/Case%20Study/2009/Jun/1278_McCarthy_Kaiser_case_study_624_update.pdf.

APPENDIX B

The EHR at the heart of KP HealthConnect (purchased from vendor Epic Systems Corp.) provides a longitudinal record of member encounters across clinical settings and includes laboratory, medication, and imaging data. HP HealthConnect also incorporates

- Electronic prescribing and test ordering (computerized physician order entry) with standard order sets to promote evidence-based care.
- Population and patient-panel management tools such as disease registries to track patients with chronic conditions.
- Decision support tools such as medication-safety alerts, preventive care reminders, and online clinical guidelines.
- Electronic referrals that directly schedule patient appointments with specialty care physicians.
- Performance monitoring and reporting capabilities.
- Patient registration and billing functions.

KP HealthConnect is designed to electronically connect members to their health care team, to their personal health information, and to relevant medical knowledge to promote integrated health care. For example, members can complete an online health risk assessment, receive customized feedback on behavioral interventions, participate in health behavior change programs, and choose whether to send results to KP HealthConnect to facilitate communication with their physician.

To more fully engage patients in their care, physicians and staff encourage them to sign up for enhanced online services. As a result, more than one-third of health plan members nationwide (and nearly one-half of members in Northern California) are using a web portal called My Health Manager to track selected medical information from the EHR, view a history of physician visits and preventive care reminders, schedule and cancel appointments, refill prescriptions, and send secure electronic messages to their care team or pharmacist. Online laboratory test results—the most popular online function—include links to a knowledge base of information on test results and related self-care strategies. A pilot project is testing the capability for members (initially Kaiser employees) to transfer information securely from My Health Manager to Microsoft Corporation's HealthVault personal health record application.

Physician leaders report that access to the EHR in the exam room is helping to promote compliance with evidence-based guidelines and treatment protocols, eliminate duplicate tests, and enable physicians to handle multiple complaints more efficiently within one visit. A study in the Northwest region found that patient satisfaction with physician encounters increased after the introduction of the EHR in exam rooms there. Early findings from ongoing hospital implementations suggest that the combination of computerized physician-order entry, medication bar coding, and electronic documentation tools is helping to reduce medication administration errors.

Use of the EHR and online portal to support care management and new modes of patient encounters appears to be having positive effects on utilization of services and patient engagement. For example, three-quarters or more of online users surveyed agreed that the portal enables them to manage their health care effectively and that it makes interacting with the health care team more convenient. Patients in the Northwest region who used online services made 10 percent fewer primary or urgent care visits than before they had online access (7 percent fewer visits compared with a control group of patients).

HIT in Practice: Care Coordination and Transitions

Having a broad spectrum of services available within one organization and, in many cases, in one location, makes it easier to coordinate care for patients. Kaiser Permanente's integrated model of care focuses not only on the spectrum of medical care that a patient may need at any one time, but also on members' interactions with the organization across time and the continuum of care—clinic, hospital, home, hospice, or extended care.

The Northern California region uses a population and patient-panel management strategy to improve care and outcomes for patients who have—or who are at risk for developing— chronic diseases. This approach is built on the philosophy that a strong primary care system offers the most efficient way to interact with most patients most of the time, while recognizing that some patients need additional support and specialty care to achieve the best possible outcomes. Patients are stratified into three levels of care:

1. Primary care with self-care support for the 65 percent to 80 percent of patients whose conditions are generally responsive to lifestyle changes and medications.
2. Assistive care management to address adherence problems, complex medication regimens, and comorbidities for the 20 percent to 30 percent of patients whose diseases are not under control through care at level 1.
3. Intensive case management and specialty care for the 1 percent to 5 percent of patients with advanced disease and complex comorbidities or frailty.

Level 1 emphasizes a proactive team approach that conserves physician time for face-to-face encounters by enhancing the contributions of ancillary staff (medical assistants and also nurses and pharmacists in some locations) to conducting outreach to patients between visits. The team uses a population database and decision support tools built into the EHR to track patients with chronic conditions such as diabetes or heart disease, develop action plans to engage them in self-care, ensure that they are taking appropriate medications, and remind them to get preventive care and other tests when needed.

Outreach to patients with chronic conditions typically occurs as follows: The physician reserves a weekly appointment slot to meet with his or her staff and review a computer-generated list of 10 to 20 patients who are not achieving treatment goals. The physician indicates follow-up instructions for each patient, such as increasing medication dosage or ordering a test. The medical assistant or nurse then contacts the patient to relay the physician's instructions, using prepared scripts to ensure consistent communication. Contact is typically made by telephone but may occur by letter in some cases.

At level 2, care managers (specially trained nurses, clinical social workers, or pharmacists) support the primary care team to help patients gain control of a chronic condition. Interventions may include providing self-care education, titrating medications according to protocol, and making referrals to educational classes (e.g., for smoking cessation). The goal is to move patients back to level 1 after an intervention period of several months to a year. Successful transitions require that primary care teams be prepared to follow up with patients and prevent them from relapsing. Care managers may be part of the local primary care team or may be centrally located at a medical center, depending on local resources.

An example of intensive case management (level 3) is a cardiac rehabilitation program called Multifit for patients with advanced heart disease, such as those recovering from a heart attack or heart surgery. Nurse case managers provide telephonic education and support for up to 6 months to help patients make lifestyle changes and reduce their risk of future cardiac events. Aided by the EHR and a patient registry, the Colorado region enhanced the program by adding a telephonic cardiac medication management service provided by clinical pharmacy specialists, with ongoing follow-up until patients achieve treatment goals and can be transferred to primary care for maintenance. Results for patients participating in the Colorado program included the following:

- Cholesterol screening increased from 55 percent to 97 percent of patients, while cholesterol control has almost tripled from 26 percent to 73 percent of patients.
- Relative risk of death declined by 89 percent among those enrolled in the program within 90 days of a cardiac event, and by 76 percent for those with any contact with the program.

HIT as an Engine for Continuous Innovation

Developing Improved Modes of Care Delivery

The 21st Century Care Collaborative is using KP HealthConnect to develop innovations that will transform the ability of primary care teams to improve patient care delivery and member experience while also promoting a sustainable work environment for clinicians and staff. A prototype change package—developed from the experience of several pilot-test sites—is being spread regionally using a flexible approach that lets facilities and teams test elements to determine what works best in their circumstances. Principles and examples include the following:

1. Understand the needs of your population: Design the work and build the care team to meet the needs; for example, maximize team roles and optimize team communication.
2. Develop relationship-based care and demonstrate that we know members; for example, convene member councils, complete after-visit summaries.
3. Provide alternatives to traditional office visits; for example, offer telephone visits and group visits, use secure messaging.
4. Embrace total panel ownership; for example, conduct outreach to patients with chronic conditions, follow up with patients on new medicines.
5. Engage members in collaborative care planning; for example, use goal sheet with diabetic patients, convene chronic care support groups.

These changes have synergistic effects. For example, replacing face-to-face visits with telephone visits saves time and increases convenience for members. It also frees time for the care team to conduct proactive panel-management activities, address urgent-care needs, and look for other opportunities to make things easier for patients, such as by calling those on the appointment schedule to resolve problems over the phone. Pilot sites reported improved quality and increased satisfaction for members and staff.

Pursuing Advances in Medicine

In Northern California, Kaiser Permanente's Division of Research conducts epidemiological and health services research to improve the health and medical care of members and the population at large. A major current project is assembling one of the world's largest biobanks of genetic, environmental, and health data. The biobank will enable research on the causes of diseases that eventually may lead to advances in diagnosis, treatment, and prevention. Almost 400,000 Northern California members have volunteered to participate in the program by completing a health survey and are being asked to contribute saliva samples for DNA analysis.

Lessons Learned

The Right People at the Table

It's imperative that clinicians play a significant role in the planning, design and implementation of an EHR system. They use the system day in and day out, so they need to be involved in the decision-making process. If not, you end up with just a fancier version of the paper record. In designing HealthConnect, hundreds of stakeholders and IT experts worked together for months to figure out the functions the system needed to best serve its members.

Training Is Integral to Success

A large portion of costs were attributable to training and workflow re-design. A great deal of time and energy was spent to accommodate the ramping-up process after the system was implemented. Kaiser has continued with the training and exchanges of best practices and believes it must be an ongoing process.

Don't Underestimate the Desire to Do the Right Thing

It would be unrealistic to say that every doctor switched over to electronic records without any issue. The transition was much more of a culture shock for doctors who had been using paper records for 30 or 40 years. Some were more resistant to change than others, which can be expected in a project of this size. At the end of the day, though, clinicians understood that what was being done was in the best interest of the patient.

THE SMART GRID[3]

Conception

The Smart Grid was mandated at the federal level. Title XII of The Energy Independence and Security Act of 2007 stated that the National Institute for Standards and Technology has "primary responsibility to coordinate development of a framework that includes protocols and model standards for information management to achieve interoperability of smart grid devices and system."

Vision

As conceived, the Smart Grid will

- Enable active participation by consumers
- Accommodate all generation and storage options
- Enable new products, services, and markets
- Provide power equality for the digital economy
- Optimize asset utilization and operate efficiently
- Anticipate and respond to system disturbances (self-heal)
- Operate resiliently against attack and natural disaster

Governance

At the recommendation of the Federal Energy Regulatory Commission, a profit-neutral organization known as an independent system operator or regional transmission organization will be charged with coordinating and managing the operations of the grid. The scale of these organizations is variable (e.g., local, state, regional).

Consumers Energy

In response to a request from Consumers Energy's president and chief executive officer, Dave Joos, a small company team started investigating the smart grid in early 2007. Since then, Consumers Energy has created the Smart Services Learning Center, a smart-grid testing and demonstration facility, to assess vendor products and provide product and integration testing. The company performs product field tests by using strategically deployed off-grid meters that are tied back wirelessly to the center.

Consumers Energy's initial testing and assessment has revealed a clear

---

[3] Prepared by Roundtable staff.

lack of product standardization and integration throughout the industry. With this in mind, the company believes more standardization must be achieved before beginning a full-scale smart-grid system implementation. Company officers, managers, and directors understand the risks involved with deploying systems too quickly and support efforts to further assess and improve vendor products.

Consumers Energy is working with other industry experts to help establish standards and guidelines for an integrated, secure smart-grid systems environment. For example, the company helped create the SAP Lighthouse Council, a group of leading utilities and vendors that collaborate with SAP to develop standardized software and interfaces for smart-grid systems and devices.

Employees also are helping ensure that standardized interfaces are built into customer and grid-based devices to allow for easy connectivity with new utility systems and devices. They have been actively involved with other utilities, vendors, standards organizations, and regulators to ensure that appropriate security capabilities are built into the systems, and that systems can be updated easily when new security threats arise. Upgradability, standard interfaces, and vigorous testing are the best methods for minimizing risks, avoiding product obsolescence, and lowering product costs.

The Model

Fundamentally, the Smart Grid is a long-term, complex systems development project of nationwide scale and implications. It uses the engineering approach of accommodating a wide variety of legacy nodes that are organic—constantly growing and evolving like a biological system. This continuous evolution is desirable, so that the Smart Grid's architecture can preserve, and indeed encourage, the capacity of every node to innovate locally and deal with complexity in a way that suits local and grid needs.

The Smart Grid development methodology is not based on comprehensive internal design and operating standards for each node on the grid to follow. There is no need for consensus among the nodes on how they should operate within local boundaries. Instead, the approach accommodates highly diverse nodes connecting to the Smart Grid using open data translation protocols that standardize information management, rather than using the internal workings of each node. The grid becomes a communications bus to which each node must be able to write, and from which each node must be able to read. This architecture preserves capacities for local operating autonomy and innovation throughout the Smart Grid. It is also manages a standardized communications capacity among complex, and otherwise noninteroperable, legacy nodes on the grid. These features are all characteristics of ultra-large-scale (ULS) software intensive systems.

VISA AND THE "CHAORDIC" GOVERNANCE MODEL[4]

> By Chaord, I mean any self-organizing, adaptive, non-linear, complex system, whether physical, biological, or social, the behavior of which exhibits characteristics of both order and chaos or, loosely translated to business terminology, cooperation and competition.—Dee Hock

Background

In the 1960s, the nascent credit card industry witnessed rapid growth, quickly outgrowing the governance structure of most companies. Although membership and participation were booming, companies were losing money. As the decade neared a close, a lack of organizational regulation and control left the industry with estimated losses in the tens of millions.

Foundations of a New Model

In an attempt to regain control of the industry, Bank of America formed a small committee to devise solutions to operational problems. In his role as chair of this committee, Dee Hock began to construct a new governance model. According to Hock, what emerged from the meeting was a set of several principles, framed as "what if" questions:

- What if the organization were cooperatively and equitably owned, with all relevant and affected parties eligible to participate in functions, governance and ownership?
- What if power and function were distributive, with no power vested in or function performed by any part that could reasonably be exercised by any more peripheral part?
- What if it were self-organizing, with participants having the right to self-organize at any time, for any reason, at any scale, with irrevocable rights of participation in governance at any greater scale?

---

[4] Prepared by Roundtable Staff using the following sources:

Fowler, J. Gone chaordic: Dee Hock, the mastermind behind VISA, has some ideas about reorganizing health care. *Health Forum Journal*.
Hock, D. W. 1995. The chaordic organization: Out of control and into order. *World Business Academy Perspectives* 9(1).
Waldrop, M. M. 1996. Dee Hock on organizations. *Fast Company*. http://www.fastcompany.com/magazine/05/dee3.html.
Waldrop, M. M. 1996. The Trillion-Dollar Vision of Dee Hock. *Fast Company*. http://www.fastcompany.com/magazine/ 05/deehock.html?page=0%2C0.

APPENDIX B   275

- What if governance were distributive, with no individual, institution, or combination of either or both, particularly management, able to dominate deliberations or control decisions at any scale?
- What if it could seamlessly blend cooperating and competing, with all parts free to compete in unique, independent ways, yet could yield self-interest and cooperate when necessary to the inseparable good of the whole?
- What if it could be infinitely malleable, yet extremely durable, with all parts capable of constant, self-generated, modification without sacrificing its essential nature, thus releasing human ingenuity and spirit?

VISA—A Novel, Chaordic Organization

As envisioned by Hock, the governance model that emerged from that meeting, and would become the structure behind VISA, defied previously well-established tenets of corporate organization. VISA was a nonstock, for-profit membership corporation with ownership in the form of nontransferable rights of participation. VISA was highly decentralized and highly collaborative and functioned, as Hock believed, as "an enabling organization" above all else. Similar to a Jeffersonian governmental structure, everything possible (authority, initiative, decision making, wealth) was relegated to the periphery, with only standards and the most large-scale operational issues remaining under centralized control. The center-and-periphery model posed a logical solution to a fundamental problem within the credit card industry: member financial institutions were all competitors (issuing their own cards) but, in order to have a sustainable system, needed to all cooperate (regardless of which bank issues cards, all VISA cards must be accepted by all merchants).

According to Hock, the success of this business model is best demonstrated by the fact that, although VISA is an enormous corporation, few know of its organizational structure. However, at the same time, the core of the enterprise has no knowledge of or authority over a vast number of the constituent parts. No part knows the whole, the whole does not know all the parts and none has any need to. The entirety is largely self-regulating.

Core Tenets of Chaordic Organizations

Hock has long insisted that the VISA model cannot be transposed successfully onto any other industry. It is the notion of a chaordic governance model, not anything specific to VISA's history, that can be used across institutions. However, inherent in toeing the line between chaos and order, designing and implementing such a governance model is an organic and dynamic process unique to the institution attempting it. Although the product will be drastically different in each case, there are certain core tenets of the chaordic model. Some examples include

- *Maximize human ingenuity.* Hock argues that the most abundant, least expensive, most underutilized, and frequently abused resource in the world was human ingenuity; the source of that abuse was archaic, Industrial Age institutions and the management practices they spawned.
- *Organizations must have clarity of a shared purpose, common principles, and strength of belief.* According to Hock, organizations are merely conceptual embodiments of a very old, very basic idea—the idea of community. An organization's success has enormously more to do with clarity of a shared purpose, common principles and strength of belief in them than to assets, expertise, operating ability, or management competence.
- *Push all possible operations to the periphery.* No function should be performed by any part of the whole that could reasonably be done by any more peripheral part, and no power vested in any part that might reasonably be exercised by any lesser part.
- *Foster and tolerate evolution.* The organization must be adaptable and responsive to changing conditions, while preserving overall cohesion and unity of purpose. The governing structure must not be a chain of command, but rather a framework for dialogue, deliberation, and coordination among equals.

C

Example Stakeholder Responsibilities and Opportunities

Organization	HIT-Related Activities
Federal agencies	
Health and Human Services:	
ONC	Coordinate federal efforts in HIT adoption and use
AHRQ	Program management, content development, communication
CDC	Public health monitoring/population health improvement
CMS	Implement HIT to reduce costs and improve quality of care
FDA	Postmarket drug/device surveillance; data reuse
HRSA	Improve access/coordination for underserved populations
NIH	Collaborative research and rapid translation from study to clinic
Other departments:	
Commerce/NIST	Standards and interoperability
DOD/Health Affairs	Telehealth research and design, patient care system
FCC	National Broadband Plan
NSF	Fund digital infrastructure research and development
Veterans Affairs/VHA	EHR/PHR system design and use for patient care and research

Organization	HIT-Related Activities
IT Companies—e.g., Allscripts, Epic, Cerner, GE, Google, Microsoft, Dossia	Software systems supporting integrated clinical and business functions and patient portals
Healthcare delivery—e.g., Geisinger, Kaiser Permanente, Virginia Mason, Group Health Cooperative, Mayo, Partners HealthCare	Use of digital capacity to improve patient care, increase patient involvement, and speed research insights
Academic medical centers—e.g., Duke, MD Anderson, Vanderbilt	Use of digital capacity to speed research insights from clinical care and apply research findings to improve clinical care
Cooperation capacity resources—e.g., ACOs, HMORN, PEDSNET	Implementation and use of data sharing and distributed datasets
Stakeholder organizations—e.g., ACP, ACC, AMIA, eHI, NeHC, NPWC, STS	Advance stakeholder interest in HIT system development and use
Independent sector—e.g., CDISC, CHcF, Markle, NCQA, NQF, RWJF	Funding and facilitating innovation in the HIT field

NOTE: Sample list, neither definitive nor complete. See page xxiii for list of acronyms.

D

Summary Overview of Meaningful Use Objectives

Summary Overview of Meaningful Use Objectives

Objective	Measure
Core set of objectives to be achieved by all eligible professionals, hospitals, and critical access hospitals to qualify for incentive payments	
Record patient demographics (sex, race, ethnicity, date of birth, preferred language, and in the case of hospitals, date and preliminary cause in the event of death)	Over 50% of patients' demographic data recorded as structured data
Record vital signs and chart changes (height, weight, blood pressure, body mass index, growth charts for children)	Over 50% of patients 2 years of age or older have height, weight, and blood pressure recorded as structured data
Maintain up-to-date problem list of current and active diagnoses	Over 80% of patients have at least one entry recorded as structured data
Maintain active medication list	Over 80% of patients have at least one entry recorded as structured data
Maintain active medication allergy list	Over 80% of patients have at least one entry recorded as structured data
Record smoking status for patients 13 years of age or older	Over 50% of patients 13 years of age or older have smoking status recorded as structured data

continued

Summary Overview of Meaningful Use Objectives

Objective	Measure
For individual professionals, provide patients with clinical summaries for each office visit; for hospitals, provide an electronic copy of hospital discharge instructions on request	Clinical summaries provided to patients for over 50% of all office visits within 3 business days; over 50% of all patients who are discharged from the inpatient department or emergency department of an eligible hospital or critical access hospital and who request an electronic copy of their discharge instructions are provided with it
On request, provide patients with an electronic copy of their health information (including diagnostic-test results, problem list, medication lists, medication allergies, and for hospitals, discharge summary and procedures)	Over 50% of requesting patients receive electronic copy within 3 business days
Generate and transmit permissible prescriptions electronically (does not apply to hospitals)	Over 40% are transmitted electronically using certified EHR technology
Computer provider order entry (CPOE) for medication orders	Over 30% of patients with at least one medication in their medication list have at least one medication ordered through CPOE
Implement drug–drug and drug–allergy interaction checks	Functionality is enabled for these checks for the entire reporting period
Implement capability to electronically exchange key clinical information among providers and patient-authorized entities	Perform at least one test of EHR's capacity to electronically exchange information
Implement one clinical decision support rule and ability to track compliance with the rule	One clinical decision support rule implemented
Implement systems to protect privacy and security of patient data in the EHR	Conduct or review a security risk analysis, implement security updates as necessary, and correct identified security deficiencies
Report clinical quality measures to CMS or states	For 2011, provide aggregate numerator and denominator through attestation; for 2012, electronically submit measures

Reproduced with permission from Blumenthal, D., and M. Tavenner. 2010. The "meaningful use" regulation for electronic health records. *New England Journal of Medicine* 363(6):501-504.

E

PCAST Report Recommendations[1]

The Chief Technology Officer of the United States should

- In coordination with the Office of Management and Budget (OMB) and the Secretary of HHS, and using technical expertise within ONC, develop within 12 months a set of metrics that measure progress toward an operational, universal, national health IT infrastructure. Research, prototype, and pilot efforts should not be included in this metric of operational progress.
- Annually, assess the Nation's progress in health IT by the metrics developed, and make recommendations to OMB and the Secretary of HHS on how to make more rapid progress.

The Office of the National Coordinator should

- Move more boldly to ensure that the Nation has electronic health systems that are able to exchange health data in a universal manner based on metadata-tagged data elements. In particular, ONC should signal now that systems will need to have this capability by 2013 in order to be deemed as making "meaningful use" of electronic health information under the HITECH Act.

---

[1] *Excerpted from*: PCAST (President's Council of Advisors on Science and Technology). 2010. Realizing the Full Potential of Health Information Technology to Improve Healthcare for Americans: The Path Forward. http://www.whitehouse.gov/sites/default/files/microsites/ostp/pcast-health-it-report.pdf.

- Act to establish initial minimal standards for the metadata associated with tagged data elements, and develop a roadmap for more complete standards over time.
- Facilitate the rapid mapping of existing semantic taxonomies into tagged data elements, while continuing to encourage the longer-term harmonization of these taxonomies by vendors and other stakeholders.
- Support the development of reference implementations for the use of tagged data elements in products. Certification of individual products should focus on interoperability with the reference implementations.
- Set standards for the necessary data element access services (specifically, indexing and access control) and formulate a strategic plan for bringing such services into operation in an interoperable and intercommunicating manner. Immediate priority should be given to those services needed to locate data relating to an individual patient.
- Facilitate, with the Small Business Administration, the emergence of competitive companies that would provide small or under-resourced physician practices, community-based long-term care facilities, and hospitals with a range of cloud-based services.
- Ensure that research funded through the SHARP (Strategic Health IT Advanced Research Projects) program on data security include the use of metadata to enable data security.

The Centers for Medicare & Medicaid Services should

- Redirect the focus of meaningful use measures as rapidly as possible from data collection of specified lists of health measures to higher levels of data exchange and the increased use of clinical decision supports.
- Direct its efforts under the Patient Protection and Affordable Care Act toward the ability to receive and use data from multiple sources and formats.
- In parallel with (i.e., without waiting for) the NRC study on IT modernization, begin to develop options for the modernization and full integration of its information systems platforms using modern technologies, and with the necessary transparency to build confidence with Congress and other stakeholders.
- When informed by the preliminary and final NRC study reports, move rapidly to implement one or more of the options already formulated, or formulate new options as appropriate, with the goal of making substantial progress by 2013 and completing implemen-

tation by 2014. CMS must transition into a modern information technology organization, allowing integration of multiple components and consistent use of standards and processes across all the provider sectors and programs it manages.
- Exercise its influence as the Nation's largest healthcare payer to accelerate the implementation of health information exchange using tagged data elements. By 2013, meaningful use criteria should include data submitted through reference implementation processes, either directly to CMS or (if CMS modernization is not sufficiently advanced) through private entities authorized to serve this purpose.
- By 2013, provide incentives for hospitals and eligible professionals to submit meaningful use clinical measures that are calculated from computable data. By 2015, encourage or require that quality measures under all of its reporting programs (the Physician Quality Reporting Initiative, hospitals, Medicare Advantage plans, nursing homes, etc.) be able to be collected in a tagged data element model.

The Department of Health and Human Services should

- Develop a strategic plan for rapid action that integrates and aligns information systems through the government's public health agencies (including FDA, CDC, NIH, and AHRQ) and benefits payment systems (CMS and VA).
- Convene a high-level task force to align data standards, and population research data, between private and public sector payers.
- Convene a high-level task force to develop specific recommendations on national standards that enable patient access, data exchange, and de-identified data aggregation for research purposes, in a model based on tagged data elements that embed privacy rules, policies and applicable patient preferences in the metadata traveling with each data element.
- As the necessary counterpart to technical security measures, propose an appropriate structure of administrative, civil, and criminal penalties for the misuse of a national health IT infrastructure and individual patient records, wherever such data may reside.
- Appoint a working group of diverse expert stakeholders to develop policies and standards for the appropriate secondary uses of healthcare data. This could be tasked to the Interagency Coordinating Council for Comparative Effectiveness Research.
- With FDA, bring about the creation of a trusted third-party notification service that would identify and implement methods for re-identification of individuals when data analysis produces important new findings.

Other or multiple agencies

- AHRQ should be funded to develop a test network for comparative effectiveness research. The FDA, and also other HHS public health agencies, should enable medical researchers to gain access to de-identified, aggregated, near-real-time medical data by using data element access services.
- HHS should coordinate ONC activities with CDC, FDA, and any other entities developing adverse event and syndromic surveillance networks.
- The Department of Defense and the Department of Veteran Affairs should engage with ONC and help to drive the development of standards for universal data exchange of which they can become early adopters.

F

Workshop Agendas

**Digital Infrastructure for the Learning Health System:
The Foundation for Continuous Improvement in Health and Health Care**

*An Institute of Medicine Workshop Series
Sponsored by the Office of the National Coordinator for
Health Information Technology*

Series objectives

1. Foster a shared understanding of the vision for the electronic infrastructure for continuous learning and quality-driven health and healthcare programs.
2. Explore current capacity, approaches, incentives, and policies; and identify key technologic, organizational, policy, and implementation priorities.
3. Discuss the characteristics of potentially disruptive, breakthrough developments.
4. Consider strategy options and priorities for accelerating progress on the approach to the infrastructure, and for moving beyond to a more seamless learning enterprise.

Issues motivating the discussion
- Rapid developments in information technology that substantially facilitate potential use of health data for knowledge generation, and expedited application of new knowledge for clinical care.
- Policy initiatives that will lead in the near future to the electronic capture and storage of virtually all clinical data, as well as data from several related areas of health—health care, public health, clinical research—to realize the system's full potential for individuals and populations.

- Promising potential in federated/distributed approaches that allow data to remain local while still enabling querying and pooling of summary data across systems.
- Ongoing innovation in search technologies with the potential to accelerate use of available data from multiple sources for new insights.
- Meaningful use criteria and health reform provisions that provide starting points and incentives for the development of a learning system for quality improvement and population health, while underscoring the need to be strategic on issues and opportunities, while maintaining flexibility to accommodate breakthrough capacities.
- Need for careful attention to limiting the burden for health data collection to the issues most important to patient care and knowledge generation.
- Requirement for governance policies that foster the data utility for the common good, cultivate the trust fabric with the public and between data sharing entities, and accelerate collaborative progress.
- Availability of standards for aggregation of large pools of data for purposes such as CER, biomarker validation, disease modeling, and improving research processes.

❖

WORKSHOP #1: OPPORTUNITIES, CHALLENGES, PRIORITIES

❖

July 27–28, 2010

Venable Conference Facility
575 Seventh Street NW, Washington, DC 20001

Day One: Tuesday, July 27

8:00am   Coffee and light breakfast available

8:30am   **Welcome, introductions, and overview**
Welcome, framing of the meeting and workshop series, agenda overview
- o Michael McGinnis (Institute of Medicine)
- o Charles Friedman (Office of the National Coordinator for Health IT)
- o Laura Adams (Planning Committee Chair, Rhode Island Quality Institute)

APPENDIX F

9:00am   Session 1: Visioning perspectives on the electronic health utility
National leader/decision maker from each of several key areas will offer a perspective on the vision and opportunities for the electronic health utility, briefly describe the current state of the infrastructure, its use relative to the potential, and the key actions and priorities moving forward.
Moderator: Laura Adams (Rhode Island Quality Institute)
➢ Individual and patient perspective
Adam Clark (Lance Armstrong Foundation)
➢ Practicing clinician perspective
James Walker (Geisinger)
➢ Quality and safety perspective
Janet Corrigan (National Quality Forum)
➢ Clinical research perspective
Christopher Chute (Mayo Clinic)
➢ Population health perspective
Martin LaVenture (Minnesota Department of Health)

OPEN DISCUSSION

11:00am   Session 2: Technical strategies: data input, access, use—and beyond
Presentations to consider issues, needs, and approaches related to data input, access and use—as well as infrastructure requirements to foster web-mediated remote-site interventions—for continuous learning and improvement in health and health care.
Moderator: Chris Greer (Office of Science and Technology Policy)
➢ Building on the foundation of meaningful use
Doug Fridsma (Office of the National Coordinator for Health IT)
➢ Interoperability for the learning healthcare system
Rebecca Kush (Clinical Data Interchange Standards Consortium)
➢ Grids, federations, and clouds
Jonathan Silverstein (University of Chicago)
➢ Querying heterogeneous data
Shaun Grannis (Regenstrief Institute)

A panel of responders from the quality, clinical research, and population health communities to respond to presentations, share their experiences, and propose solutions.
    Ida Sim (University of California, San Francisco)
    John Halamka (Beth Israel Deaconess Medical Center)
    Robert Kahn (Corporation for National Research Initiatives)

OPEN DISCUSSION

1:00pm   **Lunch**

1:30pm   **Session 3: Ensuring engagement of population and patient needs**
Presentations to consider issues, needs, and approaches in use of the electronic infrastructure to address compelling priorities in patient and population health improvement.
- **Transparency on cost/outcomes at individual and population levels**
Mark McClellan (Brookings Institution)
- **Integrated use of personal and population-wide data sources**
Kenneth Mandl (Harvard University)
- **Optimizing chronic disease care and control**
Sophia Chang (California HealthCare Foundation)
- **Targeting population health disparities**
Christopher Gibbons (Johns Hopkins University)

A panel of responders to respond to presentations, share their experiences, and propose solutions.
    Don Kemper (Healthwise)
    Eric Larson (Group Health)
    Patricia Brennan (University of Wisconsin)

OPEN DISCUSSION

3:30pm   **Session 4: Weaving a strong trust fabric**
Presentations to consider issues, needs, and approaches related to building the broad-scale confidence necessary for operation of the electronic infrastructure for continuously learning and improving health and healthcare programs.
Moderator: Mark Frisse (Vanderbilt University)

➢ Facilitating and chronicling data use for better health/health care
Edward Shortliffe (American Medical Informatics Association)
➢ Privacy and consent strategies
Deven McGraw (Center for Democracy and Technology)
➢ HIPAA and a learning healthcare system
Bradley Malin (Vanderbilt)
➢ System security
Ian Foster (Argonne National Lab)

A panel of responders from ongoing collaborative efforts and experts with big-picture perspectives to respond to presentations, share their experiences, and propose solutions.
    Robert Shelton (Private Access, Inc.)
    Kristen Rosati (Coppersmith Schermer & Brockelman PLC)
    Richard Platt (Harvard Pilgrim)

OPEN DISCUSSION

5:30pm **Concluding Keynote**

David Blumenthal (National Coordinator for Health IT)

6:00pm **Adjourn to reception**

Day Two: Wednesday, July 28

8:30am **Welcome and Recap of First Day**

9:00am **Session 5: Stewardship and governance in the learning health system**
Presentations on issues, needs, approaches, and arrangements—formal and informal, public and private, national and international—necessary to steward the development of a digital infrastructure to deliver health data and information that is timely, user-friendly, secure, reliable, research-ready, supports continuous learning and accelerated improvements in health and health care.
Moderator: Michael Kahn (Children's Hospital Denver)
➢ Governance coordination, needs, and options
Laura Adams (Rhode Island Quality Institute)

➤ Harmonizing compliance, and enforcement requirements
Theresa Mullin (Food and Drug Administration)
➤ Research access and prioritization issues
Shawn Murphy (Partners Healthcare)
➤ A case study in governance: The National Information Governance Board for Health and Social Care (UK)
Harry Cayton (National Information Governance Board)

A panel of responders from ongoing efforts and experts with big-picture perspectives to respond to presentations, share their experiences, and propose solutions.
Rachel Nosowsky (University of California)
Don Detmer (University of Virginia)
Meryl Bloomrosen (American Medical Informatics Association)
Doug Peddicord (Oldaker, Belair & Wittie)

OPEN DISCUSSION

11:00am Session 6: Fostering the global dimension of the health data trust
Presentations to consider issues, needs, and approaches related to setting the stage for evolution of an electronic infrastructure that can serve as a global resource for continuous learning and improvement for health and healthcare programs.
Moderator: Michael Ibara (Pfizer)
➤ **Transform**
Brendan Delaney (Kings College London)
➤ **HealthGRID/SHARE**
Tony Solomonides (University of the West England, Bristol)
➤ **Global collaborative safety strategies**
Ashish Jha (Harvard University)
➤ **Global public health strategies**
David Buckeridge (McGill University)

OPEN DISCUSSION

12:30pm Lunch

1:00pm Session 7: Perspectives on Innovation
Thought leader participants from across stakeholder groups as well as from outside the health field to reflect on the

meeting's discussions, respond to questions, and offer unique insights and novel perspectives on innovation strategies for the electronic infrastructure supporting continuous learning and improvement in health and health care.
    Daniel Friedman (Population and Public Health Information Services)
    Molly Coye (Public Health Institute)
    Matthew Holt (Health 2.0)
    Michael Liebhold (Institute for the Future)

OPEN DISCUSSION

2:30pm   **Session 8: Breakout sessions**
Five small groups will assemble with representation spanning the affinity groups of interest—individual and patient, practicing clinician, quality improvement experts, clinical researchers, and population health—to identify key principles and strategies for development of the electronic infrastructure envisioned—including identification of questions addressed to the panel of responders.

4:00pm   **Session 9: Reporting back to the group**
This session will feature reports back from small groups on proposed strategic approaches, followed by discussion across groups, and identification of common themes across approaches, challenges, and solutions.

OPEN DISCUSSION

5:30pm   **Summary, Next Steps, and Concluding Remarks**

6:00pm   **Adjourn**

❖

WORKSHOP #2: THE SYSTEM AFTER NEXT

❖

September 7–8, 2010

Keck Center, The National Academies
500 Fifth Street NW, Washington, DC 20001

Day One: Tuesday, September 7

8:00am   Coffee and light breakfast available

8:30am   **Welcome, introductions, and overview**
Welcome, framing of the meeting and workshop series, agenda overview
- o Harvey Fineberg (Institute of Medicine)
- o Charles Friedman (Office of the National Coordinator for Health IT)
- o Laura Adams (Planning Committee Chair, Rhode Island Quality Institute)
- o Michael McGinnis (Institute of Medicine)

9:30am   **Three breakout groups: patient and public, technical issues, governance**
Three breakout groups clustered according to participant expertise/interest with respect to technical advancement, governance and patient/public engagement. Each group will be tasked with using the preparatory group's proposed categories and component issues as a starting point to develop and present the framework and most important relevant options for a national strategy. A 10- to 15-minute presentation by a representative of the relevant breakout group will lead off the corresponding plenary session.

12:00pm   **Lunch/Poster session**

1:00pm   **System requirements for technical advancement and innovation**
Technical issues constitute the basic starting point for progress in the electronic infrastructure for health improvement. These include the overlapping sets of issues related to information

processing models, vocabulary value sets, human–computer interaction, and security frameworks. Progress is dependent not only on identifying and engaging the specific elements within each set, but on achieving the right balance between the potential for facilitative standardization and the need for adaptive flexibility and innovation. The session will begin with a 10- to 15-minute presentation from a representative from the "Technical advancement and innovation" breakout group. Moderated discussion based on the prioritized questions and solutions presented will follow, including, if/as appropriate, brief input from resource people for the case studies identified.

OPEN DISCUSSION

3:00pm   **Break**

3:15pm   **Requirements for establishment of stewardship and governance**
Stewardship and governance provisions are intimately related to the pace at which the developing technical capacity of the electronic infrastructure emerges and is applied for continuous improvement in health and health care. The trust and cooperative environment engendered in the existence, nature, stakeholder representation, and implementation of such provisions will determine the availability and impact of this electronic utility. The session will begin with a 10- to 15-minute presentation from a representative from the "Stewardship and governance" breakout group. Moderated discussion based on the prioritized questions and solutions presented will follow, including, if/as appropriate, brief input from resource people for the case studies identified.

OPEN DISCUSSION

5:30pm   **Concluding comments**

6:00pm   **Adjourn to reception**

Day Two: Wednesday, September 8

8:30am Welcome

9:00am **Requirements for patient and public engagement**
Where stakeholder acceptance is involved, it generally comes down to "What's in it for me?" A precondition for progress in the e-health utility is the appreciation and acceptance—the understanding and demand for the delivery of the benefits, and trust and confidence related to safeguards against risks. The session will begin with a 10- to 15-minute presentation from a representative from the "Patient and public engagement" breakout group. Moderated discussion based on the prioritized questions and solutions presented will follow, including, if/as appropriate, brief input from resource people for the case studies identified.

OPEN DISCUSSION

11:00am **Summary, next steps, and concluding remarks**
Discussion will be summarized, priorities identified, and the plan for the progression to the final workshop laid out.

12:00pm **Adjourn**

❖

WORKSHOP #3: STRATEGY SCENARIOS

❖

October 5, 2010

House of Sweden
2900 K Street NW, Washington, DC 20007

Tuesday, October 5

8:00am Coffee and light breakfast available

8:30am **Welcome, introductions, and overview**
Welcome, framing of the meeting and workshop series, agenda overview

APPENDIX F 295

           o Charles Friedman (Office of the National Coordinator for Health IT)
           o Laura Adams (Planning Committee Chair, Rhode Island Quality Institute)
           o Michael McGinnis (Institute of Medicine)

9:00am **Review of strategic options from Workshops 1 and 2**
Overview of strategic options identified to accelerate development of the electronic ecosystem necessary for a continuously learning and improving health system.
- Technical and knowledge generation issues and options
Christopher Chute (Mayo Clinic)
- Individual engagement issues and options
Robert Shelton (Private Access, Inc.)
- Governance issues and options
Laura Adams (Rhode Island Quality Institute)

OPEN DISCUSSION

10:00am **Review of practical considerations**
A discussion of the existing efforts and accompanying considerations that will be relevant to the development of strategy options.
- Emerging communities of excellence
James Walker (Geisinger Health System)
- Emerging drivers of interoperability, scale, and utility
Daniel Masys (Vanderbilt University)
- Implications inherent ULS system dynamics
William Knaus (University of Virginia)
- Levers for government and ONC as change agent
Charles Friedman (Office of the National Coordinator for Health IT)

OPEN DISCUSSION

11:00am **Breakout groups**
Participants are broken into three groups, each focused one of the following groups of issues: technical, knowledge generation and use, governance, and individual engagement.

For their respective areas, groups are asked to
—Propose basic principles for approach

--Consider and revise, as indicated, strategic options from overview, including alternative scenarios
—Identify key stakeholders and responsibilities
—Postulate timetables and expectations—and related assumptions

12:30pm Lunch

1:00pm   Technical options, responsibilities, and expectations

         OPEN DISCUSSION

2:00pm   Knowledge generation and use options, responsibilities, and expectations

         OPEN DISCUSSION

3:00pm   Break

3:15pm   Governance options, responsibilities, and expectations

         OPEN DISCUSSION

4:15pm   Individual engagement options, responsibilities, and expectations

         OPEN DISCUSSION

5:15pm   Concluding comments

G

Workshop Participants

❖

WORKSHOP #1: OPPORTUNITIES, CHALLENGES, PRIORITIES

❖

July 27–28, 2010

Venable Conference Facility
575 Seventh Street NW, Washington, DC 20001

Amy Abernethy
Duke Cancer Care Research
 Program

Laura Adams
Rhode Island Quality Institute

Daniel Armijo
Altarum Institute

Leslie Ball
Food and Drug Administration

Elmer Bernstam
University of Texas

Cynthia Bero
Partners Healthcare

Meryl Bloomrosen
American Medical Informatics
 Association

David Blumenthal
Office of the National Coordinator
 for Health IT

Jim Bodenbender
McKesson Corporation

Jennifer Bordenick
eHealth Initiative

Patricia Brennan
University of Wisconsin

William Bria
Shriners Hospital for Children

Jeff Brown
Harvard Pilgrim Healthcare
    Institute

David Buckeridge
McGill University

Harry Cayton
The National Information
    Governance Board for Health
    and Social Care

John Ceccatti
Conceptual Research

Sophia Chang
California HealthCare Foundation

Basit Chaudhry
Independent

Christopher Chute
Mayo Clinic

Adam Clark
Lance Armstrong Foundation

Elaine Collier
National Institutes of Health

Laura Conn
Centers for Disease Control and
    Prevention

Janet Corrigan
National Quality Forum

Molly Coye
Public Health Institute

Art Davidson
Denver Public Health

Brendan Delaney
Kings College

Don Detmer
University of Virginia

Tim Elwell
Misys Open Source Solutions

Deborah Estrin
University of California, Los
    Angeles

John Feikema
Visionshare

Kevin Fickenscher
Dell

Jonathan Fielding
Los Angeles County Public Health

Ian Foster
Argonne Lab

Douglas Fridsma
Office of the National Coordinator
    for Health IT

Charles Friedman
Office of the National Coordinator for Health IT

Daniel Friedman
Population and Public Health Information Services

Mark Frisse
Vanderbilt University

Jennifer Garvin
University of Utah

Douglas Gentile
Allscripts

M. Chris Gibbons
Johns Hopkins Medical Institutions

Shaun Grannis
Regenstrief Institute

Chris Greer
Office of Science and Technology Policy

Carl Gunter
University of Illinois

John Halamka
Beth Israel Deaconess Medical Center

Jim Hansen
Dossia Consortium

David Hardison
Science Applications International Corporation

Yael Harris
Health Resources Services Administration

Haym Hirsch
National Science Foundation

Matthew Holt
Health 2.0

George Hripcsak
Columbia University

Michael Ibara
Pfizer

Ashish Jha
Harvard University

Michael Kahn
Children's Hospital Denver

Robert Kahn
Corporation for National Research Initiatives

Erin Karnes
The Brookings Institution

Mohit Kaushal
Federal Communications Commission

Donald Kemper
Healthwise

Carl Kesselman
University of Southern California

Todd Ketch
The American Health Quality Association

William Knaus
University of Virginia

Isaac Kohane
Harvard University

Robert Kolodner
Open Health Tools

Wayne Kubick
Phase Forward

Joel Kupersmith
Veterans Administration

Rebecca Kush
Clinical Data Interchange
    Standards Consortium

Eric Larson
Group Health

Martin LaVenture
Minnesota Department of Health

Lisa Lee
Centers for Disease Control and
    Prevention

Bettijoyce Lide
National Institute of Standards and
    Technology

Michael Liebhold
Institute for the Future

Herb Lin
National Research Council

Ravi Madduri
Argonne National Laboratory

Subha Madhavan
Georgetown University

Bradley Malin
Vanderbilt University

Kenneth Mandl
Harvard University

Janet Marchibroda
Office of the National Coordinator
    for Health IT

Mark McClellan
Engelberg Center for Health Care
    Reform

Kathleen McCormick
Science Applications International
    Corporation

Clement McDonald
National Institutes of Health

Michael McGill
Internet2

Deven McGraw
Center for Democracy and
    Technology

Anne McIntyre
Centers for Disease Control and
    Prevention

Karen Milgate
Centers for Medicare & Medicaid
    Services

Joyce Mitchell
University of Utah

APPENDIX G *301*

Donald Mon
American Health Information
 Management Association

Rick Moore
National Committee for Quality
 Assurance

Theresa Mullin
Food and Drug Administration

Julie Murchison
Health 2.0 Accelerator

Sharon Murphy
Institute of Medicine

Shawn Murphy
Partners HealthCare

Rachel Nelson
Office of the National Coordinator
 for Health IT

Chalapathi Neti
IBM

Joshua Newman
Salesforce.com

Rachel Nosowsky
University of California

J. Nwando Olayiwola
Community Health Center, Inc.

Robin Osborn
Commonwealth Fund

Doug Peddicord
Oldaker, Belair & Wittie

Richard Platt
Harvard Pilgrim Healthcare
 Institute

Doug Porter
Blue Cross and Blue Shield

Eva Powell
National Partnership for Women
 and Families

Marc Probst
Intermountain Health

Judith Racoosin
Food and Drug Administration

Stephanie Reel
Johns Hopkins University

Karin Remington
National Institutes of Health

Wes Rishel
Gartner

Roberto Rocha
Partners Healthcare System, Inc.

Kristen Rosati
Coppersmith Schermer &
 Brockelman PLC

David Ross
Public Health Informatics Institute

Joshua Rubin
Kanter Family Foundation

Joel Saltz
Emory University

Jim Scanlon
Department of Health and Human Services

Aaron Seib
National eHealth Collaborative

Raj Shah
CTIS, Inc.

Robert Shelton
Private Access

Edward Shortliffe
American Medical Informatics Association

Jonathan Silverstein
University of Chicago

Ida Sim
University of California, San Francisco

Tony Solomonides
University of the West of England

Michael Stebbins
Office of Science Technology and Policy

Walter Suarez
Kaiser Permanente

Paul Tang
Palo Alto Medical Foundation

Jonathan Teich
Elsevier

Jim Traficant
Harris Healthcare Solutions

Howard Wactlar
National Science Foundation

James Walker
Geisinger Health Systems

Ed Walters
The Brookings Institution

Gio Wiederhold
Stanford University

Janet Woodcock
Food and Drug Administration

Janet Wright
American College of Cardiology

Peter Yu
Palo Alto Medical Foundation

Wil Yu
Office of the National Coordinator for Health IT

JiaJie Zhang
University of Texas

APPENDIX G *303*

❖

WORKSHOP #2: THE SYSTEM AFTER NEXT

❖

September 7–8, 2010

Keck Center, The National Academies
500 Fifth Street NW, Washington, DC 20001

Amy Abernethy
Duke Cancer Care Research
    Program

Laura Adams
Rhode Island Quality Institute

Aneel Advani
Indian Health Service

Cheryl Austein-Casnoff
National Opinion Research Center

Landen Bain
Board of Directors, Clinical
    Data Interchange Standards
    Consortium

Elmer Bernstam
University of Texas

Jim Bodenbender
McKesson Corporation

Jennifer Bordenick
eHealth Initiative

Jeff Brown
Harvard Pilgrim Healthcare
    Institute

Kenneth Buetow
National Institutes of Health

David Carell
Group Health

Justine Carr
Caritas Christi

John Ceccatti
Conceptual Research

Basit Chaudhry
Independent

Christopher Chute
Mayo Clinic

Elaine Collier
National Center for Research
    Resources

Janet Corrigan
National Quality Forum

Greg Downing
Department of Health and Human
    Services

Margo Edmunds
Institute of Medicine

Jon Eisenberg
National Academy of Sciences

Tim Elwell
Misys Open Source Solutions

Deborah Estrin
University of California, Los Angeles

Lynn Ethredge
George Washington University

John Feikema
Visionshare

Kevin Fickenscher
Dell

Charles Friedman
Office of the National Coordinator for Health IT

Jennifer Garvin
University of Utah

Pierce Grahm-Jones
Office of the National Coordinator for Health IT

Tina Grande
Healthcare Leadership Council

Shaun Grannis
Regenstrief Institute

Chris Greer
Office of Science and Technology Policy

Carl Gunter
University of Illinois

Jim Hansen
Dossia Consortium

David Hardison
SAIC, Inc.

Betsy Humphreys
National Library of Medicine

John Hurdle
University of Utah

Michael Kahn
Children's Hospital Denver

Sean Kassim
Food and Drug Administration

Mohit Kaushal
Federal Communications Commission

Joy Keeler
The MITRE Corporation

Donald Kemper
Healthwise

William Knaus
University of Virginia

Robert Kolodner
Open Health Tools

Wayne Kubick
Phase Forward

Rebecca Kush
Clinical Data Interchange Standards Consortium

Martin LaVenture
Minnesota Department of Health

APPENDIX G

David Ledbetter
Emory University

Lisa M. Lee
Centers for Disease Control and Prevention

Herb Lin
National Research Council

Ravi Madduri
Argonne National Laboratory

Richard Marks
Patient Command, Inc.

Robert Marotta
WebMD

Joseph Mayer
Columbia University Medical Center

Kathleen McCormick
National Institutes of Health

Michael McGill
Internet2

Deven McGraw
Center for Democracy and Technology

Donald Mon
American Health Information Management Association

Rick Moore
National Committee for Quality Assurance

Theresa Mullin
Food and Drug Administration

Sharon Murphy
Institute of Medicine

Rachel Nelson
Office of the National Coordinator for Health IT

Stephen Ondra
Department of Veterans Affairs

John Orwat
Blue Cross Blue Shield Association

Doug Peddicord
Association of Clinical Research Organizations

Judith Racoosin
Food and Drug Administration

Stephanie Reel
Johns Hopkins

Mitra Rocca
Food and Drug Administration

Roberto Rocha
Partners Healthcare System

Josh Rubin
Kanter Family Foundation

Tom Savel
Centers for Disease Control and Prevention

Mary Shaw
Carnegie Mellon University

Robert Shelton
Private Access

Jonathan Silverstein
University of Chicago

Ida Sim
University of California, San Francisco

Richard Singerman
TrustNetMD.com

Jamie Skipper
Office of the National Coordinator for Health IT

Tony Solomonides
University of West England

William Stead
Vanderbilt University

Kevin Sullivan
University of Virginia

Latanya Sweeney
Carnegie Mellon University

Jonathan Teich
Elsevier

Micky Tripathi
Massachusetts eHealth Collaborative

Reed Tuckson
UnitedHealth Group

Howard Wactlar
National Science Foundation

James Walker
Geisinger Health System

Paul Wallace
Kaiser Permanente

Ed Walters
The Brookings Institution

Jon White
Agency for Healthcare Research and Quality

Janet Wright
American College of Cardiology

William Yasnoff
Health Record Banking Alliance

Peter Yu
Palo Alto Medical Foundation

Wil Yu
Office of the National Coordinator for Health IT

JiaJie Zhang
University of Texas

APPENDIX G

❖

WORKSHOP #3: STRATEGY SCENARIOS

❖

OCTOBER 5, 2010

HOUSE OF SWEDEN
2900 K Street NW, Washington, DC 20007

Laura Adams
Rhode Island Quality Institute

Landen Bain
Clinical Data Interchange
 Standards Consortium

Meryl Bloomrosen
American Medical Informatics
 Association

Jim Bodenbender
McKesson Corporation

Jeff Brown
Harvard Pilgrim Healthcare
 Institute

David Buckeridge
McGill University

Christopher Chute
Mayo Clinic

Adam Clark
FasterCures

Janet Corrigan
National Quality Forum

Don Detmer
American Medical Informatics
 Association

Greg Downing
Department of Health and Human
 Services

Charles P. Friedman
Office of the National Coordinator
 for Health IT

Jennifer Hornung Garvin
University of Utah

Jim Hansen
Dossia Consortium

Craig Jones
The Vermont Blueprint for Health

Robert Kahn
Corporation for National Research
 Initiatives

William A. Knaus
University of Virginia

Rebecca Kush
Clinical Data Interchange
 Standards Consortium

Lisa M. Lee
Centers for Disease Control and Prevention

Ravi Madduri
Argonne National Laboratory

Kenneth D. Mandl
Harvard Medical School

Richard D. Marks
Patient Command, Inc.

Daniel Masys
Vanderbilt University

David McCallie. Jr.
Cerner Corporation

J. Michael McGinnis
Institute of Medicine

Richard Moore
National Committee for Quality Assurance

Theresa M. Mullin
Food and Drug Administration

Douglas Peddicord
Association of Clinical Research Organizations

Judith A. Racoosin
Food and Drug Administration

Roberto A. Rocha
Partners Healthcare System

Robert Shelton
Private Access

Edward H. Shortliffe
American Medical Informatics Association

Jonathan C. Silverstein
University of Chicago

Richard Singerman
TrustNetMD.com

Walter G. Suarez
Kaiser Permanente

James Walker
Geisinger Health System

Peter Yu
Palo Alto Medical Foundation

Wil Yu
Office of the National Coordinator for Health IT

OTHER PUBLICATIONS IN THE LEARNING HEALTH SYSTEM SERIES

The Learning Healthcare System

Evidence-Based Medicine and the Changing Nature of Health Care

Leadership Commitments to Improve Value in Health Care: Finding Common Ground

Value in Health Care: Accounting for Cost, Quality, Safety, Outcomes, and Innovation

Redesigning the Clinical Effectiveness Research Paradigm: Innovation and Practice-Based Approaches

Clinical Data as the Basic Staple of Health Learning: Creating and Protecting a Public Good

The Healthcare Imperative: Lowering Costs and Improving Outcomes

Learning What Works: Infrastructure Required for Comparative Effectiveness Research

Engineering a Learning Healthcare System: A Look at the Future

Patients Charting the Course: Citizen Engagement and the Learning Health System